1997
YEAR BOOK OF
ORTHOPEDICS®

Statement of Purpose

The YEAR BOOK Service

The YEAR BOOK series was devised in 1901 by practicing health professionals who observed that the literature of medicine and related disciplines had become so voluminous that no one individual could read and place in perspective every potential advance in a major specialty. In the final decade of the 20th century, this recognition is more acutely true than it was in 1901.

More than merely a series of books, YEAR BOOK volumes are the tangible results of a unique service designed to accomplish the following:

- to *survey* a wide range of journals of proven value
- to *select* from those journals papers representing significant advances and statements of important clinical principles
- to provide *abstracts* of those articles that are readable, convenient summaries of their key points
- to provide *commentary* about those articles to place them in perspective

These publications grow out of a unique process that calls on the talents of outstanding authorities in clinical and fundamental disciplines, trained literature specialists, and professional writers, all supported by the resources of Mosby, the world's preeminent publisher for the health professions.

The Literature Base

Mosby and its editors survey nearly 1,000 journals published worldwide, covering the full range of the health professions. On an annual basis, the publisher examines usage patterns and polls its expert authorities to add new journals to the literature base and to delete journals that are no longer useful as potential YEAR BOOK sources.

The Literature Survey

The publisher's team of literature specialists, all of whom are trained and experienced health professionals, examines every original, peer-reviewed article in each journal issue. More than 250,000 articles per year are scanned systematically, including title, text, illustrations, tables, and references. Each scan is compared, article by article, to the search strategies that the publisher has developed in consultation with the 270 outside experts who form the pool of YEAR BOOK editors. A given article may be reviewed by any number of editors, from one to a dozen or more, regardless of the discipline for which the paper was originally published. In turn, each editor who receives the article reviews it to determine whether or not the article should be included in the YEAR BOOK. This decision is based on the article's inherent quality, its probable usefulness to readers of that YEAR BOOK, and the editor's goal to represent a balanced picture of a given field in each volume of the YEAR BOOK. In addition, the editor indicates

Year Book of Obstetrics, Gynecology, and Women's Health: Drs. Mishell, Herbst, and Kirschbaum

Year Book of Occupational and Environmental Medicine®: Drs. Emmett, Frank, Gochfeld, and Hessl

Year Book of Oncology®: Drs. Ozols, Cohen, Glatstein, Loehrer, Tallman, and Wiersma

Year Book of Ophthalmology®: Drs. Wilson, Augsburger, Cohen, Eagle, Flanagan, Grossman, Laibson, Maguire, Nelson, Penne, Rapuano, Sergott, Spaeth, Tipperman, Ms. Gosfield, and Ms. Salmon

Year Book of Orthopedics®: Drs. Sledge, Poss, Cofield, Dobyns, Griffin, Springfield, Swiontkowski, Wiesel, and Wilson

Year Book of Otolaryngology–Head and Neck Surgery®: Drs. Paparella and Holt

Year Book of Pathology and Laboratory Medicine: Drs. Mills, Bruns, Gaffey, and Stoler

Year Book of Pediatrics®: Dr. Stockman

Year Book of Plastic, Reconstructive, and Aesthetic Surgery®: Drs. Miller, Cohen, McKinney, Robson, Ruberg, Smith, and Whitaker

Year Book of Podiatric Medicine and Surgery®: Dr. Kominsky

Year Book of Psychiatry and Applied Mental Health®: Drs. Talbott, Ballenger, Breier, Frances, Meltzer, Schowalter, and Tasman

Year Book of Pulmonary Disease®: Dr. Petty

Year Book of Rheumatology®: Drs. Sergent, LeRoy, Meenan, Panush, and Reichlin

Year Book of Sports Medicine®: Drs. Shephard, Alexander, Drinkwater, Eichner, George, and Torg

Year Book of Surgery®: Drs. Copeland, Bland, Deitch, Eberlein, Howard, Luce, Seeger, Souba, and Sugarbaker

Year Book of Thoracic and Cardiovascular Surgery®: Drs. Ginsberg, Wechsler, and Williams

Year Book of Urology®: Drs. Andriole and Coplen

Year Book of Vascular Surgery®: Dr. Porter

1997

The Year Book of ORTHOPEDICS®

Editor

Clement B. Sledge, M.D.

Chairman Emeritus, Department of Orthopaedic Surgery, Brigham and Women's Hospital; John B. and Buckminster Brown Professor of Orthopaedic Surgery, Harvard Medical School, Boston, Massachusetts

Co-Editor

Robert Poss, M.D.

Department of Orthopaedic Surgery, Brigham and Women's Hospital; Professor of Orthopaedic Surgery, Harvard Medical School, Boston, Massachusetts

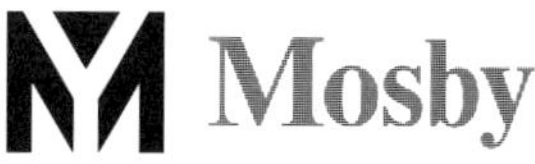

St. Louis Baltimore Boston Carlsbad Naples New York Philadelphia Portland London
Madrid Mexico City Singapore Sydney Tokyo Toronto Wiesbaden

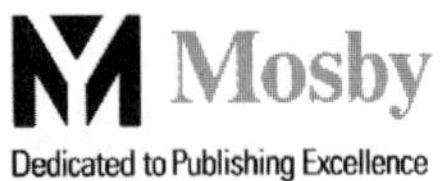

Mosby

Dedicated to Publishing Excellence

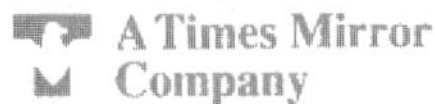

A Times Mirror
Company

Vice President and Publisher: Carol Trumbold
Director, Editorial Development: Gretchen C. Murphy
Assistant Developmental Editor, Continuity: Catherine Flanagan/Brenda Orf
Acquisitions Editor: Linda Sheehan
Illustrations and Permissions Coordinator: Steven J. Ramay
Project Manager, Editing: Jill C. Waite/Kirk Swearingen
Senior Project Manager, Production: Max F. Perez
Director, Editorial Services: Edith M. Podrazik, R.N.
Information Specialist: Kathleen Moss, R.N.
Circulation Manager: Lynn D. Stevenson

1997 EDITION
Copyright © November 1997 by Mosby–Year Book, Inc.

Printed in the United States of America
Composition by Reed Technology and Information Services, Inc.
Printing/binding by Maple-Vail

Mosby–Year Book, Inc.
11830 Westline Industrial Drive
St. Louis, MO 63146

International Standard Serial Number: 0276-1092
International Standard Book Number: 0-8151-9715-2

Associate Editors

Robert H. Cofield, M.D.
Professor of Orthopedic Surgery, Mayo Medical School; Vice-Chairman, Department of Orthopedics, Mayo Clinic, Rochester, Minnesota

James H. Dobyns, M.D.
Emeritus Professor of Orthopedic Surgery, Mayo Foundation, Rochester, Minnesota; Clinical Professor, University of Texas Health Sciences Center, San Antonio

Paul P. Griffin, M.D.
Professor of Orthopedic Surgery, Medical University of South Carolina, Charleston

Dempsey S. Springfield, M.D.
Professor and Chairman, Leni and Peter W. May Department of Orthopaedics, Mount Sinai Medical Center, New York, New York

Marc F. Swiontkowski, M.D.
Professor and Chairman, Department of Orthopaedics, University of Minnesota, Minneapolis, Minnesota

Sam W. Wiesel, M.D.
Professor and Chairman, Department of Orthopaedic Surgery, Georgetown University Medical Center, Washington, D.C.

Michael G. Wilson, M.D.
Director, Foot and Ankle Surgery Service, Brigham and Women's Hospital; Problem Foot Service, Massachusetts General Hospital; Clinical Instructor of Orthopaedic Surgery, Harvard Medical School, Boston, Massachusetts

Table of Contents

Journals Represented

Mosby and its Editors subscribe to and survey nearly 1,000 U.S. and foreign medical and allied health journals. From these journals, the editors select the articles to be abstracted. Journals represented in this YEAR BOOK are listed below.

Acta Neurochirurgica
Acta Orthopaedica Scandinavica
Acta Radiologica
American Journal of Epidemiology
American Journal of Neuroradiology
American Journal of Roentgenology
American Journal of Sports Medicine
American Journal of Surgery
American Journal of Surgical Pathology
Annals of Internal Medicine
Annals of Plastic Surgery
Annals of the Royal College of Surgeons of England
Archives of Orthopaedic and Trauma Surgery
Archives of Physical Medicine and Rehabilitation
Arthritis and Rheumatism
Arthroscopy
British Medical Journal
Cancer
Clincial Biomechanics
Clinical Nuclear Medicine
Clinical Orthopaedics and Related Research
Clinical Radiology
Foot & Ankle International
Injury
International Journal of Radiation, Oncology, Biology, and Physics
International Orthopaedics
Journal of Arthroplasty
Journal of Bone and Joint Surgery (American Volume)
Journal of Bone and Joint Surgery (British Volume)
Journal of Bone and Mineral Research
Journal of Clinical Oncology
Journal of Computer Assisted Tomography
Journal of Hand Surgery (American)
Journal of Hand Surgery (British)
Journal of Long-Term Effects of Medical Implants
Journal of Neurosurgery
Journal of Nuclear Medicine
Journal of Orthopaedic Research
Journal of Orthopaedic Trauma
Journal of Pain and Symptom Management
Journal of Pediatric Orthopedics
Journal of Shoulder and Elbow Surgery
Journal of Surgical Oncology
Journal of the National Cancer Institute
Journal of the Royal College of Surgeons of Edinburgh
Lancet
Neurosurgery

New England Journal of Medicine
Orthopedics
Pain
Pediatric Radiology
Plastic and Reconstructive Surgery
Prosthetics and Orthotics International
Radiology
Scandinavian Journal of Rheumatology
Skeletal Radiology
Southern Medical Journal
Spinal Cord
Spine
Surgical Neurology

STANDARD ABBREVIATIONS

The following terms are abbreviated in this edition: acquired immunodeficiency syndrome (AIDS), cardiopulmonary resuscitation (CPR), central nervous system (CNS), cerebrospinal fluid (CSF), computed tomography (CT), deoxyribonucleic acid (DNA), electrocardiography (ECG), health maintenance organization (HMO), human immunodeficiency virus (HIV), intensive care unit (ICU), intramuscular (IM), intravenous (IV), magnetic resonance (MR) imaging (MRI), and ribonucleic acid (RNA).

NOTE

The YEAR BOOK OF ORTHOPEDICS® is a literature survey service providing abstracts of articles published in the professional literature. Every effort is made to assure the accuracy of the information presented in these pages. Neither the editors nor the publisher of the YEAR BOOK OF ORTHOPEDICS® can be responsible for errors in the original materials. The editors' comments are their own opinions. Mention of specific products within this publication does not constitute endorsement.

To facilitate the use of the YEAR BOOK OF ORTHOPEDICS® as a reference tool, all illustrations and tables included in this publication are now identified as they appear in the original article. This change is meant to help the reader recognize that any illustration or table appearing in the YEAR BOOK OF ORTHOPEDICS® may be only one of many in the original article. For this reason, figure and table numbers will often appear to be out of sequence within the YEAR BOOK OF ORTHOPEDICS®

Publisher's Preface

Publication of the 1997 YEAR BOOK OF ORTHOPEDICS marks the end of a 9-year period of exceptional editorship by Clement B. Sledge, M.D. He and his board have provided the readers of the YEAR BOOK with discerning and informative literature and editorial commentary of the highest caliber. We extend our sincere thanks to Dr. Sledge for his valuable contributions and commitment to the YEAR BOOK OF ORTHOPEDICS.

With the 1998 edition, we wish to welcome Bernard F. Morrey, M.D., from the orthopedic surgery division of the Mayo Clinic. We look forward to working with him.

Introduction

This is my last year as editor of the YEAR BOOK OF ORTHOPEDICS, and I would like to dedicate this edition to the associate editors who have helped with this project since 1988. My co-editor, Robert Poss, and the associate editors, Robert Cofield, Jim Dobyns, Paul Griffin, Dempsey Springfield, Marc Swiontkowski, Sam Wiesel, and Mike Wilson, have made this an enjoyable adventure.

I would also like to thank the editors at Mosby–Year Book, Inc., who have been so helpful over the years, including Linda S. Sheehan and Catherine Flanagan.

I succeeded Mark Coventry, chairman of orthopedic surgery at the Mayo Clinic, as editor of the YEAR BOOK OF ORTHOPEDICS in 1988, and it is entirely appropriate that I now turn this enjoyable task over to Bernie Morrey, who is currently the chairman of orthopedic surgery at the Mayo Clinic.

Clement B. Sledge, M.D.

1 Shoulder, Arm, and Elbow

Introduction

We have had another fruitful year of investigations. Skiing-related shoulder injuries and the frequent association of alcoholism with shoulder fractures are now defined. In addition, an unusual injury, fracture of the coracoid, has been assessed, and some clarity has emerged regarding treatment recommendations.

Technical improvements are suggested: use of a reconstruction plate on clavicle fracture nonunions, supplemental use of external fixation for complex proximal humeral fractures, use of an intramedullary bone peg as an adjunct to proximal humeral fracture nonunions, modification of technique during distal clavicle excision to preserve ligament integrity, use of intra-articular injections for reduction of acute shoulder dislocations, effectiveness of capsular tightening for managing recurrent shoulder instability, arthroscopic use of capsule releases for shoulder tightness related to previous injuries or surgery, and the effectiveness of arthroscopically assisted rotator cuff repair, particularly for smaller tears. Additionally, we are reminded of modern cement techniques and their effectiveness relative to total shoulder and total elbow arthroplasty.

Magnetic resonance imaging is continually being studied. We understand its role in the diagnosis of glenoid labrum tears better (and how this does not supersede physical examination), how degenerative changes and traumatic changes in the rotator cuff may show similar changes with subtle differences, how distal biceps tears can be further defined, and interestingly, how ulnar nerve entrapment can be confirmed.

The two major areas of emphasis this year have been shoulder instability and rotator cuff disease. Examination under anesthesia has again surfaced as a useful diagnostic tool. The long head of the biceps tendon does play a role in shoulder instability—or at least seemingly so. A study this year has shown us that acute repair of a first-time anterior shoulder dislocation may not be all that effective when done arthroscopically. This is in deference to the recent supposition that arthroscopic shoulder dislocation repair is indeed effective. The article again offers some balance to our thinking on this subject. If one applies arthroscopic techniques (as well as open techniques) to an overall group of patients with recurrent instability, the success rate will not be as high as if the technique were applied to those with classic, traumatic anterior instability. Please note, instability may develop from lateral, that is, humeral, detachment of the capsule and rotator cuff rather than detachment at the glenoid rim. This lateral detachment may be more common in older people.

The acromion and its relationship to rotator cuff tearing has been further studied. The acromion has various morphological types and, superimposed on this, are degenerative changes associated with the coracoacromial ligament and the acromioclavicular joint. Rotator cuff tearing is associated with acromial changes, at least on the bursal side and for full-thickness tears, but this relationship is much less secure for articular-side tearing. In spite of all these fine studies, it is clear that our clinical classification for acromial morphology is at best imprecise. Calcium in the rotator cuff and impingement can be related, but typically are not. We should pay increasing attention to the subscapularis as a component of rotator cuff tearing. We should also beware of its use for transposition during repair of large rotator cuff tears when preoperative function is good. The role of the latissimus dorsi in the repair of larger rotator cuff tear is becoming better defined. The results are somewhat variable, and there are limitations in terms of result expectations. Strength after surgical repair of a rotator cuff tear generally improves, depending on healing time and the size of the tear.

How we do research is still somewhat confusing. Scoring systems are many and are really different. Correlation among scoring systems is rather poor, and of particular note, correlation among the various rated items within the scoring system is also rather poor. We need to direct more attention to this and not only the construction of scoring systems but also the study of their validity.

Robert H. Cofield, M.D.

Fractures

Shoulder Injuries During Alpine Skiing

Kocher MS, Feagin JA Jr (Harvard Med School, Boston; Duke Univ, Durham, NC)

Am J Sports Med 24:665–669, 1996   1–1

Objective.—Possible reasons for the increase in upper extremity injuries among alpine skiers include changes in equipment, environment, and behavior. Although shoulder injuries account for 4.5%–10% of all alpine skiing injuries, they have not been well studied. Results of an investigation to characterize the incidence and types of shoulder injuries during alpine skiing are presented.

Methods.—A retrospective review of records from 1990 to 1993 at the Jackson Hole Ski Resort ski clinic was conducted to determine the population at risk and the number of injuries per 1,000 skier-days.

Results.—There were 3,451 injuries in 3,247 patients for an incidence of 4.44 injuries per 1,000 skier-days. Upper extremity injuries represented 29.1% (n = 1,004) of all injuries, with the most common injury being a sprained thumb. Shoulder injuries accounted for 11.4% of all injuries and 39.1% of the upper extremity injuries for an incidence of 0.51 injuries per 1,000 skier-days. The most common shoulder injuries were rotator cuff strains (24.2%), anterior glenohumeral dislocations or subluxations (21.6%), acromioclavicular separations (19.6%), and clavicle fractures (10.9%), and most were due to falls (93.9%). The average age at injury was 35.4 years, and the male-to-female ratio was 3 to 1. The incidence and total number of shoulder injuries are higher than in previous studies.

Conclusion.—Because the incidence and number of shoulder injuries appear to be increasing among alpine skiers and because of the morbidity that can occur as a result of such injuries, additional studies should examine skiing surfaces, technique, education, exercise, and bracing.

▶ It is recognized that somewhere around one third of all ski injuries involve the upper extremity. Most attention has focused on injuries at the base of the thumb. This article nicely outlines the types of injuries seen in the shoulder and, importantly, identifies that rotator cuff injuries are more common than recognized.

R.H. Cofield, M.D.

Shoulder Injuries Common in Alcoholics: An Analysis of 413 Injuries
Nordqvist A, Petersson CJ (Malmö Univ, Sweden)
Acta Orthop Scand 67:364–366, 1996   1–2

Introduction.—An association has been previously reported between alcoholism and lower limb fractures. The association between alcoholism and shoulder injuries was investigated in a case-control study.

Methods.—All patients who had fractures of the proximal end of the humerus, clavicle, and scapula or who had primary, traumatic shoulder dislocations and acromioclavicular dislocations during 1987 were matched for age and gender with 2 controls who had other injuries, in a university hospital in Sweden. The names of case patients and controls were identified in the records of the Department of Alcohol Diseases.

Results.—There were records in the Department of Alcohol Diseases for 12% of patients who had shoulder injuries and only 3% of the controls. There was an even greater difference in the prevalence of alcoholism between case patients and controls among men than among women. Among men aged 30–64 years, alcohol abusers composed 71% of patients who had a lateral clavicle fracture, 40% of those who had a proximal humerus fracture, 40% of those who had a shoulder dislocation, and 29% of those who had a mid-clavicular fracture.

Conclusions.—Shoulder injuries were strongly correlated with alcohol abuse. The strongest correlations were in men who had lateral clavicle fractures. This injury in men may be a marker of alcohol abuse.

▶ One of the difficulties in treating patients who have shoulder fractures is the presence of negative patient characteristics in a substantial number of them. I think most physicians and surgeons have been impressed over time that many injuries occur in alcoholics who do not always care for themselves very well after fracture, do not protect their arms early, and do not participate fully in rehabilitation programs. This nice, short article confirms for us that a substantial number of injuries in this anatomical region do indeed occur in alcohol abusers. A review of outcome after treatment of patients who have these injuries probably should incorporate information about the proportion of alcohol abusers in the series, as this is quite likely to affect outcome adversely.

R.H. Cofield, M.D.

Clavicular Nonunion: 31/32 Healed After Plate Fixation and Bone Grafting
Bradbury N, Hutchinson J, Hahn D, et al (Univ Hosp, Nottingham, England; Queen's Med Centre, Nottingham, England)
Acta Orthop Scand 67:367–370, 1996   1–3

Background.—Factors that contribute to nonunion of the clavicle include high energy trauma, degree of displacement, lateral third fractures, soft-tissue interposition, and refracture. Most surgical treatments have been only moderately successful and have left 75% of patients with pain and 33% with shoulder dysfunction. The long-term results of plate fixation and bone grafts for nonunion of the clavicle were reported.

Methods.—Of 32 patients (mean age, 33 years) with clavicular nonunion, 15 were treated with a 3.5 mm AO dynamic compression plate and 17 were treated with a 3.5 mm AO reconstruction plate; all patients were also treated with autologous cancellous bone graft. The majority of fractures resulted from high-velocity trauma. The mean displacement of bone ends was 10 mm in patients treated with the dynamic compression plate and 18 mm in those treated with the reconstruction plate. Operations were performed at a mean of 12 months after injury. Patients completed a pain questionnaire at 18 months. Long-term follow-up occurred for a mean of 6 years.

Results.—All patients had presurgical pain, but at follow-up 13 of 15 patients and 15 of 17 patients had no pain, 1 patient had less pain, and 3 reported no change in pain. Patients returned to work an average of 6.4 and 6.6 weeks postoperatively. Six dynamic compression plates and 6 reconstruction plates were removed because of aching discomfort or cosmesis. No plates broke. Two compression plates loosened and were removed. A total of 14 of 15 nonunions treated with a compression plate

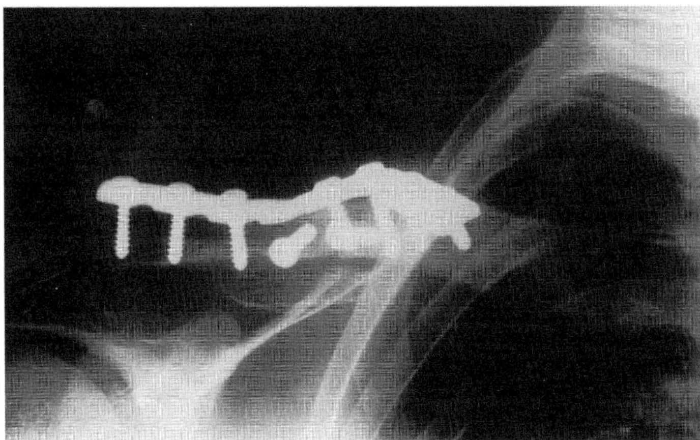

FIGURE 3.—Reconstruction plate contoured to fit angulated nonunion. (Courtesy of Bradbury N, Hutchinson J, Hahn D, et al: Clavicular nonunion: 31/32 healed after plate fixation and bone grafting. *Acta Orthop Scand* 67:367–370, 1996.)

and 15 of 17 nonunions treated with a reconstruction plate were clinically and radiologically united. There were no major complications. Overall long-term outcome was excellent.

Conclusions.—The 3.5 mm reconstruction plate is easier to contour to the sigmoid shape of the clavicle and is stronger than semi-tubular plates. Many of these nonunions treated with a reconstruction plate had a degree of angulation or displacement that did not allow the use of a compression plate because contouring would not have been possible (Fig 3). The difficulty of contouring dynamic compression plates may have caused 2 of the compression plates to cut out. The use of an AO plate with an autologous bone graft is recommended to treat nonunited fractures or nonunions of the clavicle.

▶ This nice study demonstrates that material failure of the reconstruction plate seems unlikely when applied to the treatment of nonunion of clavicle fractures. Certainly, it is much more satisfactory to use this plate than the usual dynamic or impression plate because it is difficult to bend the latter plate in various directions. Thanks to this article, we can rest assured that use of the reconstruction plate is a very reasonable option.

R.H. Cofield, M.D.

Fractures of the Coracoid Process

Ogawa K, Yoshida A, Takahashi M, et al (Keio Univ, Tokyo)
J Bone Joint Surg Br 78B:17–19, 1996   1–4

Background.—Coracoid injuries are increasing. A review of 67 consecutive patients with fractures of the coracoid process was presented and a simple clinical classification system proposed.

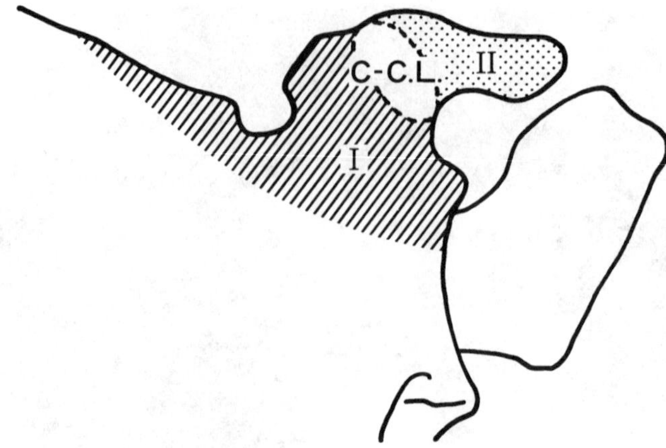

FIGURE 1.—The proposed anatomical classification of glenoid fractures into type I and type II. *C-CL* is the attachment of the coracoclavicular ligament. (Courtesy of Ogawa K, Yoshida A, Takahashi M, et al: Fractures of the coracoid process. *J Bone Joint Surg Br* 78B:17–19, 1996.)

Methods.—Between 1974 and 1994, 67 patients (12 females) aged 14 to 72 years were treated operatively and nonoperatively for coracoid fractures. Patients were followed for at least 1 year.

Results.—There were 53 type I, 11 type II, and 3 unclassified fractures (Fig 1). Sixty patients had acromioclavicular dislocations, 15 had posterolateral or lateral deltoid lacerations or abrasions, and 14 had clavicular fractures. Surgery was usually performed on patients with multiple shoulder injuries. All type I fractures, 3 type II fractures, and 1 unclassified fracture were treated operatively by open reduction and internal fixation. Of the 45 patients available for follow-up, 39 had excellent results and 6 had fair results.

Conclusion.—There were no significant differences in results between operated and nonoperated patients. Only patients with multiple shoulder injuries should be considered for operative treatment.

▶ This article is 1 of the few to collect a large series of fractures of the coracoid process, to define them relative to the coracoclavicular ligament, and to recommend a treatment approach. The recommendation of the authors for conservative treatment—unless there is a type I fracture with associated shoulder injuries and claviculoscapular discontinuity—is a sound one that quite likely will stand the test of time.

R.H. Cofield, M.D.

Surgical Treatment of Complex Fracture of the Proximal Humerus

Ko J-Y, Yamamoto R (Chang Gung Mem Hosp, Kaohsiung, Taiwan; Showa Univ, Yokohama, Japan)
Clin Orthop 327:225–237, 1996   1–5

Background.—The treatment of complex displaced fractures of the proximal humerus is challenging. Authorities disagree on which treatment is best. Open reduction, minimal soft tissue dissection, and internal fixation with or without external fixation were performed in 16 patients with complex displaced fractures of the proximal humerus.

Technique.—The patients were given general anesthesia and placed in beach-chair position. Through the deltopectoral approach, the cephalic vein was retracted laterally without interruption, and the fracture site was exposed with minimal soft tissue dissection. Dislocated humeral heads were directly reduced. When tuberosities remained with the dislocated humeral head, the surgeon made a small splitting incision in the rotator cuff between tuberosities, allowing head reduction into a normal position. The fractured greater or lesser tuberosities were reduced to align with the humeral shaft, usually with the long head of the biceps tendon serving as a guide. Kirschner wires were inserted for temporary fixation. Hoffmann external fixation was performed when the fracture geometry and bone quality were suitable. Heavy sutures or wire were used to repair the torn rotator cuff and bony fragments. The surgeon then stabilized the fracture fragments with the Hoffmann external fixation and removed the Kirschner wires (Fig 1). When the fragments were too small for Hoffmann pin fixation, the

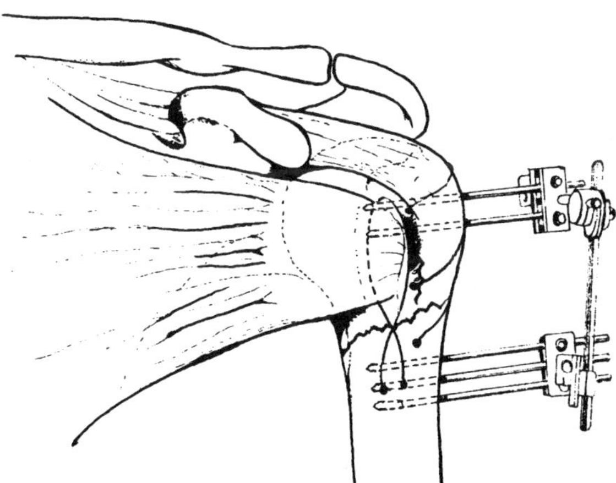

FIGURE 1.—Schematic diagram showing open reduction and suture repair of the fractured tuberosities, shaft, and rotator cuff tendon with Hoffmann external fixation. (Courtesy of Ko J-Y, Yamamoto R: Surgical treatment of complex fracture of the proximal humerus. *Clin Orthop* 327:225–237, 1996.)

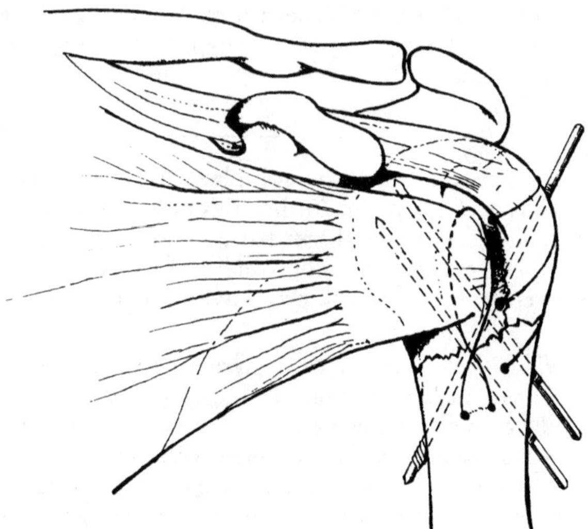

FIGURE 2.—Schematic diagram showing open reduction and suture repair of the fractured tuberosities, shaft, and rotator cuff tendon with threaded pin fixation. (Courtesy of Ko J-Y, Yamamoto R: Surgical treatment of complex fracture of the proximal humerus. *Clin Orthop* 327:225–237, 1996.)

surgeon used adjuvant multiple threaded Steinmann pin fixation to fix the bony fragments (Fig 2). A triangular bandage or simple Velpeau bandage was used for temporary immobilzation after surgery.

Conclusion.—Fracture stability was good with this technique, and a high percentage of outcomes were satisfactory. However, this procedure is not appropriate for patients who cannot tolerate anesthesia; older patients with osteoporotic bone unable to hold pins or external fixation; older patients with 4-part fracture dislocations in which avascular necrosis of the humeral head occurs often and in which a subsequent endoprosthesis insertion is not appropriate if osteosynthesis fails; and patients with head-splitting fractures.

▶ These authors have identified some adjunctive methods for maintenance of position during reduction and fixation of complex proximal humeral fractures. The results they report are excellent, and certainly these adjunctive techniques should be considered and quite likely included in the armamentarium of fracture surgeons treating these injuries.

R.H. Cofield, M.D.

Nonunions of the Surgical Neck of the Humerus: Surgical Treatment With an Intramedullary Bone Peg, Internal Fixation, and Cancellous Bone Grafting
Walch G, Badet R, Nové-Josserand L, et al (Clinique de Chirurgie Orthopédique Emilie de Vialar, Lyon, France)
J Shoulder Elbow Surg 5:161–168, 1996   1–6

Background.—Pseudarthrosis of the upper humerus is rare but causes great pain and loss of active shoulder motion. Direct surgical correction is difficult. Surgeons must immobilize the fracture by internal and external means while allowing early joint mobilization to restore muscle function and prevent stiffness. There have been problems with failure rates, complications, and poor functional results with methods such as open reduction and internal plate fixation, fixation with a tension band and intramedullary nail or T-plate, and hemiarthroplasty of the shoulder.

Methods.—In 20 patients with nonunion of the proximal humerus, surgery with the intramedullary bone peg technique was performed. The average patient age was 58 years. In 12 patients, the dominant side was involved. Eleven patients had prior operations.

Technique.—In these patients, a deltopectoral approach was used. A 6- to 10-cm corticocancellous autogenous bone graft was impacted into the distal humerus and plugged into the head (Fig 1).

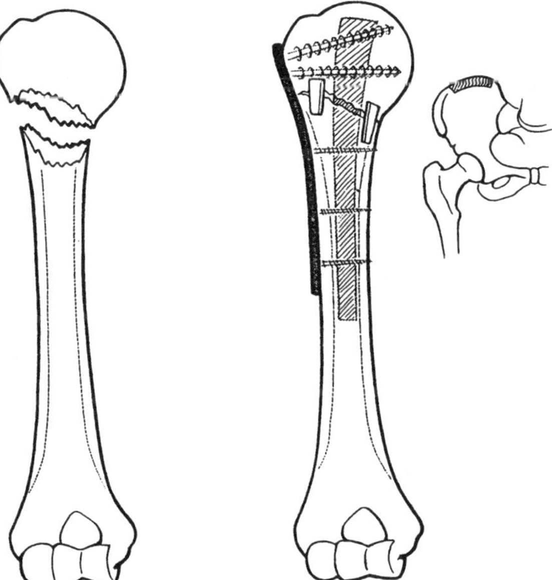

FIGURE 1.—Technique for osteosynthesis associated with intramedullary bone peg. (Courtesy of Walch G, Badet R, Nové-Josserand L, et al: Nonunions of the surgical neck of the humerus: Surgical treatment with an intramedullary bone peg, internal fixation, and cancellous bone grafting. *J Shoulder Elbow Surg* 5:161–168, 1996.)

An external T-plate was placed on the outer humerus and fixed with cortical and cancellous screws bored into the bony cortico-cancellous peg graft. A complementary cancellous graft was applied to the fracture.

Results.—The time between fracture and surgery was between 6 and 72 months. Follow-up ranged from 12 to 120 months. In 19 patients, union was confirmed. In the last patient, no peripheral callus was observed. There was no necrosis of the humeral head. Active anterior elevation of the shoulder improved from 60 degrees to 131 degrees. The results averaged 81.2%. The patients subjectively rated their results: 65% were very satisfied, 30% were satisfied, and 5% were disappointed.

Discussion.—In these patients, treatment with the intramedullary bone peg method resulted in 96% bone union. The goal was to achieve bone union. No postoperative necrosis was observed. Results were better than those seen after humeral head prosthetic replacements in fracture malunions.

▶ This article nicely demonstrates that, internal fixation of the fracture and the usual, external bone grafting can be supplemented by an internal bone graft strut and, quite likely, enhance the frequency of healing of this non-union. This has been a particularly problematic nonunion, and as such, this adjunctive technique may, in fact, be a reasonable addition to contemporary surgical technique.

R.H. Cofield, M.D.

Operative Treatment of Nonunions of the Surgical Neck of the Humerus

Duralde XA, Flatow EL, Pollock RG, et al (New York Orthopaedic Hosp)
J Shoulder Elbow Surg 5:169–180, 1996   1–7

Objective.—Nonunions of the proximal humerus, although uncommon, can result in pain and disability for the patient. Treatment by open reduction and internal fixation or hemiarthroplasty carries the potential for increased morbidity. The operative treatment of symptomatic nonunions of the surgical neck of the humerus was reviewed.

Methods.—Nonunions of the surgical neck of the humerus in 20 patients (7 men) aged 23–96 years, were treated either by open reduction and internal fixation (n = 10) or shoulder arthroplasty (n = 10). Twelve fractures were originally treated with closed reduction, and 8 fractures initially treated operatively did not heal because of inadequate fixation. Pain scores and daily function were evaluated before and after surgery.

Technique.—The deltopectoral approach was used (Fig 3). When necessary, the humeral head was replaced with a bone graft. The humeral component was cemented into the medullary canal, and the wound was closed. Passive motion was started after surgery.

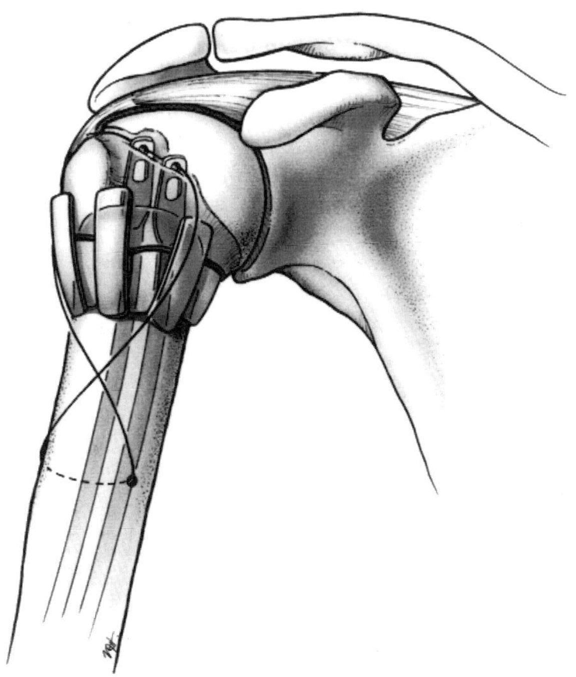

FIGURE 3.—Open reduction and internal fixation with modified Enders rods and figure-of-eight wire for surgical neck nonunion. The nonunion site is bone grafted. (Courtesy of Duralde XA, Flatow EL, Pollock RG, et al: Operative treatment of nonunions of the surgical neck of the humerus. *J Shoulder Elbow Surg* 5:169–180, 1996).

Results.—Patients were followed for an average of 51 months. Results were excellent in 5 patients, satisfactory in 6, and unsatisfactory in 9. Average pain scores were significantly diminished after surgery (3.9 vs. 1.4). Before surgery 16 patients had severe pain, 1 had moderate pain, and 3 had minimum pain. After surgery 3 patients had severe pain, 4 had moderate pain, and 13 had minimum pain. Before surgery all patients had severe functional restriction. After surgery 11 patients had satisfactory functional gains at or above the horizontal, 4 had satisfactory functioning below 90 degrees, and 5 did not improve. Satisfactory or excellent results were achieved in 8 of the 12 fractures originally treated nonoperatively but in only 3 of the fractures initially treated with internal fixation.

Conclusion.—Only 55% of the patients had excellent or satisfactory results. Pain was reduced significantly but function improved only moderately. Reconstruction of nonunions of the humerus should be reserved for patients with more severe disability and pain.

▶ This manuscript offers information on the outcomes of the rather classic approaches to the treatment of proximal humeral nonunions. Good results can be achieved, but heterogeneity of the outcome is unfortunately what we have come to expect. There may be ways to improve the outcome of these fractures (Abstract 1–6); however, the importance of this article is the emphasis on attention to detail and the recognition that these are very difficult problems to treat successfully.

R.H. Cofield, M.D.

Dislocations and Joint Instability

The Role of the Acromioclavicular Ligaments and the Effect of Distal Clavicle Resection

Branch TP, Burdette HL, Shahriari AS, et al (Emory Univ, Atlanta, Ga)
Am J Sports Med 24:293–297, 1996   1–8

Background.—Several researchers have studied the function of the clavicle-scapula complex. However, none has specifically described the role of the acromioclavicular ligaments in controlling scapular rotation around the distal clavicle or the effects of surgical intervention.

Methods.—Thirteen fresh cadaver shoulders, consisting of the clavicle, acromioclavicular ligaments, coracoclavicular ligaments, and scapula, were used. A goniometer was specially designed to measure range of motion in each of the 3 orthogonal axes of rotation of the scapula (anterior-posterior axial rotation, protraction-retraction, and abduction-adduction) with reference to the clavicle. Sequential sectioning was done in 2 experiments. Range of motion was determined in the intact shoulder and after each sectioning cut.

Findings.—Only 5 mm of the distal clavicle needed to be resected to ensure that no bone-to-bone contact occurred in rotation after resection. The end result for range of motion in the 3 axes did not depend on whether the inferior acromioclavicular ligament or the superior acromioclavicular ligament was cut before 5 mm of the distal clavicle was removed.

Conclusion.—The coracoclavicular ligaments alone clearly do not control scapular rotation around the distal clavicle. The findings of this study suggest that, if all the ligaments are injured at the time of distal clavicle resection, the distal clavicle-scapula complex will become rotationally unstable. These findings also suggest that the acromioclavicular ligaments remaining after distal clavicle resection are important adjuncts to rotational stability.

▶ This study offers some new light on technical variations in excising the distal clavicle. The acromioclavicular ligaments are important for claviculo-scapular stability. If the coracoclavicular ligaments are normal, only a small amount of bone needs to be excised. When excising the distal clavicle, it is useful to preserve as many ligaments around the articulation as possible. As a corollary to this, it seems wise to bring additional soft tissue into the defect and to effect a firm closure when performing this surgery by standard open methods. Also, it will be useful to protect the joint to allow these tissues to heal firmly before instituting substantial passive or active movement of the shoulder girdle.

R.H. Cofield, M.D.

Diagnosis of Glenoid Labral Tears: A Comparison Between Magnetic Resonance Imaging and Clinical Examinations

Liu SH, Henry MH, Nuccion S, et al (Univ of California, Los Angeles)
Am J Sports Med 24:149–154, 1996
1–9

Background.—Several diagnostic modalities have been described in the evaluation of glenoid labral tears. A high degree of intraobserver and interobserver variability has been reported, and some authorities have questioned the value of these modalities in preoperative planning. To date, no one has directly compared MRI with other diagnostic modalities. The accuracy of MRI and physical examination in establishing the diagnosis of glenoid labral tears was determined.

Methods.—Fifty-four patients with a mean age of 34 years who had pain caused by anterior instability or glenoid labral tears unresponsive to 6 months of conservative treatment were studied retrospectively. None of the patients had signs of rotator cuff lesions. Sixty-four percent of the patients were athletes engaged in throwing activities. Sixty-one percent could recall specific trauma to the shoulder. The clinical examination included history-taking with special attention to pain with overhead activity, clicking, and shoulder instability. Apprehension, relocation, load and shift, inferior sulcus sign, and crank tests were performed. The efficacies of physical examination and MRI in predicting the presence of glenoid labral tears were compared, with confirmation by arthroscopy.

Findings.—The presence of labral tears was confirmed arthroscopically in 76% of patients. The sensitivity and specificity of MRI were 59% and 85%, respectively. The corresponding values for physical examination were 90% and 85%.

Conclusion.—Physical examination predicts the presence of glenoid labral tears more accurately than MRI. Thus, the diagnostic workup can be completed in the clinic, saving the patient time and expense.

▶ Congratulations to the authors on studying not only imaging methodology but also comparing it with physical examination in reference to arthroscopy as the standard. I think many orthopedic surgeons have long suspected that the physical examination parameters for the diagnosis of shoulder instability are very reasonable, and, in fact, that is confirmed by this study, as well as by much, less specific information in the literature. It is interesting that when comparing physical examination to MRI, physical examination is clearly superior. Magnetic resonance imaging will often not be necessary and, when used, is an adjunct rather than the key to exclusion or inclusion of the diagnosis.

R.H. Cofield, M.D.

Translation of the Glenohumeral Joint With the Patient Under Anesthesia

Hawkins RJ, Schutte JP, Janda DH, et al (Univ of Colorado, Vail; Steadman Hawkins Clinic, Vail, Colo; Inst for Preventative Sports Medicine, Ann Arbor, Mich; et al)
J Shoulder Elbow Surg 5:286–292, 1996

1–10

Background.—Shoulder instability is currently evaluated with a careful history, dynamic physical examination, and static radiographic analysis. Unlike instability of the knee, standards have not been established for defining radiographic instability in the shoulder. In an attempt to establish such standards, radiographic humeral head translation during general anesthesia was characterized in normal individuals and in patients with either anterior or multidirectional shoulder instability.

Methods.—Eighteen patients with no history of shoulder problems, 10 patients with recurrent anterior shoulder dislocation, and 10 patients with multidirectional shoulder instability underwent radiographic evaluation under general anesthesia. The load and shift test was used to determine the degree of anterior and posterior translation of the humeral head, which was measured radiographically.

Results.—In the control group, anterior translation was 17%, posterior translation was 26%, and inferior translation was 29%. The patients with anterior instability had humeral head translation of 29% anteriorly (1.9 times that of the controls), 21% posteriorly (0.8 times that of the controls), and 49% inferiorly (1.7 times that of the controls). The patients with multidirectional instability had humeral head translation of 28% anteriorly (1.8 times that in the control group), 52% posteriorly (1.9 times that in the control group), and 46% inferiorly (1.6 times that in the control group).

Conclusion.—There were trends toward greater passive humeral translation among patients with clinical instability compared with patients with normal shoulder function. However, passive laxity varied widely in both the normal group and the shoulder instability groups, with significant overlap between them. Therefore, excessive laxity or translation alone cannot be assumed to be related to instability. Joint laxity must be considered within the context of the patient's history and physical examination to establish a diagnosis.

▶ This study used radiographs and standard measurement techniques to assess translation of the glenohumeral joint with the shoulder in near neutral position. The findings indicated that those with instability have more translation but that there is considerable overlap between normal and abnormal when testing is performed in this manner. This work nicely documents that the clinical assessment by drawer testing and sulcus sign testing does often show increased translation in patients with clinical instability, but one cannot use this method alone for making the diagnosis; it is 1 more piece of information to diagnose shoulder instability.

R.H. Cofield, M.D.

Role of the Long Head of the Biceps Brachii in Glenohumeral Stability: A Biomechanical Study in Cadavera

Pagnani MJ, Deng X-H, Warren RF, et al (Lipscomb Clinic/Columbia Sports Medicine, Nashville, Tenn; Hosp for Special Surgery, New York)
J Shoulder Elbow Surg 5:255–262, 1996   1–11

Background.—It is generally believed that contraction of the rotator cuff muscles causes compression of the humeral head into the glenoid fossa, increasing the force needed to translate the humeral head. The biceps brachii muscle is thought to be a supinator of the forearm and flexor of the elbow. However, it has been hypothesized that the long head of the biceps stabilizes the glenohumeral joint. The effect of simulated contraction of the long head of the biceps brachii on glenohumeral translation in multiple shoulder positions was studied.

Methods.—Ten cadaveric shoulders were mounted on a special apparatus attached to a servo-controlled hydraulic testing device. The shoulders were subjected to sequential 50-newton anterior, posterior, superior, and inferior forces and a 22-newton joint compressive load. An air cylinder was used to apply a constant force to the tendon of the long head of the biceps brachii. Testing was done with the shoulders in 7 positions of glenohumeral elevation and rotation.

Findings.—The application of a force to the long head of the biceps brachii significantly reduced humeral head translation. The long head of the biceps had a more marked influence at middle and lower elevation angles. The application of a 55-newton force to the biceps tendon with the shoulder in 45 degrees of elevation and neutral rotation decreased anterior translation by 10.4 mm, inferior translation by 5.3 mm, and superior translation by 1.2 mm (Fig 3).

Conclusions.—The long head of the biceps brachii seems to contribute to shoulder stability. The application of a force to the biceps tendon decreases anteroposterior and superoinferior translations.

▶ This biomechanical study reinforces that if, in fact, the long head of the biceps brachii is active during shoulder movements, it does contribute significantly to shoulder stability. The clinical implication is that unless there is a clear reason to tenodese the long head of the biceps to the proximal humerus (this is relatively uncommon), it should remain in place and will serve some function around the shoulder in addition to its functions of elbow flexion and forearm supination.

R.H. Cofield, M.D.

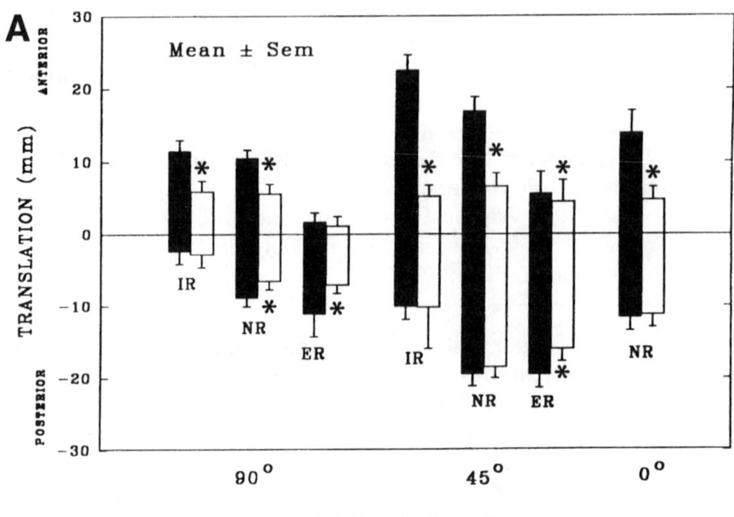

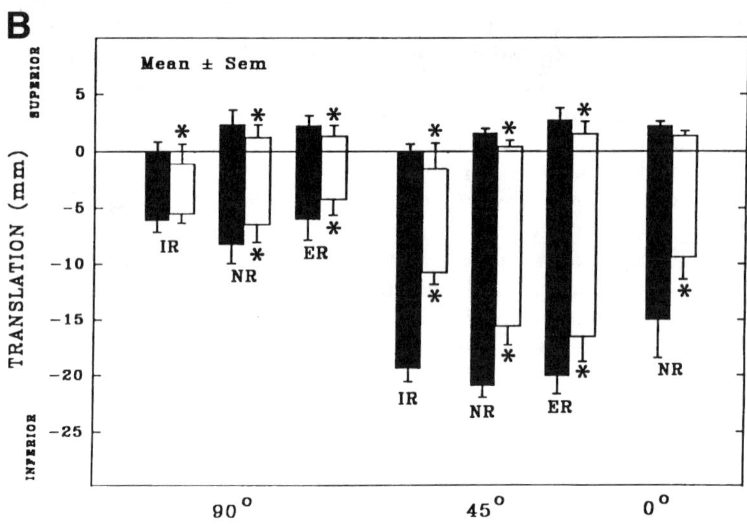

FIGURE 3.—Effect of 55-newton force applied to long head of biceps brachii on glenohumeral translation. Joint compressive load of 22-newton and 50-newton anterior, posterior, superior, and inferior displacement forces were applied. *Solid* bars represent mean translations in vented condition before application of biceps force. *Open* bars represent mean translations after application of biceps force. Statistically significant decreases in translation resulted from application of biceps force and are indicated by *asterisks*. *Abbreviations: IR,* internal rotation: *NR,* neural rotation; *ER,* external rotation. **A,** anteroposterior translation; **B,** superinferior translation. (Courtesy of Pagnani MJ, Deng X-H, Warren RF, et al: Role of the long head of the biceps brachii in glenohumeral stability: A biomechanical study in cadavera. *J Shoulder Elbow Surg* 5:255–262, 1996.)

Intraarticular Lidocaine Versus Intravenous Analgesic for Reduction of Acute Anterior Shoulder Dislocations: A Prospective Randomized Study

Matthews DE, Roberts T (Univ of Mississippi, Jackson)
Am J Sports Med 23:54–58, 1995

1–12

Background.—It is generally agreed that muscle spasm is the greatest impediment encountered in reducing a dislocation of the shoulder. Therefore, sedative or analgesic medication is generally used. However, intra-articular lidocaine was recently introduced to provide analgesia for reduction of anterior shoulder dislocations. The efficacy of intra-articular lidocaine was compared with that of parenteral analgesic and sedation during reduction of anterior shoulder dislocations in a prospective, randomized study.

Methods.—Thirty consecutive patients with acute anterior shoulder dislocations were randomly assigned to receive either intra-articular lidocaine or parenteral morphine sulfate and midazolam before undergoing reduction with 1 of 2 techniques: the traction-countertraction technique or scapular rotation with traction on the arm in the prone position. The patients rated their pain during the procedure on a scale of 1 to 10. The physicians rated the difficulty of performing the reduction maneuver. Complications, the need for monitoring, and the time between admittance and discharge were noted for each patient.

Results.—Pain and the difficulty of the maneuvers were similar in the 2 groups, with adequate anesthesia and relief of muscle spasm demonstrated in all patients. There were no complications in the lidocaine group, whereas 3 patients in the IV sedation group had nausea and 2 patients required pulse oximeter monitoring and reversal agents. The mean length of stay was 78 minutes in the lidocaine group and 186 minutes in the IV sedation group.

Conclusion.—Intra-articular lidocaine is a safe and effective analgesic agent for reducing pain and preventing muscle spasm in patients undergoing reduction of acute anterior shoulder dislocations.

▶ In many emergency rooms, local injection for musculoskeletal injuries has become a less common practice. It is interesting and useful to see this small but prospective and randomized study indicating that local injection for reduction of acute anterior shoulder dislocation is apparently quite effective and safe.

R.H. Cofield, M.D.

Primary Anterior Dislocation of the Shoulder in Young Patients: A Ten-Year Prospective Study

Hovelius L, Augustini BG, Fredin H, et al (Gävle Hosp, Sweden; Regionsjukhuset, Örebro, Sweden; Malmö Allmänna sjukhus, Sweden; et al)
J Bone Joint Surg Am 78A:1677–1684, 1996   1–13

Methods.—In a prospective, multicenter study at 27 Swedish hospitals of 257 dislocations of the glenohumeral joint (52 female), patients were treated by mobilization for 3 to 4 weeks (group 1), with use of a sling until comfortable (group 2), or were given varied treatment (group 3). At 10 years, 245 patients (247 shoulders) were interviewed and examined and the shoulders assessed radiographically. Comparisons were analyzed statistically.

Results.—There were no recurrent dislocations in 129 shoulders although 8 were considered by the patients to be unstable, 11 shoulders had 1 recurrent dislocation, 58 with recurrent dislocations were operated on, and 49 with recurrent dislocations were not treated operatively. Arthropathy was mild in 23 shoulders, moderate in 16, and severe in 2. There was articular incongruity in 32 shoulders, 23 of which also had arthropathy ($P< 0.0001$). These 23 shoulders had at least 1 recurrent dislocation compared with 79 of the 176 with a congruent joint ($P=0.01$). Of 189 patients with bilateral radiographs, 24 had dislocation or subluxation of the contralateral shoulder. Four of these shoulders had evidence of moderate or severe arthropathy compared with 3 of 165 stable contralateral

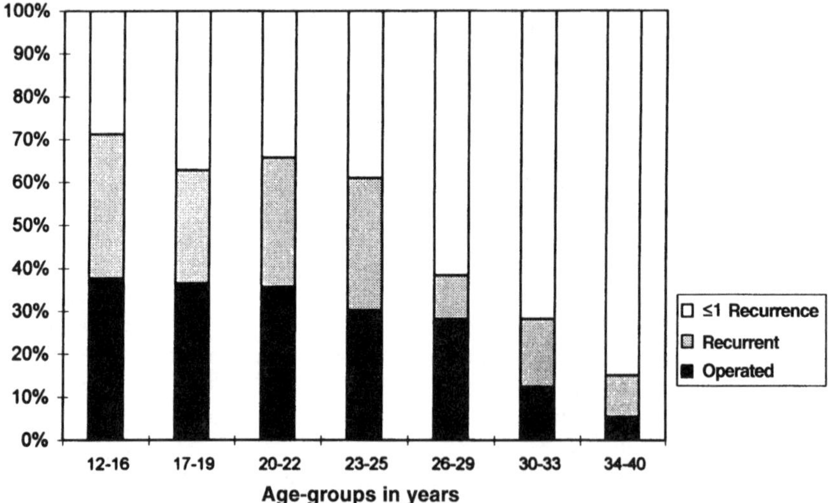

FIGURE 4.—Histogram shows the percentages of shoulders that had no or only 1 recurrence of dislocation, those that had recurrence leading to operative treatment, and those that had 2 or more recurrences but no operative treatment, according to the various age groups, at the 10-year follow-up evaluation. Shoulders that had a fracture of the greater tuberosity are excluded. (Courtesy of Hovelius L, Augustini BG, Fredin H, et al: Primary anterior dislocation of the shoulder in young patients: A ten-year prospective study. *J Bone Joint Surg Am* 78A:1677–1684, 1996.)

shoulders ($P<$ 0.001). A significant number of patients over age 25 needed surgery (Fig 4). When dislocation recurred within 2 to 5 years after initial injury, operative intervention was not necessary in 24 shoulders (22%). Dislocation of the contralateral shoulder occurred in 16% of 12- to 22-year-olds, 21% of shoulders in 23- to 29-year-olds and 3% of shoulders in 30- to 40-year-olds. A Hermodsson lesion, present on the initial radiograph in 99 of 185 shoulders, was significantly associated with a worse prognosis at 10 years than shoulders with no lesion.

Conclusion.—At 10-year followup, 23 shoulders showed mild arthropathy, 16 had moderate arthropathy, and 2 had severe arthropathy. Some of these shoulders had not had recurrent dislocations. Most recurrent dislocations occurred between years 2 and 5. Patients older than age 25 had a higher operation rate.

▶ This study again reinforces what a few other studies have found; recurrent rates are moderate in younger individuals. The need for subsequent surgery occurs in one quarter to one third of patients. It is very appealing to consider treating traumatic first-time dislocations with surgery (typically arthroscopic), but this article reminds us that in doing so, we would operate on many more patients initially than would subsequently require surgery. Of special note is the fact that the youngest patient group (12 to 16 years of age) has a recurrence rate similar to those in the upper teenage years and in the early 20s and that the frequency of recurrent dislocations falls off dramatically at about age 25.

R.H. Cofield, M.D.

The Capsular Imbrication Procedure for Recurrent Anterior Instability of the Shoulder

Wirth MA, Blatter G, Rockwood CA Jr (Univ of Texas, San Antonio)
J Bone Joint Surg (Am) 78–A:246–259, 1996   1–14

Background.—Many operative techniques have been described for the stabilization of anterior glenohumeral instability in patients with recurrent instability unresponsive to physician-directed rehabilitation. A number of these procedures, however, do not address the pathologic condition in the glenohumeral capsule and labrum, and complications result. An operative approach designed to repair the capsulolabral injury and decrease the overall capsular volume was described.

Methods and Findings.—One hundred thirty-eight patients with 142 affected shoulders underwent an anatomical capsular imbrication reconstruction. Capsulolabral injury was repaired, and the anteroinferior capsular ligaments were reinforced with an imbrication method that reduced the overall capsular volume. In 108 shoulders (group 1), the recurrent instability was associated with a defined traumatic episode. In the remaining 34 (group 2), there was no distinct history of trauma. Anatomical capsular imbrication was the main procedure performed in 90 shoulders. The remaining 52 shoulders had been treated unsuccessfully at least once before. Outcomes were good or excellent in 93% of the shoulders at 2 to 12 years after surgery. The results were excellent in 40 of the 52 shoulders that had previously failed reconstruction, good in 5, fair in 4, and poor in 3.

Conclusion.—To be effective, anterior shoulder reconstruction must restore premorbid function and stability while maintaining a physiologic range of motion. Anatomical capsular imbrication is an effective technique for reconstructing recurrent anterior instability of the shoulder, regardless of the cause.

▶ This article nicely reinforces that Bankart lesions are common in those with trauma, and that direct suture repair of the lesion is desirable. More important, though, it lets us know that capsular tensioning is an important part of the procedure, that there are a number of patients with capsular laxity and instability who do not have a Bankart lesion, and that both the former and the latter group benefit greatly by adjustment of the capsular tension as a part of the operative repair.

R.H. Cofield, M.D.

Arthroscopic Anterior Labral Reconstruction Using a Transglenoid Suture Technique: Results in Active-duty Military Patients

Mologne TS, Lapoint JM, Morin WD, et al (Naval Med Ctr, San Diego, Calif)
Am J Sports Med 24:268–274, 1996   1–15

Background.—Ideally, surgical treatment of traumatic anterior glenohumeral instability would repair the torn or detached labrum and reestablish the integrity of the inferior glenohumeral ligament. Historically, the open Bankart procedure has been the gold standard in surgical management of these lesions. However, arthroscopic stabilization of the glenohumeral joint is now possible. A 3-year experience with arthroscopic transglenoid suture reconstruction of the anteroinferior glenoid labrum in athletic military patients was reviewed in a retrospective study.

Operative Technique.—A diagnostic arthroscopic examination is performed, using standard anterior and posterior shoulder arthroscopic portals. The frayed labral or rotator cuff muscular tissue is débrided and the scapular neck is abraded to bleeding bone in the area of labral attachment. Polydioxanone sutures are placed in the labrum. One or two 2-mm Beath pins are placed through the glenoid, drilled across the scapular neck, and placed through the infraspinatus muscle. Then, 0-PDS labral sutures are delivered through the holes with the Beath pins and tied posteriorly over the infraspinatus fascia. Postoperatively, the shoulder is immobilized for 6 weeks before passive motion is begun. Active motion is begun at 8 weeks, and resistive exercises are begun after full motion is achieved.

Methods.—The inpatient and outpatient records of 48 patients undergoing 49 arthroscopic procedures were reviewed. The patients had 3 types of injuries: a history of traumatic glenohumeral dislocation (29 patients), traumatic recurrent glenohumeral subluxation (12 patients), and shoulder pain and apprehension on testing, but no subjective instability (7 patients). Follow-up data included the occurrence of recurrent instability, functional outcome, and return to athletic participation. Predictors of recurrent instability were analyzed.

Results.—Recurrent instability was reported during follow-up in 45% of the patients with a history of glenohumeral dislocations and 33% of the patients with a history of glenohumeral subluxations. In the dislocation group, the functional results were good or excellent in 52%, fair in 14%, and poor in 34%. Functional results in the subluxation group were good or excellent in 50%, fair in 25%, and poor in 25%. In the shoulder pain group, functional results were good or excellent in 63% and poor in 37%. Return to full athletic participation was achieved in 48% of the dislocation group, 33% of the subluxation group, and 71% of the shoulder pain group. Compliance with postoperative immobilization for 6 weeks was the only significant predictor of outcome. There was a complication rate of 14%, with 7 complications in 5 patients. The complications included suprascapular nerve palsy in 3 patients and traction-induced musculocutaneous nerve palsy, septic shoulder, portal abscess, and adhesive capsulitis in 1 patient each.

Conclusion.—Arthroscopic transglenoid suture for anterior labral reconstruction was associated with a high rate of recurrent instability in athletic military patients, although the risk of recurrent instability was reduced in patients with immobilized shoulders for a full 6 weeks postoperatively. Suprascapular nerve palsy emerged as a significant potential complication of the procedure. Therefore, this arthroscopic technique is not recommended for the management of glenohumeral instability in young athletic patients.

▶ Unlike arthroscopically assisted rotator cuff repair, arthroscopically mediated anterior capsule repair has a great variation in results, according to reports. This report is an example of those in which the results have not been favorable compared with the more standard, traditional, open suturing techniques. It appears that unless new arthroscopic techniques are developed, the traditional open methods are preferrable.

R.H. Cofield, M.D.

An Arthroscopic Technique for Anterior Stabilization of the Shoulder With a Bioabsorbable Tack

Speer KP, Warren RF, Pagnani M, et al (Duke Univ, Durham, NC; Hosp for Special Surgery, New York; Univ of Pittsburgh, Pa)
J Bone Joint Surg Am 78A:1801–1807, 1996   1–16

Background.—Arthroscopy can be used to re-establish a functional inferior glenohumeral ligament and stabilize the shoulder after injury. A technique for arthroscopic stabilization of the shoulder using a bioabsorbable tack was described.

Study Group.—The records of the first 52 patients who were managed athroscopically for the anterior stabilization of the glenohumeral joint with a bioabsorbable tack were reviewed. There were 47 male and 5 female patients in the study group. The average age of these patients was 28 years, and the dominant shoulder was affected in 29 of the participants. The injury mechanism was traumatic dislocation in 36 patients, of whom 25 sustained the injury playing contact sports.

Surgical Technique.—A complete glenohumeral arthroscopic examination was performed before surgery. A Bankart lesion was present in 50 patients and a chondral Hill-Sachs lesion in 44. The osseous glenoid rim was abraded. A grasper was inserted and used to reduce the labrum and shift it 0.5 to 1.0 cm superiorly on the glenoid rim. A cannulated drill was inserted, and the bioabsorbable tack was impacted over the drill wire and inserted under arthroscopic visualization. Two or 3 tacks were used for each procedure. The patient used a sling for 4 weeks and performed pendulum, range-of-motion, and isometric forearm exercises. After 4 weeks, patients were permitted passive forward flexion and elevation of the shoulder and external rotation. At 6 weeks, progression to full range of motion was permitted. Participation in contact sports was not allowed for 5 months. Follow-up of 49 patients took place at 24 to 64 months, with the remaining 3 patients interviewed by telephone.

Results.—At follow-up, 79% of patients were asymptomatic and were participating in sports. The repair was considered a failure in 21%. In 4 cases, the failure was caused by traumatic reinjury during a contact sport, but the remaining 7 failures were atraumatic. Because of recurrent instability, 8 patients had an open glenoid-based capsulorrhaphy. There was no evidence of tacks in these patient and the Bankart lesions were completely healed.

Conclusion.—This retrospective study indicates that this technique is useful for patients with a traumatic injury and a thick mobile Bankart lesion. It is best suited for repair of detachment of the anterior aspect of the labrum. This procedure will not be successful if anatomical reattachment of a displaced Bankart lesion will not restore shoulder stability, and such patients should be treated with open capsulorrhaphy or a capsular shift-type procedure.

▶ This well-balanced report probably tells it like it is. If one is quite careful in patient selection and selects the optimal situation for the use of arthroscopic repair—and does it well—it is often effective in eliminating the instability. Of the 21% who failed in this series, many failed because of continuing capsule laxity. Certainly, the Bankart lesion and capsule laxity co-exist in many patients—if not most or all patients. It is useful to know that in about 80% of patients, fixation of the Bankart lesion alone will solve the problem.

I think we are getting closer and closer to understanding the role of the arthroscopic technique for anterior stabilization. As techniques evolve and improve, no doubt this will ease more and more toward the standard for a typical, traumatically induced, recurrent anterior instability problem.

R.H. Cofield, M.D.

Arthroscopic Bankart Repair Using a Degradable Tack: A Followup Study Using Optimized Indications
Laurencin CT, Stephens S, Warren RF, et al (Cornell Univ, New York)
Clin Orthop 332:132–137, 1996   1–17

Objective.—Arthroscopic Bankart repair using degradable polymeric tacks is a fairly new technique for correcting shoulder instability. Initial results showed that 21% of patients had recurrent anterior instability. According to the authors of that study, this was the result of faulty patient selection. Results for patients selected using more stringent criteria were reported.

Methods.—A total of 22 arthroscopic Bankart repair procedures were performed in 21 patients (2 women), aged 19 to 69 years. The dominant arm was injured in 9 patients. After surgery, the patients' arms were placed in a sling for 4 weeks and the patients performed passive motion exercises followed by assisted exercise. The patients achieved their fullest range of motion by 3 months and participated in sports at 5 months.

Results.—Intraoperatively, 10 shoulders had a 3+ anterior laxity, 9 had a 2+ anterior laxity, 1 had a 1+ anterior laxity, 2 had a 2+ posterior laxity, 9 had a 1+ posterior laxity, and 9 had a 0+ posterior laxity. Five shoulders had a 1+ sulcus sign. There were no perioperative complications. At a mean follow-up of 35 months, 17 shoulders were rated excellent, 1 was rated fair, and 2 were rated poor. Seventeen patients (18 shoulders) had no recurring instability. One had 3 dislocation episodes and 1 had 3 episodes of shoulder subluxation. The patient with a fair result had shoulder weakness. Patients reported satisfaction in 90% of shoulders.

Conclusion.—There was 10% recurrent instability in this group of patients compared with 21% recurrent instability in the first group of patients treated with arthroscopic Bankart repair.

▶ Indications for the use of arthroscopically mediated repair for shoulder instability are becoming refined. The success of the procedure is increasing. Now the frequency of failure is probably only about twice that of standard open repair, whereas it was once much higher.

R.H. Cofield, M.D.

Recurrent Instability of the Shoulder After Age 40

Neviaser RJ, Neviaser TJ (George Washington Univ, Washington, DC)
J Shoulder Elbow Surg 4:416–418, 1995   1–18

Introduction.—Typically, recurrent dislocation of the shoulder occurs in patients younger than 40 years of age. There has been little study of the tissue injuries causing recurrent dislocation of the shoulder with onset after age 40. A series of patients older than 40 years of age with a first occurrence of recurrent instability of the shoulder were studied retrospectively.

Methods.—Twelve patients were studied in whom instability of the shoulder occurred between the ages of 52 and 83 years. There was recurrent anterior instability in 11 patients and recurrent posterior dislocation in 1 patient. In all cases, the onset was traumatic, and the recurrent episodes occurred early, sometimes immediately, after the injury. All of the patients with anterior instability had the subscapularis and underlying anterior capsule torn from the lesser tuberosity; they were mobilized and sutured to the lesser tuberosity. In the patient with posterior dislocation, the infraspinatus, upper teres minor, and underlying capsule were torn from the greater tuberosity; these tendons and the capsule were mobilized and sutured to the greater tuberosity. No patients had labral detachment.

Results.—All the patients ultimately achieved stability and range of motion equal to those of their other shoulder. One of the patients with anterior instability required a repeated procedure to resuture the capsule and subscapularis to the tuberosity, and a modified postoperative rehabilitation strategy.

Conclusion.—In patients experiencing recurrent anterior and posterior dislocations after the age of 40 years, the injury may be related to torn rotator cuff tendon and shoulder capsule detachment with intact labral attachments. Repairing the tendon and capsule attachments can restore stability and motion.

▶ When considering patients with recurrent instability, we now focus on the capsule and rotator cuff. These authors remind us that in older patients (where instability is not all that common), we must consider lateral detachment of the rotator cuff and capsular structures carefully. Fortunately, physical examination is usually reliable in doing this. If that does not suffice, MRI should be a useful adjunct to diagnosis in this setting.

R.H. Cofield, M.D.

Capsulitis

The Clinical Course of Shoulder Pain: Prospective Cohort Study in Primary Care
Croft P, for the Primary Care Rheumatology Society Shoulder Study Group (Univ of Keele, Stoke on Trent, England)
BMJ 313:601–602, 1996
1–19

Objective.—Although shoulder pain is common, few patients see a specialist. Little is known about the outcome of these injuries. Results of a prospective cohort study to determine the outcome of shoulder pain in primary care were presented.

Methods.—Disability questionnaires were sent to 166 patients with shoulder pain 6 and 18 months after they consulted 12 general practitioners. The questionnaire contained 22 disability items in 5 categories: sleeping problems, physical problems, problems dressing, psychological symptoms, and dependency. There was a 75% response at 6 months and a 57% response at 18 months. Most patients were treated by injection (58%). Capsulitis was the most common diagnosis (39%). A prior incidence of shoulder pain was reported by 22% of patients.

Results.—At the initial visit, patients gave positive responses to 11 of 22 of the disability items. At 6 months, patients gave positive responses to an average of 4.1 items. Only 21% reported full recovery. Most complaints were the same as those reported at baseline. Patients with a baseline disability score > 10, symptoms lasting longer than a month, receiving an injection for pain, having severe restricted passive elevation, and a history of shoulder pain had a significantly poorer outcome at 6 months.

Conclusion.—Shoulder problems are longer lasting than previously thought. About 25% of patients had a previous episode of shoulder pain. After 6 months, only 20% of episodes had resolved, and after 18 months, only 50% of patients had recovered completely. Patients treated by injection had a poorer prognosis, possible because their symptoms were worse at baseline. The relationship between duration of symptoms and outcome suggests that delay in seeking medical help may have adverse prognostic consequences.

▶ This interesting study of patients seen with shoulder pain at a general medical practice reinforces for us the fact that symptoms often last a long time. It also allows us to appreciate the fact that a substantial number of patients will improve with time and that prolonged conservative treatment has merit. This study also argues for more exact diagnoses to try to establish who will improve, and who will not improve, over time.

R.H. Cofield, M.D.

Arthroscopic Release for Chronic, Refractory Adhesive Capsulitis of the Shoulder

Warner JJP, Allen A, Marks PH, et al (Univ of Pittsburgh, Pa)
J Bone Joint Surg Am 78A:1808–1816, 1996   1–20

Introduction.—Most patients with idiopathic adhesive capsulitis improve with gentle physical therapy. If not, they may undergo closed manipulation under anesthesia. Some patients who still have limited mobility may undergo open soft-tissue release. A new surgical alternative for refractory adhesive capsulitis of the shoulder—arthroscopic capsular release—is described.

Methods.—Arthroscopic capsular release was performed in 23 patients with idiopathic adhesive capsulitis during a 3-year period. All patients had persistent pain and limitation of motion after supervised physical therapy and closed manipulation. There were 12 women and 11 men (mean age, 43 years). Arthroscopic anterior capsular release, was followed by 48 hours of intensive, inpatient physical therapy. The physical therapy was done with interscalene regional analgesic, achieved with either repeated nerve blocks or continuous infusion via interscalene catheter. Impingement in 6 patients was treated with arthroscopic acromioplasty.

Results.—There were no treatment complications. When evaluated at a mean follow-up of 39 months, the patients averaged a 48-point increase in the score of Constant and Murley. All patients were pain free or had only mild discomfort when using the shoulder forcefully. Shoulder motion improved by a mean of 49 degrees of flexion, 42 degrees of external rotation in adduction, and 53 degrees of external rotation in abduction. Internal rotation improved by 8 spinous process levels in adduction and 33 degrees in abduction. All of these improvements were significant, and brought the operated shoulder to within a mean of 7 degrees of the values recorded for the unaffected shoulder.

Conclusions.—In patients with idiopathic adhesive capsulitis of the shoulder that does not respond to other treatments, arthroscopic capsular release offers a new treatment alternative. This operation improves motion and reduces pain with little operative morbidity. A controlled capsular release can be performed, and any concomitant lesions can be treated at the same time. After arthroscopic release, the manipulation required to restore motion is much reduced.

► I must say that I have never encountered a patient with idiopathic adhesive capsulitis of the shoulder who did not eventually undergo self resolution and regain a large amount of the pre-existent motion. In line with this, the patients forming the larger group from which these operative patients were selected had loss of motion after an operative procedure or loss of motion after some form of trauma. These events then precipitated the inflammatory response and the shoulder stiffness. I concur that there are some patients within these groups who do not regain their movement over time, and occasionally, capsular release will be necessary. This article demonstrates that arthroscopic capsular release can be safe and effective. The worry, of course, is that the shoulder may then become unstable. Fortunately, this has not become an issue—to date...

R.H. Cofield, M.D.

Rotator Cuff and Other Tendon Injuries

The Acromion: Morphologic Condition and Age-related Changes. A Study of 420 Scapulas

Nicholson GP, Goodman DA, Flatow EL, et al (Orthopaedics Indianapolis Inc, Ind; Orthopaedics South, Riverdale, Ga; Columbia-Presbyterian Med Ctr, New York)

J Shoulder Elbow Surg 5:1–11, 1996   1–21

Background.—There have been several reports of the variability in the shape, slope, and size of the acromion and of the incidence of os acromiale. However, there have been no longitudinal studies of acromial morphology. The impact of aging on acromial morphology was investigated.

Methods.—A total of 420 scapulas from 210 skeletal specimens were studied from equal numbers of female and male and black and white subjects in five 10-year age groups between 21 and 70 years. Measurements of acromial length, anterior width, and anterior thickness and of the length and height of the acromial facet of the acromioclavicular joint were made with digital calipers. The inclination of the acromioclavicular joint was determined in relation to the sagittal plane. The acromial morphologic condition (flat, curved, or hooked) was determined with lateral outlet view radiographs. Visual inspection was used to detect acromial spur formation and degenerative changes at the acromioclavicular joint facet of the acromion.

Results.—Meso-acromiale was observed in 6% of the scapulas and 8% of the specimens, with bilateral involvement in 7 of 17 subjects. Of the remaining scapulas, the acromial morphologic condition was type I (flat) in 32%, type II (curved) in 42%, and type III (hooked) in 26%. Aside from a statistically significant increase in the type II and a decrease in the type III morphologic condition in the 51- to 60-year age group, there were no consistent trends in changing morphologic types with advancing age. The incidence of spur formation increased with advancing age. Acromion size differed significantly between men and women. Among women, the average dimensions were as follows: length, 40.6 mm; width, 18.4 mm; and thickness, 6.7 mm. Among men, the average dimensions were as follows: length, 48.5 mm; width, 19.5 mm; and thickness, 7.7 mm. Age did not affect acromial dimensions. The acromial facet of the acromioclavicular joint had a mean length of 17.3 mm and a mean height of 9.1 mm and was medially inclined in 49% of subjects, vertical in 48%, and laterally inclined in 3%. There were significantly more arthritic facets in specimens of subjects older than 50 years of age compared with younger subjects (70% vs. 9%).

Conclusion.—Aging is associated with significant increases in degenerative changes at the acromial facet of the acromioclavicular joint and in anterior acromial spur formation. However, aging does not affect the acromial dimensions or consistently affect the acromial morphologic condition. The normal variations in acromial morphologic condition can be independent contributors to impingement disease, in addition to the effects of age-related degenerative changes.

▶ These authors nicely define for us that there are distinct morphologic types of acromion processes and that there are also age-related and degenerative changes of the acromion. Both factors need to be considered when evaluating the acromion in a symptomatic patient.

R.H. Cofield, M.D.

Histological Analysis of the Coracoacromial Arch: Correlation Between Age-related Changes and Rotator Cuff Tears

Panni AS, Milano G, Lucania L, et al (Catholic Univ, Rome; Univ of Sassari, Italy)
Arthroscopy 12:531–540, 1996

1–22

Background.—Research has shown that patients with partial or full-thickness tears of the rotator cuff have degenerative and proliferative changes in the coracoacromial arch. However, few researchers have tried to define the relationship between rotator cuff tears and degenerative changes seen in the structures of the coracoacromial arch. Age-related changes in the coracoacromial arch were analyzed and correlated with rotator cuff tears.

Methods.—Eighty shoulders were obtained from 40 cadavers, aged a mean 58.4 years at death. The rotator cuff and acromion were examined grossly, and the coracoacromial ligament was examined histologically.

Findings.—The incidence and severity of cuff tears increased with age. Age-related degenerative changes in the coracoacromial ligament, degeneration of the acromial bone-ligament junction, and acromial spur formation were observed. Anterior acromial spur was unassociated with acromion morphologic features. The incidences of bursal-side and complete cuff tears were increased when the acromion was curved or beaked. Degenerative changes in the undersurface of the acromion also occurred in normal rotator cuffs. In all specimens, bursal-side and complete cuff tears were correlated with severe degenerative changes in the acromion. Articular side cuff tears were unassociated with acromial structure or degenerative changes in the coracoacromial arch. The relationship between cuff tears and acromial spur was more apparent when a type III acromion was present.

Conclusions.—The incidence and severity of rotator cuff tears are associated with aging and the morphologic features of the acromion. Rotator cuff tears involving the bursal side are frequently correlated with changes in the coracoacromial ligament and acromion undersurface. However, articular-side partial tears are not associated with degenerative changes in the coracoacromial arch.

▶ This straightforward study is very useful in bringing some order to the relationship between aging, the coracoacromial arch, rotator cuff tearing, and the site of rotator cuff tearing. There are many factors involved, and one is usually not sure that things are this simple and straightforward, but, if so, this article is a step forward in organizing the information about this subject.

R.H. Cofield, M.D.

Reliability of Radiographic Assessment of Acromial Morphology
Jacobson SR, Speer KP, Moor JT, et al (Southern California Ctr for Sports Medicine, Long Beach; Duke Univ, Durham, NC; Inst for Preventative Sports Medicine, Ann Arbor, Mich; et al)
J Shoulder Elbow Surg 4:449–453, 1995   1–23

Background.—In the most commonly used radiographic classification system for acromial morphology, flat (type I), curved (type II), and hooked (type III) acromial shapes are identified. The interobserver and intraobserver reliability of determinations of acromial morphology using this system were reported.

Methods.—Six shoulder surgeons independently reviewed and classified 126 supraspinatus outlet radiographs. Two surgeons classified each radiograph a second time.

Findings.—Intraobserver reliability was good to excellent, with a coefficient of 0.888. However, interobserver reliability was poor to fair, with a coefficient of 0.516. By consensus, 20.6% of the radiographs were classified as type I, 60.3% as type II, and 19.1% as type III. Reliability was lowest when observers had to delineate between type II and type III morphology.

Conclusion.—Low interobserver reliability makes it difficult to compare studies by different authors and to establish the true incidence of acromial morphologic types. Interobserver reliability may be improved by adopting a system with more objective classification criteria and one that allows for the continuous nature of acromial morphologic types.

▶ In this study using radiographs, it is apparent that classifying acromial morphology is difficult and may be inconsistent. As such, we probably need both better imaging methods and a more refined technique for measuring acromial shape. The standard radiographs and the usual observational methods give us a general sense about the acromion, but as one delves more deeply into details of acromial analysis, our contemporary methodology falls short of what we would wish it to do.

R.H. Cofield, M.D.

Rotator Cuff Strain: A Post-traumatic Mimicker of Tendinitis on MRI

Anzilotti KF Jr, Schweitzer ME, Oliveri M, et al (Thomas Jefferson Univ, Philadelphia; Orthopedic Associates, Langhorne, Pa)
Skeletal Radiol 25:555–558, 1996

1–24

Background.—Authorities have suggested that acute trauma may be a mechanism of cuff injury. However, there is little evidence supporting this. Also, no imaging criteria exist to distinguish such injury from impingement. The current study determined whether some young patients have acute, posttraumatic insults to the rotator cuff that mimic the early stages of impingement.

Methods.—One hundred ninety-seven consecutive shoulder MR images were reviewed retrospectively. The results of 83 were correlated with clinical findings. Two examiners independently assessed the location of intratendon signal and adjacent bone marrow abnormalities on T1- and T2-weighted images.

Findings.—The signal intensity of patients younger than 35 years was more localized in atypical locations (the posterior aspect of the supraspinatus tendon) and more commonly associated with marrow abnormalities and with trauma. In addition, younger patients were less likely to need surgery, especially younger patients with bone bruises. In contrast, patients older than 45 years had more widespread signal in the tendon, only rarely had bone bruises, and required surgery more frequently (Fig 1).

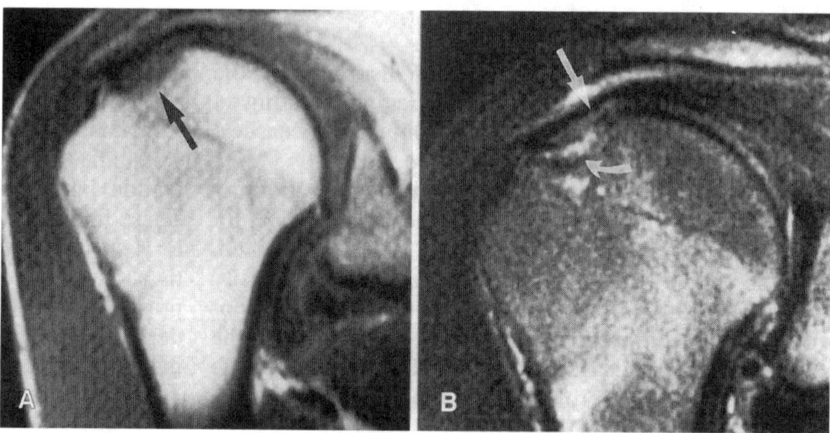

FIGURE 1.—A, B, a patient, 27 years, with a recent history of shoulder trauma. A, T1-weighted coronal oblique image (551/15, 128 × 256) shows a low signal intensity area, with moderately well defined margins in the subchondral humeral head (*arrow*). B, the corresponding T2-weighted image (3500/102, 256 × 256) shows this region in the subchondral humeral head (*curved arrow*), as well as a characteristic ill-defined high signal intensity region in the posterior aspect of the supraspinatus tendon, which is overlying the apparent bone bruise (*straight arrow*). (Courtesy of Anzilotti KF Jr, Schweitzer ME, Oliveri M, et al: Rotator cuff strain: A post-traumatic mimicker of tendinitis on MRI. *Skeletal Radiol* 25:555–558, 1996.)

Conclusions.—Some patients younger than 35 years with MR features superficially resembling those of tendinitis may have traumatic lesions. Neither isolated impingement nor findings of impingement in the posterior aspect of the cuff has been associated with bone bruises.

▶ This is 1 of what I predict will be a number of studies offering clinical correlations with MRI. It clearly indicates that degenerative changes and traumatic changes can be easily confused. In this group, strains were more commonly focal changes, and often there was an associated bone bruise. Most important, it notifies us yet again that we must be careful when interpreting imaging studies. Similar changes on the image may, in fact, be 2 completely different things: in 1 instance, a firm scar; in the second, degenerated tendons with mucoid infiltration.

R.H. Cofield, M.D.

Relationship Between Calcifying Tendinitis and Subacromial Impingement: A Prospective Radiography and Magnetic Resonance Imaging Study

Loew M, Sabo D, Wehrle M, et al (Univ of Heidelberg, Germany)
J Shoulder Elbow Surg 5:314–319, 1996   1–25

Background.—Calcifications are a common cause of shoulder pain and stiffness. A degenerative pathogenesis has been proposed for these calcifications, and they have been implicated in subacromial impingement. The coincidence of calcifying tendinitis and a narrowing of the subacromial space was investigated in a prospective radiographic and imaging study.

Methods.—Seventy-five consecutive patients with symptomatic calcific tendinitis of the rotator cuff underwent radiographic and MRI evaluation. The images were analyzed independently by the performing radiologist and 2 other investigators to assess the rotator cuff and humeral head for signs of degenerative alteration.

Results.—Radiographic studies of the 75 patients revealed 53% with type I acromions, 32% with type II acromions, and 16% with type III acromions. The MR images showed 3 types of calcium deposits: compact, homogeneous, 1-part, clearly defined structure in 54%; subdivided, homogeneous, clearly defined structure in 38%; and diffuse, poorly defined structure of low signal intensity in 7%. These calcium deposits were typically in the midportion of the tendon or under its acromial surface. There was a markedly low rate of coincidence of calcifying tendinitis and advanced rotator cuff lesions, with a partial-thickness tear of the supraspinatus tendon occurring in only 1 patient.

Conclusion.—A definite correlation between calcifying tendinitis and subacromial impingement was not found. Therefore, subacromial decompression by anterior acromioplasty is not routinely indicated in the surgical management of calcifying tendinitis.

▶ There is much consideration of whether a patient seen with calcifying tendinitis also has ongoing impingement problems. This study defines for us the fact that although these 2 conditions can co-exist, usually they do not.

R.H. Cofield, M.D.

Arthroscopic Assisted Rotator Cuff Repair: Results Using a Mini-Open Deltoid Splitting Approach

Blevins FT, Warren RF, Cavo C, et al (Univ of New Mexico, Albuquerque; Cornell Univ, New York; Cleveland Clinic Found, Ohio)
Arthroscopy 12:50–59, 1996

1–26

Background.—Although the success rate of open rotator cuff repair is high, this technique has some limitations. The importance of an intact deltoid has been emphasized. Deltoid detachment may be avoided through the use of an arthroscopic assisted deltoid splitting miniarthrotomy methods. The outcomes of the first 64 rotator cuff tears treated at 1 center using an arthroscopic assisted mini-open method were reported.

Methods.—The 64 patients were interviewed and completed a detailed questionnaire. Forty-seven returned for a physical examination. Patient ages ranged from 31 to 85 years. The average tear size was 8 cm². Follow-up ranged from 12 to 65 months.

Findings.—All patients reported pain and weakness before surgery. Positive impingement signs were present in 96% of the patients preoperatively and in 16% postoperatively. Active elevation was significantly increased from 129 to 166 degrees. At the follow-up assessment, active elevation in the operative and contralateral shoulders did not differ significantly. Weakness was detected during the physical examination in 83% of the patients initially and in 22% at the final assessment. Significant improvement was noted in mean pain and function scores. Eighty-nine percent of the patients were satisfied with their outcomes. Additional surgery was needed in 3 patients. Cuff tear size was unassociated with the final Hospital for Special Surgery shoulder score.

Conclusion.—Arthroscopic assisted rotator cuff repair is safe and effective in the treatment of cuff tears of a wide variety of sizes. The outcomes in this series are comparable to those of open repair.

▶ These authors demonstrate in an ample number of patients that arthroscopic assisted rotator cuff repair can be done consistently, and the results parallel those of traditional methods. I believe the authors have demonstrated quite nicely that this is an acceptable treatment alternative. I do not think they have shown that it represents an improvement in technique.

R.H. Cofield, M.D.

Comparison of Open and Arthroscopically Assisted Rotator Cuff Repairs

Baker CL, Liu SH (Hughston Clinic, Columbus, Ga)
Am J Sports Med 23:99–104, 1995   1–27

Background.—Although open rotator cuff repair with acromioplasty can achieve good pain relief and functional improvement, it usually results in disappointing functional status in athletes. Shoulder arthroscopy has been used in rotator cuff repair with promising results. The results of open and arthroscopically assisted miniopen rotator cuff repairs were compared in a retrospective study.

Methods.—The records of 36 patients undergoing either open (20 shoulders) or arthroscopic (17 shoulders) rotator cuff repairs over a 3-year period were reviewed. The patients were followed for an average of 3.2 years in the arthroscopic group and 3.3 years in the open repair group. Each patient was evaluated for pain and function (using the University of California, Los Angeles [UCLA] rating scale), range of motion, and manual strength before surgery and during follow-up. The size of the tear was determined intraoperatively. Hospitalization, complications, and the interval between surgery and full return to activity were compared.

Results.—The UCLA shoulder ratings indicated good or excellent results in 83% of the arthroscopic group and in 94% of the open surgery group. When analyzed by tear size, good or excellent results were achieved by all patients with small tears, 88% in the arthroscopic group and 73% in the open repair group with moderate tears, and 50% in the arthroscopic group and 80% in the open group with large tears. There were no significant differences between the 2 groups in pain reduction or functional improvement. Range of motion increased significantly in both groups, with greater flexion achieved in the arthroscopic group. All patients had increased postoperative strength, with greater abduction strength found in the arthroscopic group. The hospital stay averaged 1.2 days in the arthroscopic group and 2.3 days in the open repair group. Previous activities could be performed without restriction in an average of 4.5 months after surgery in the arthroscopic group and 5.6 months after surgery in the open repair group.

Conclusion.—Arthroscopically assisted rotator cuff repair is comparably effective to open rotator cuff repair. The arthroscopic technique has the advantages of shorter hospitalization and rehabilitation time and allows the inspection and treatment of glenohumeral joint abnormalities, subacromial decompression with treatment of the acromioclavicular joint lesions, and preserved deltoid attachment.

▶ This, as with the article by Blevins and co-authors (Abstract 1–26), reaffirms that arthroscopically assisted rotator cuff repair results seem to equal those of the open repair method when performed by surgeons very skilled in this technique. Again, it seems apparent that the results are in general not improved, but are, if not equal, nearly equal.

R.H. Cofield, M.D.

Isolated Rupture of the Subscapularis Tendon: Results of Operative Repair
Gerber C, Hersche O, Farron A (Hôpital Cantonal, Fribourg, Switzerland; Univ of Zurich, Switzerland)
J Bone Joint Surg Am 78A:1015–1023, 1996

1–28

Background.—Although recognition of isolated rupture of the tendon of the subscapularis muscle has become widespread with use of MRI, the outcome of treatment for this surgery has not been documented. The results of surgical repair of this lesion were studied in 16 consecutive patients with a complete, traumatic, isolated tear of the subscapularis tendon.

Methods.—All 16 patients were men (aged 33 to 60 years); none showed avulsion of the lesser tuberosity. Surgical treatment comprised exploration and protection of the axillary nerve, mobilization of the subscapularis, transosseus reinsertion of the tendon to a trough formed at the lesser tuberosity, closure of the rotator interval, and 6 weeks' postoperative protection of the shoulder. Mean duration of follow-up was 43 months.

Results.—Outcome was subjectively rated as good or excellent by 13 patients. Functional shoulder scores (system of Constant) averaged 82% of the normal value for age and sex. Twelve patients showed normal active flexion, 3 showed a decrease of 15 degrees or less, and 1 showed severe limitation. The patients' capacity to work in their original occupations averaged 59% full capacity before surgery and 95% after. Neither capacity for work at the time of operation, type of occupational work, state of the biceps, nor duration of follow-up was related to quality of outcome. However, a longer time interval between injury and repair was associated with a less successful outcome.

Conclusions.—Surgical treatment of isolated tears of the subscapularis muscle generally produces favorable results, including a significant gain in the patients' capacity to work (disability with regard to work decreased by 36%). Early repair consistently led to a favorable outcome, whereas delayed repair resulted in a less satisfactory outcome. Thus attempts at nonsurgical repair of these lesions may not be justified.

▶ This important paper reinforces the idea that clearly traumatically induced tears of the subscapularis (a portion of the rotator cuff) can occur in persons of various ages and that they may occur separately from associated involvement with the supraspinatus tendon. The diagnosis of the problem may therefore be somewhat subtle. Treatment when symptoms are present may not be technically simple but is quite straightforward. In these patients, it is important to investigate for concomitant problems in the supraspinatus that may or may not exist. If so, the treatment will probably vary, including not only repair of the subscapularis but also repair of the supraspinatus tendon and anterior acromioplasty.

R.H. Cofield, M.D.

Subscapularis Transfer for Reconstruction of Massive Tears of the Rotator Cuff

Karas SE, Giachello TL (New England Orthopedic Surgeons, Springfield, Mass)

J Bone Joint Surg (Am) 78–A:239–245, 1996   1–29

Background.—Several authors have proposed transposition of the proximal half to two thirds of the subscapularis tendon for the reconstruction of large rotator cuff tears that are not amenable to more traditional reconstructive procedures, especially tears associated with widespread scarring in the surrounding tissue, supraspinatus retraction, or loss of tissue available for repair. One experience with subscapularis tendon transfer in patients with chronic massive tears of the rotator cuff not amenable to direct primary repair was assessed retrospectively.

Patients and Methods.—Twenty patients aged 36 to 72 years with rotator cuff tears greater than 5 cm underwent reconstruction with the subscapularis tendon and subacromial decompression. None of the injuries could be repaired by direct tendon-to-bone or tendon-to-tendon procedures. Follow-up ranged from 23 to 70 months.

Outcomes.—Seventeen patients reported that they were satisfied with their results at the lastest follow-up. However, 9 patients reported weakness and discomfort with extended or repetitive overhead activity. Another 2 patients had substantial pain relief but had lost active elevation of the shoulder.

Conclusion.—Subscapularis transfer facilitates closure of massive rotator cuff tears that cannot be repaired adequately with simpler, more traditional reconstructive methods. However, it should be used cautiously in patients with full functional elevation before surgery, as loss of active shoulder elevation can occur.

▶ Almost all tears of the rotator cuff are treated by direct suture, either tendon-to-tendon or tendon-to-bone. In a few instances, transposition of local tendons from their usual attachment site to a site more cranial on the humeral head is used as an adjunct to the repair. It is important to recall that this is not commonly necessary. It might be most useful in some patients with rheumatoid arthritis at the time of humeral head prosthetic replacement. It is occasionally useful in other patients, but, as the authors have nicely demonstrated, if a patient has ample active elevation before surgery, one must be very hesitant to transfer any intact musculotendinous units during rotator cuff repair. This includes, of course, the subscapularis attachment.

R.H. Cofield, M.D.

Transfer of Latissimus Dorsi for Irreparable Rotator-Cuff Tears

Aoki M, Okamura K, Fukushima S, et al (Sapporo Med Univ, Japan)
J Bone Joint Surg Br 78:761–766, 1996   1–30

Objective.—Numerous methods can be used to reconstruct irreparable rotator cuff tears, but many have resulted in unacceptably high failure rates. One procedure that has yielded high success rates is transfer of the latissimus dorsi tendon. A review of the experience at 1 Japanese institution discusses and compares results with the latissimus dorsi transfer procedure with other surgical methods and presents a radiographic assessment and electromyographic analysis of risk factors influencing shoulder function.

Methods.—Latissimus dorsi transfer was performed on 12 shoulders of 10 patients (1 woman) aged 48–62 because the cuff defect was irreparable by the McLaughlin procedure with the arm at 60 degrees' abduction. The patients were monitored for an average of 35.6 months. Radiography was used to evaluate osteoarthritis and determine the extent of proximal migration of the humeral head. Pain, function, movement, and patient satisfaction were rated by the UCLA shoulder rating scale. Electromyography was used to assess neuromuscular function of the transferred latissimus dorsi and supraspinatus muscles.

Results.—With the UCLA scale, 4 shoulders were rated excellent, 4 good, 1 fair, and 3 poor. Pain scores improved from 2.4 at baseline to 7.7 after surgery, function from 3.1 to 7.8, active forward flexion from 3.1 to 4.2, and strength from 3.3 to 4.2. Average total scores improved from 11.8 to 28.0. There was no increase in osteoarthritis in 7 shoulders and progression in 5. Six shoulders showed signs of humeral head migration. Electromyographic analysis revealed electrical activity in the supraspinatus muscle for all shoulders during flexion, abduction, and external rotation, with synergistic activity observed in the transferred latissimus dorsi in 9 shoulders, particularly during external rotation. Risk factors for poor outcome included multiple operations, detachment of the deltoid, tearing of 3 or more components of the rotator cuff, and rupture of the long head of the biceps.

Conclusion.—Transfer of the latissimus dorsi for irreparable rotator cuff tears is effective in restoring shoulder function.

► This article presents a realistic picture relative to latissimus dorsi transfer; it presents material suggesting that it can be a useful adjunct for rotator cuff repair but also points out that the results can be variable and improvement is often not dramatic. The treatment of large rotator cuff tears continues to be quite difficult. This transfer may be useful in select situations as indicated by this report. There are, of course, limitations of this method, and they are becoming more clearly defined as information about this technique accrues.

R.H. Cofield, M.D.

Strength After Surgical Repair of the Rotator Cuff

Rokito AS, Zuckerman JD, Gallagher MA, et al (Hosp for Joint Diseases, New York)
J Shoulder Elbow Surg 5:12–17, 1996   1–31

Background.—Pain relief and functional improvement have been the traditional goals of rotator cuff repair. However, strength recovery and its influence on clinical outcome have recently been getting more attention. The recovery of shoulder strength, determined by comprehensive isokinetic testing, and factors correlating with it were studied prospectively after surgical repair of full-thickness rotator cuff tears.

Methods.—Over a 3-year period, 42 consecutive patients underwent repair of rotator cuff tears with a standardized surgical and rehabilitation protocol. Tear size was graded intraoperatively, and the tears were classified as either small or medium (in 24 patients, group 1) or large or massive (in 18 patients, group 2). Shoulder strength was assessed with isokinetic strength testing in flexion/extension, abduction/adduction, and external/internal rotation at 60 degrees/sec, and was calculated as a percentage of the contralateral side. Patients were also evaluated clinically, using the University of California, Los Angeles (UCLA) Shoulder Rating Scale for Pain and Function of the Shoulder.

Results.—All patients experienced a progressive improvement in strength in all 3 planes tested, with the swiftest improvement occurring in flexion and abduction. Strength recovery was similar during the first 6 months, regardless of the tear size. However, during the second 6 months, patients with large or massive tears had significantly slower recovery of strength than did patients with small or medium tears. At 12 months, the recovery of strength in flexion was 97% in group 1 and 70% in group 2; in abduction it was 112% in group 1 and 86% in group 2; and in external rotation it was 97% in group 1 and 86% in group 2. Overall, by 12 months, mean work values increased to 70% in flexion, 70% in abduction, and 90% in external rotation, with similar increases in mean power. At 1 year, the average UCLA scores were 33.5 in group 1 and 28.3 in group 2. These scores correlated significantly with the strength measurements.

Conclusion.—Strength recovery after rotator cuff repair can be adequately measured with isokinetic testing and correlates with tear size and with clinical outcome. At least 1 year of rehabilitation is required to achieve recovered strength, with more rehabilitation needed for patients with large or massive tears.

▶ Strength after rotator cuff repair has been measured by several investigators, and varying findings have been recorded. This more detailed study nicely informs us that the time from surgery to measurement is important, that the size of the rotator cuff tear is important, and, perhaps most importantly, that the recovery of strength can be quite good after the use of traditional rotator cuff repair methods.

R.H. Cofield, M.D.

Distal Rupture of the Tendon of Biceps Brachii: Evaluation by MRI and the Results of Repair

Le Huec JC, Moinard M, Liquois F, et al (Bordeaux Hosp, France)
J Bone Joint Surg Br 78:767–770, 1996   1–32

Objective.—Ruptures of the distal part of the tendon of the biceps brachii are rare and are frequently diagnosed late. The value of MRI in determining the degree of retraction of the tendon and assessing the results of surgery after at least 1 year is discussed.

Methods.—Magnetic resonance image assessment was performed on 10 male patients aged 27–58 with a rupture of the distal part of the biceps brachii tendon; 8 of the ruptures were diagnosed and treated within 6 weeks of injury and 2 were diagnosed 6 months after injury.

Operative Technique.—An incision is made on the anterior aspect of the elbow, and the tendon is located, freed of adhesions, and sutured. The tuberosity is located, two 2.9-mm holes are drilled, and anchoring pins are inserted. Sutures passed through the pinholes are attached to the distal biceps tendon, which is reinserted on the radial tuberosity (Fig 2). At 1 year, mobility, pain, strength, and range of flexion and supination were measured.

Results.—T2 sequences showed an empty sheath filled with liquid when there was complete rupture of the tendon. Recent lesions showed up as hyperintense signals. At the tendon site in older injuries there was a heterogeneous area with a liquid signal. Muscle atrophy was also present. Eight patients had reinsertion on the radial tuberosity, 1 had reinsertion on the anterior brachial muscle, and 1 refused surgery. At 1 year, all patients

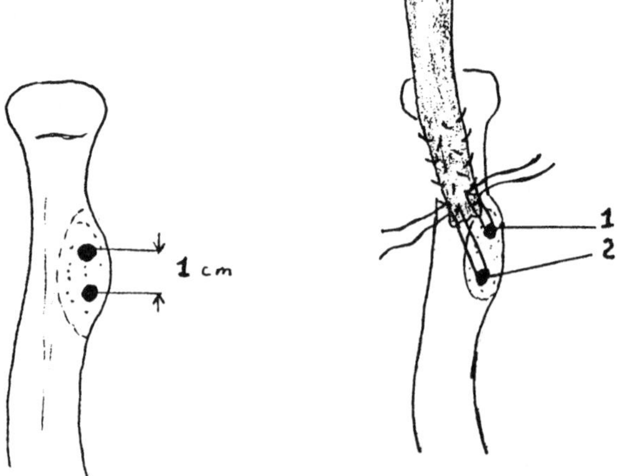

FIGURE 2.—Location of an anchor used for reinsertion of the biceps brachii tendon. (Courtesy of Le Huec JC, Mionard M, Liquois F, et al: Distal rupture of the tendon of biceps brachii: Evaluation by MRI and the results of repair. *J Bone Joint Surg Br* 78:767–770, 1996.)

had 160 degrees of flexion and 90 degrees of supination, 6 had no pain, and 4 of 8 operated patients reported slight discomfort on repeated movement. Flexion-supination muscle strength of the 8 reinsertion patients varied from 45 to 20 kg. The patient with reinsertion on the anterior brachial muscle had a strength of 15 kg, and the patient who refused surgery had a strength of 12 kg. Loss of power in the 8 reinsertion patients was 11% when compared with the unoperated arm and 50% in the patient with reinsertion on the brachial muscle.

Conclusion.—Based on mobility, strength, supination, and flexion measurements 1 year after surgery, repair of rupture of the distal part of the biceps brachii tendon by reinsertion on the radial tuberosity gave better results than reinsertion on the anterior brachial muscle. Magnetic resonance imaging was useful in defining the lesions and in distinguishing between recent and long-standing injuries.

▶ This article combines modern technology for detection, repair, and measurement of the effectiveness of repair of a rupture of the distal aspect of the biceps brachii. In summary, MRI seems effective for preoperative assessment. The use of suture anchors facilitates repair, and muscle strength measurements document almost 90% return of strength. The authors are to be commended for organizing this material so well.

R.H. Cofield, M.D.

Arthritis and Arthroplasty

Modern Cement Technique and the Survivorship of Total Shoulder Arthroplasty
Norris BL, Lachiewicz PF (Univ of North Carolina, Chapel Hill)
Clin Orthop 328:76–85, 1996   1–33

Background.—Total shoulder athroplasty effectively relieves pain and improves motion in patients with debilitating pain from glenohumeral arthritis. However, many researchers have reported increased loosening of the glenoid component with time. The extent to which modern cement technique reduces the incidence of radiographic loosening of the glenoid component was studied.

Methods.—One surgeon performed 38 consecutive Neer II total shoulder arthroplasties in 35 patients using the modern cement technique. The patients were followed for 2 to 9.5 years. Before surgery, 22 shoulders had osteoarthritis or avascular necrosis, 10 had rheumatoid arthritis, and 6 had posttraumatic arthritis. Cement fixation techniques initially described for total hip arthroplasty were used to implant 26 metal-backed and 12 polyethylene glenoid components. In 32 shoulders, humeral components were implanted with cement.

Findings.—No intraoperative fractures or postoperative neurapraxias occurred. At the most recent follow-up, patients reported no or slight pain with activity for 36 shoulders. The average increase in active forward elevations was 38 degrees. In active external rotation, the increase was 29 degrees. No revisions have been necessary. All components are still in place. Survival of the arthroplasty was 97% at 5 and 93% at 8 years: failure was defined as definite radiographic component loosening. Only 3 shoulders showed radiolucent lines around more than half the bone cement interface of the humeral component. Only 2 shoulders showed radiolucent lines around more than half the bone cement interface of the glenoid component. A complete radiolucent line and a change in position were observed in both components in 1 severely osteopenic shoulder.

Conclusions.—The improved arthroplasty survival and low rate of component loosening were probably associated with the use of the new cement technique. With meticulous attention to cement technique, glenoid resurfacing may be performed with a low rate of loosening, even when the rotator cuff has been torn.

▶ This much-needed article informs us about something we believed but were not quite sure would be true: that is, attention to the more modern cement techniques developed for hip and knee surgery and applied to the shoulder will improve the outcome and the radiographic appearance of the interfaces of particularly the glenoid component in total shoulder arthroplasty. Thus, without changing fundamental concepts but applying modern technology carefully, the outcome of shoulder arthroplasty can be improved.

R.H. Cofield, M.D.

Neurologic Complications After Total Shoulder Arthroplasty

Lynch NM, Cofield RH, Silbert PL, et al (Mayo Clinic and Mayo Found, Rochester, Minn)
J Shoulder Elbow Surg 5:53–61, 1996
1–34

Background.—Little attention has been given to the neurologic complications of total shoulder arthroplasty. The incidence of these complications, associated factors, and prognosis were determined in 1 series of patients.

Methods and Findings.—Of 368 patients undergoing 417 total shoulder arthroplasties between 1975 and 1989, 17 had a neurologic problem postoperatively. The most common diagnoses were osteoarthritis and rheumatoid arthritis. In 12 patients, the neurologic deficits were localized to the brachial plexus. The upper and middle trunks were affected in most patients. Idiopathic brachial plexopathy was documented in 3 patients. In 1 patient, pre-existing dysesthesias in the lower trunk and medial cord distribution were exacerbated, and 1 patient had a median neuropathy at the wrist. In 4 patients, lesions significantly hindered shoulder rehabilitation and general activity. Six patients had lesions that temporarily impaired their scheduled rehabilitation program. At 1 year, neurologic recovery was graded as good in 11 shoulders and fair in 5. Risk factors for the development of postoperative neurologic complications were the use of the long deltopectoral approach with the deltoid attached to the clavicle and acromion and the use of methotrexate. Operative time was correlated with postarthroplasty neurologic complications. Shorter operative times were related to more neurologic complications. The presumed mechanism of injury in most patients was traction on the plexus during surgery.

Conclusion.—The incidence of neurologic complications after total shoulder arthroplasty was 4%. One percent had deficits that significantly impaired shoulder rehabilitation. More than half the patients receiving methotrexate had neurologic complications, and all such complications occurred in patients whose deltoid attachment was maintained during the surgical approach. Neurologic assessment is indicated in the early postoperative period in all patients with total shoulder arthroplasty. The prognosis for neurologic recovery was generally good.

▶ It has long been thought and taught that nerve injury associated with shoulder arthroplasty represented a traumatic injury to the local nerves—the musculocutaneous and axillary nerves. This article demonstrates that neurologic injury after a total shoulder arthroplasty does occur; that recovery is usual; and that the neurologic injury is one of a contusion or stretch, quite likely the latter, and usually located at some point in the brachial plexus. As such, prevention is directed toward careful positioning before surgery and care in arm positioning and traction during the procedure. With these methods, neurologic complications can quite likely be reduced; however, it seems unlikely that they will be completely eliminated. Fortunately, recovery is the rule.

R.H. Cofield, M.D.

Advanced Cement Technique Improves Fixation in Elbow Arthroplasty
Faber KJ, Cordy ME, Milne AD, et al (Univ of Western Ontario, London, Canada)
Clin Orthop 334:150–156, 1997   1–35

Background.—Total elbow arthroplasty is used for the reconstruction of joints damaged by arthritis but with a lower success rate than hip or knee arthroplasty. This may be the result of deficits in the initial cementing technique. An in vitro model was used to compare advanced cementing techniques with the conventional techniques presently in use for fixation in elbow arthroplasty.

Methods.—Sixteen fresh frozen cadaveric distal humeri were randomized to either conventional or advanced cementing techniques. The conventional technique consisted of canal irrigation, manual insertion, and thumb packing of doughy bone cement. The advanced cementing technique consisted of canal preparation by irrigation, brushing, and drying with gauze, followed by plugging 12 cm proximal to the trochlea center. A delivery system was used to add low viscosity cement under pressure. After polymerization for at least 2 hours, all humeri were radiographed and then cut into 10-mm-thick sections. These sections were photographed and then digitized to quantify cement filling. An Instron 8501 material testing machine was used to determine the maximum load to failure.

Results.—The amount of cement filling was significantly greater in those humeri filled with the advanced technique than in those filled with the conventional technique. The failure load and the failure stress were also significantly greater in the humeri filled with the advanced technique.

Conclusion.—Application of advanced cementing techniques—including proper cleaning of bone surfaces, canal plugging, and pressurization of low viscosity cement—resulted in significant improvement in fixation of the humeral stem. Development of an effective cement restrictor and in vivo application of the advanced cementing techniques described should improve initial humeral fixation. This could help to decrease the failure rate of elbow arthroplasty.

▶ A number of times people have suggested that cement technique in the upper extremity is not as important a factor as in the lower extremity. This may, in fact, be true but, in reality, cement technique is important everywhere. One should not neglect the details of cement utilization. This article nicely illustrates that more advanced cement techniques improve the characteristics of the interface and, presumably, the longevity of implant fixation.

R.H. Cofield, M.D.

Nerve Entrapment and Injury

Suprascapular Nerve Entrapment: Experience With 28 Cases
Antoniadis G, Richter H-P, Rath S, et al (Univ of Ulm, Guenzburg, Germany)
J Neurosurg 85:1020–1025, 1996   1–36

Introduction.—A wide variety of disorders may lead to shoulder pain. One cause that is seldom considered in the differential diagnosis is entrapment neuropathy of the suprascapular nerve (SN). The 28 consecutive cases of SN entrapment reviewed here were evaluated over a 10-year period.

Patients and Methods.—Patients were 21 men and 6 women with a mean age at operation of 32.8 years. Twenty-one had an operation on their dominant side and 5 on their nondominant side; 1 patient was affected bilaterally. The problem was related to athletic activities in 16 patients, and 5 had a history of trauma to the shoulder region. The mean duration of symptoms before surgery ranged from 9 months in the 3 patients with ganglion cysts to 41 months in trauma cases. Pain over the suprascapular notch was reported by 21 patients, and 17 had paresis and atrophy of both the supraspinatus (SS) and infraspinatus (IS) muscles. Electromyography showed signs of denervation in all cases. After several weeks of conservative therapy proved unsuccessful, surgical decompression of the nerve was done. The patient is placed prone and a skin incision (6–8 cm) is made slightly above the spine of the scapula (Fig 2).

Results.— Twenty-four cases (25 patients) were available for evaluation at a mean of 20.8 months after surgery. Sixteen of 19 patients with

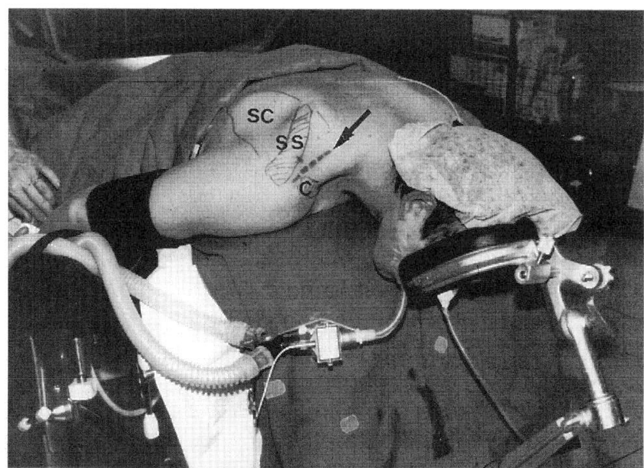

FIGURE 2.—A patient placed prone for the posterior approach. A skin incision *(arrow)* is made above the spine of the scapula *(SSC)*. Abbreviations: C, clavicle; SC, scapula. (Courtesy of Antoniadis G, Richter H-P, Rath S, et al: Suprascapular nerve entrapment: Experience with 28 cases. *J Neurosurg* 85:1020–1025, 1996.)

preoperative pain were completely free of pain and 3 reported improvement. Improvements in motor function were achieved in the SS muscle (86.7% of cases) and the IS muscle (70.8% of cases). Muscle atrophy improved more slowly, but it resolved in 80.7% of cases involving the SS muscle and in 50% of cases involving the IS muscle. No postoperative complications occurred.

Discussion.—Surgery is indicated for patients with SN entrapment when pain fails to respond to conservative treatment or when atrophy of the SS and IS muscles is present. The posterior surgical approach yields good results while minimizing risks and complications.

▶ This article details a rather large series. Treatment was directed at dividing the superior transverse scapular ligament. It is interesting that many cases recovered with a reduction in pain and significant improvement in motor function. I think it behooves us all not to forget in this day of MRI and ganglions that SN entrapment is in the literature most consistently related to entrapment in the suprascapular notch. This fact is reinforced by this article.

R.H. Cofield, M.D.

Ulnar Nerve Entrapment at the Elbow: Correlation of Magnetic Resonance Imaging, Clinical, Electrodiagnostic, and Intraoperative Findings
Britz GW, Haynor DR, Kuntz C, et al (Univ of Washington, Seattle)
Neurosurgery 38:458–465, 1996   1–37

Background.—Ulnar nerve entrapment at the elbow is the second most commonly diagnosed entrapment neuropathy after carpal tunnel syndrome. Its diagnosis is traditionally based on clinical and electrodiagnostic data. Magnetic resonance imaging has recently been reported to be useful in documenting nerve signal and configuration changes in peripheral nerve entrapment disorders. Magnetic resonance imaging findings were correlated with clinical, electrodiagnostic, and operative results in patients with ulnar nerve entrapment at the elbow.

Methods.—Twenty-seven patients with nerve entrapment in 31 elbows were studied, together with 10 asymptomatic subjects. The patients had numbness and parasthesia of the fourth and fifth digits and weakness and clumsiness of the hand, symptoms that were considered compatible with the diagnosis of ulnar nerve entrapment.

Findings.—Ulnar neuropathy was confirmed by electrodiagnostic assessment in 77% of the elbows. Neuropathy was localized to the elbow region in 68%. MRI showed an increased signal of the ulnar nerve in 97% of the 31 elbows and enlargement of the ulnar nerve in 74%. There were no abnormalities on MRI in the control group. The increased signal was noted at a mean of 27 mm proximal to the distal humerus, extending distally a mean of 4 mm below the distal humerus, with a mean total length of 34 mm. Ulnar nerve enlargement occurred at a mean of 19 mm proximal to the distal humerus, extending distally a mean of 8 mm above the distal humerus, with a mean total length of nerve enlargement of 12 mm (Fig 1A, B).

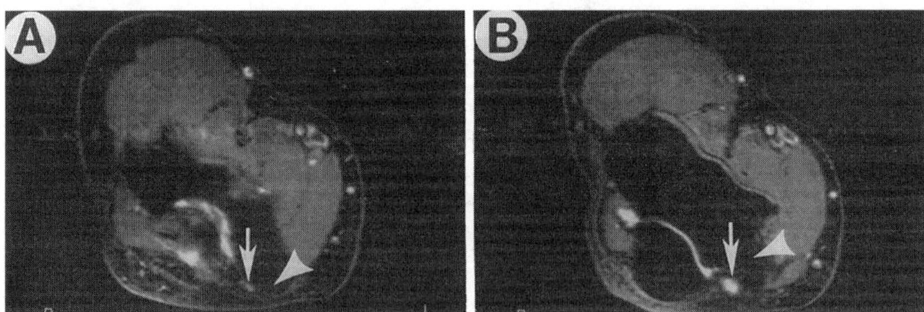

FIGURE 1A-B.—Magnetic resonance imaging axial sections using a short term inversion recovery pulse sequence across the elbow in a patient with left cubital tunnel syndrome. The ulnar nerve (*white arrows*) is posterior to the medial epicondyle (*white arrowheads*). Note the increase in signal and size of the ulnar nerve across the cubital tunnel (**B**) and then a decrease in signal and size proximally (**A**). (Courtesy of Britz GW, Haynor DR, Kuntz C, et al: Ulnar nerve entrapment at the elbow: Correlation of magnetic resonance imaging, clinical, electrodiagnostic, and intraoperative findings. *Neurosurgery* 38:458–465, 1996.)

Conclusion.—Magnetic resonance imaging is sensitive and specific in the diagnosis of ulnar nerve entrapment at the elbow. The finding of increased signal of the ulnar nerve is more sensitive than nerve enlargement.

▶ This very detailed and carefully performed study using MRI to document image changes in nerves may, in fact, be a useful adjunct to the diagnosis of ulnar nerve entrapment at the elbow. No doubt, there will be some patients with substantial symptoms but few confirmatory signs in whom this will prove useful. To confirm the diagnosis correspondingly, it may also be useful in excluding significant ulnar nerve entrapment in patients with symptoms with few confirmatory signs and a normal image. Exactly how this fits into the diagnostic sequence is yet to be determined, but the findings are rather convincing.

R.H. Cofield, M.D.

Transfer of the Levator Scapulae, Rhomboid Major, and Rhomboid Minor for Paralysis of the Trapezius
Bigliani LU, Compito CA, Duralde XA, et al (Columbia Presbyterian Med Ctr, New York City)
J Bone Joint Surg (Am) 78A:1534–1540, 1996   1–38

Background.—Paralysis of the trapezius muscle resulting from spinal accessory nerve injury leads to disabling pain, deformity, and loss of function. Although several reconstructive procedures have been described, the long-term outcomes have been generally unsatisfactory because of progressive stretching of the reconstruction. The Eden-Lange procedure, which provides substitution for all 3 components of the trapezius muscle through transfer of the levator scapulae and rhomboid major and minor muscles, has yielded successful results. The long-term outcomes of this procedure in 1 group of patients were assessed.

Methods and Findings.—Twenty-two patients underwent transfer of the levator scapulae and rhomboid major and minor muscles for trapezius muscle paralysis resulting from injury of the spinal accessory nerve (Fig 1). The injury occurred during biopsy of a cervical node in 13 patients, trauma in 7, and radical neck dissection in 2. Trapezius function had not improved with physical therapy or surgical attempts at neurolysis or reconstruction of the spinal accessory nerve in any of the patients. In 14 patients, the clinical diagnosis had been incorrect. In 12, electromyographic examination was inaccurate or incomplete. In 3 patients, a long thoracic nerve palsy developed. The mean follow-up was 7.5 years, with a range of 2–14 years. Operative outcomes were determined on the American Shoulder and Elbow Surgeons Shoulder Evaluation Form. Results were excellent in 13 patients, satisfactory in 6, and unsatisfactory in 3. Pain relief was adequate and function improved in all but 3 patients.

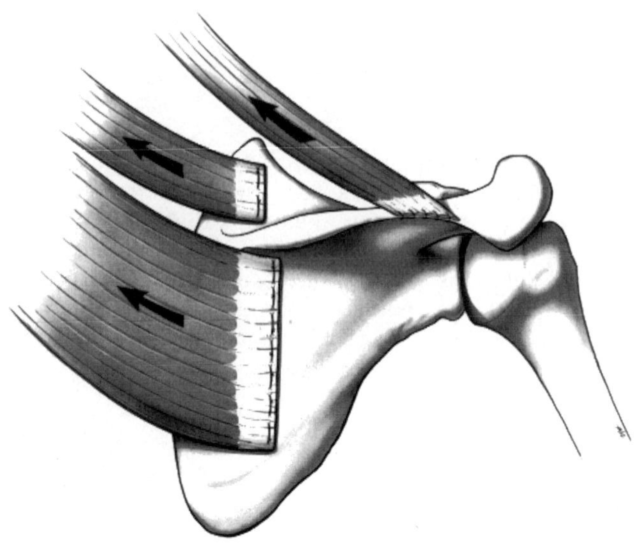

FIGURE 1.—Illustration demonstrating lateral transfer of the levator scapulae to the scapular spine and transfer of the rhomboid minor to the supraspinatus fossa and the rhomboid major to the infraspinatus fossa. The transfer of the rhomboid minor cephalad to the scapular spine is a modification of the original procedure. Placement of the muscle in this position more efficiently substitutes for the middle portion of the trapezius, stabilizes the superior angle of the scapula, and closes the gap between the levator scapulae and the rhomboid minor. The *arrows* indicate the direction of pull of the muscles that were transferred. (Courtesy of Bigliani LU, Compito CA, Duralde XA, et al: Transfer of the levator scapulae, rhomboid major, and rhomboid minor for paralysis of the trapezius. *J Bone Joint Surg [Am]* 78A:1534–1540, 1996.)

Conclusions.—Transfer of the levator scapulae and rhomboid muscles is a valuable orthopedic reconstructive procedure for patients with trapezius paralysis. Although it is not appropriate as a primary procedure when neurolysis or repair of the spinal accessory nerve is indicated, it can be used as a salvage procedure in patients with pain, deformity, and reduced function of the shoulder girdle resulting from irreparable injury of the spinal accessory nerve.

▶ The authors kindly introduced the Eden-Lange technique to many of us in North America in their 1985 report.[1] This expanded study with longer follow-up evaluation indicates very reasonable results, and as one would expect, following a muscle transfer procedure.

R.H. Cofield, M.D.

Reference

1. Bigliani LU, Perez-Sanz JR, Wolfe IN: Treatment of trapezius paralysis. *J Bone Joint Surg (Am)* 67A:871–877, 1985.

Clinical Research

Scoring Systems for Shoulder Conditions

Romeo AA, Bach BR Jr, O'Halloran KL (Rush-Presbyterian St Luke's Med Ctr, Chicago; Oconomowoc, Wis)
Am J Sports Med 24:472–476, 1996   1–39

Introduction.—The various shoulder scoring systems lack validity, correlation, and interrater reliability. A standard shoulder system is needed. Four shoulder scoring systems were used to evaluate the results of 53 shoulder stabilization procedures performed on 52 patients.

Methods.—A single physician performed 34 open Bankart-type repairs, 15 capsular shifts, and 4 arthroscopic stabilizations. The 4 scoring scales were Rowe, modified-Rowe, University of California at Los Angeles (UCLA), and the pre-1994 American Shoulder and Elbow Surgeons scale.

Results.—Remarkably different results were observed with the 4 scoring scales. The UCLA scoring system indicated 85% of patients had excellent results. Only 38% of patients had an excellent score when the modified-Rowe was used. Overall, 89% to 95% of patients had good or excellent results and 5% to 11% had fair or poor results. Correlation between the Rowe, modified Rowe, and the American Shoulder and Elbow Surgeons scores was fair. The correlation with the UCLA score was rated poor. Interrater reliability was poor between the 4 systems.

Conclusion.—Scoring systems for patients who underwent shoulder stabilization procedures showed remarkable variability, poor correlation, and poor interrater reliability. Without a widely accepted scoring system for the shoulder, clinicians are not able to compare management of shoulder conditions. Investigations can be biased based on selection of a particular scoring system. A system is needed that is well-accepted and based on the functional status of the patient.

▶ Enough shoulder systems to measure outcome have now been constructed so that we can more fully measure the outcomes of treatment or nontreatment. Unfortunately, the systems are not exactly congruent or interchangeable. This article is included to help us recognize this fact and to appreciate that over the next few years it is quite likely that scoring systems will be modified, and some of those now in place will not be as frequently used.

R.H. Cofield, M.D.

Relationships Between Measurements of Impairment, Disability, Pain, and Disease Activity in Rheumatoid Arthritis Patients With Shoulder Problems

Boström C, Harms-Ringdahl K, Nordemar R (Karolinska Inst, Stockholm)
Scand J Rheumatol 24:352–359, 1995   1–40

Background.—A number of separate instruments exist for evaluating physical pain, function, physical and psychosocial functioning, and disability. For patients with rheumatoid arthritis of the shoulder, the relationships among measurements of shoulder movement impairment, disability, shoulder pain intensity, and disease activity were studied.

Methods.—Over 3 years, 67 women followed for rheumatoid arthritis that included shoulder symptoms entered the study. Shoulder movement impairment was measured by physiotherapists for 5 common shoulder movements. Patients answered a shoulder-arm disability questionnaire and appropriate portions of the Health Assessment Questionnaire (HAQ), the Sickness Impact Profile (SIP), and the Functional Status Questionnaire (FSQ). Disease activity was measured by upper extremity joint examination and by erythrocyte sedimentation rate. Results were compared statistically to seek correlations.

Results.—Although there was a significant relationship among shoulder movement impairment, shoulder-arm disability, pain, HAQ, SIP, and FSQ, none was more than moderate. Disease activity, measured by joint swelling and erythrocyte sedimentation rate, did not correlate significantly with any of the other measurements or the questionnaires.

Conclusion.—Although there is some overlap in their measurement, impairment, disability, pain intensity, and disease activity remain separate areas and must be individually evaluated.

▶ There is a pernicious tendency to combine various measured factors into a rating system, to compare rating systems, or to look for 1 key factor that will explain the patient's situation relative to the shoulder. This manuscript nicely outlines that many factors used to measure shoulder disease are related, but each has importance and represents a slightly different aspect of the situation. As such, it is probably key to measure several different variables, to report them separately, and then, if desired, to combine them into some rating system—but not to jump to the last step and use that alone.

R.H. Cofield, M.D.

2 Hip Replacement, Osteoporosis, and Related Issues

Introduction

In 1997, the literature on total hip arthroplasty provided new information regarding a variety of subjects. Areas of particular interest in this chapter include assessment of the effectiveness of various treatments for osteonecrosis, long-term results in revision total hip arthroplasty of various grafting techniques that augment deficient bone, strategies for the detection and prophylaxis of venous thromboembolism, and evaluation of possible infection in total hip replacements.

A number of factors that adversely affect the results of total hip arthroplasty were reported this year, as well as surgical techniques that address difficult reconstructive situations. A number of new issues have been raised by recent reports: the efficacy of erythropoietin, advantages of autologous blood donation, the use of preoperative irradiation in patients who are at risk for heterotopic ossification, the novel use of bioactive glass powder in bone cement, and new information regarding the emerging clinical applications of autologous cartilage transplantation. Finally, two papers are reviewed that seek to evaluate the effectiveness of outcomes assessment instruments.

On a personal note, it has been my pleasure to serve as coeditor of the YEAR BOOK OF ORTHOPEDICS and as editor of the section on total hip arthroplasty since 1989. During these 8 years I have received much favorable comment from readers of the YEAR BOOK, and I have been enriched by the wide spectrum of literature I reviewed to prepare these volumes. The YEAR BOOK is a most worthwhile endeavor, both to its readers and its editors, and I am confident that the new editors will successfully carry this effort forward.

Robert Poss, M.D.

Radiographic Techniques

Evaluation of the Singh Index for Measuring Osteoporosis

Koot VCM, Kesselaer SMMJ, Clevers GJ, et al (Univ Hosp, Utrecht, The Netherlands)
J Bone Joint Surg [Br] 78B:831–834, 1996   2–1

Background.—Determining the degree of osteoporosis in elderly patients with proximal femoral fractures may help clinicians choose the best treatment. The Singh index is often used to measure osteoporosis. The degree of osteoporosis is based on the appearance of the trabecular bone structure of the proximal femur on a plain anteroposterior radiograph. The gold standard for measuring osteoporosis is dual-energy x-ray absorptiometry, which gives a precise evaluation of bone mineral density. The interobserver and intraobserver agreement of readings of the Singh index of osteoporosis was evaluated, and the results of evaluation of osteoporosis using dual-energy x-ray absorptiometry and the Singh index were compared.

Methods.—The preoperative radiographs of 80 consecutive patients older than 55 years with a fracture of the femoral neck or trochanteric region were evaluated by 6 observers to determine the Singh index. A week later, 10 of those radiographs were reviewed again by the 6 observers. In 77 of the 80 patients, dual-energy x-ray absorptiometry was used to measure bone mineral density.

Results.—There was low interobserver agreement. Of the 72 radiographs, only 3 were given the same Singh classification by all 6 observers. The kappa values were 0.15–0.54. There was substantial intraobserver agreement. Kappa values were 0.63–0.88. Comparison of results of dual-energy x-ray absorptiometry and the Singh index of bone mineral density showed absolutely no correlation.

Conclusions.—Interobserver agreement of readings of the Singh index was unacceptable. Intraobserver agreement of readings of the Singh index showed substantial strength. There was no correlation between the Singh index and bone mineral density as measured by dual-energy x-ray absorptiometry. On the basis of these findings, it is concluded that the Singh index has no value in evaluating osteoprosis.

► The Singh index for measuring osteoporosis has been found to have little value in assessing the degree of osteoporosis. The authors found large interobserver variation and, although intraobserver variations showed strong agreement, these differences suggest that the interpretation of radiographs using this index is highly variable and highly subjective. Most strikingly there was little correlation between the Singh index and bone density as measured by dual-energy x-ray absorptiometry. The usefulness of the Singh index has been supplanted by more reliable and objective measurements of bone density.

R. Poss, M.D.

Early Radiographic Results Comparing Cemented and Cementless Total Hip Arthroplasty

Mulliken BD, Nayak N, Bourne RB, et al (Univ Hosp, London, Ont, Canada)
J Arthroplasty 11:24–33, 1996   2–2

Background.—The comparative efficacy of cemented and cementless fixation in total hip arthroplasty is unclear. Early results of cemented total hip arthroplasty have shown high rates of long-term failure. There have been encouraging long-term results of Charnley total hip arthroplasty in more recent reports. Improved cementing methods have decreased aseptic loosening on the femoral side, but long-term socket loosening still occurs. Lysis with cementless implants has been a problem. Thigh pain, instability, and resorptive bone remodeling have occurred with cementless femoral stems. Early radiographic results of cemented and cementless total hip arthroplasty in a randomized, double-blind trial were evaluated.

Methods.—Total hip arthroplasty was performed in 147 patients; 76 were cemented and 71 were cementless. In both groups, the average patient age was 65 years, and the number of male and female patients was similar. Follow-up was 3, 6, and 12 months postoperatively, and annually thereafter. Radiographs were taken at each follow-up visit. Patients and observers were blinded to the type of fixation during the follow-up period.

Results.—At 4–6 years, no revisions had been made in either group. Two cemented acetabular components were definitely loose and 18 were probably loose. Seven cemented stems were possibly loose. One cementless socket was unstable. In 10 cases, cementless femoral component subsidence occurred, although the sinkage stabilized within 6 months; at last follow-up, no stem was unstable. There was very little significant femoral bone resorption. "Spot welds" with this titanium stem were uncommon. Distal cortical hypertrophy was common, although the cause was unknown. Osteolysis occurred with 6 cemented and 10 cementless sockets. In 15 cemented and 1 cementless stems, a small area of lysis was seen in the proximal medial femoral neck. There was no distal femoral lysis in either group.

Discussion.—Osteolysis continues to be a major problem with cemented and cementless fixation in total hip arthroplasty. The use of this cemented metal-backed acetabulum should be reevaluated because of a high rate of early radiographic failure. A porous-coated titanium socket fixed with peripheral fins and screws provides excellent short-term stability. A cementless tapered titanium stem provides excellent stability; radiographic evaluation for this stem differs from the evaluation for a chrome-cobalt stem.

▶ At a relatively early radiographic follow-up of patients who had cemented and uncemented total hip arthroplasties, significant changes in component fixation and the appearance of osteolysis were observed. This paper points to the importance of frequent and continuing radiographic and clinical follow-up of all patients who have undergone total joint arthroplasty.

R. Poss, M.D.

Early Migration Predicts Late Aseptic Failure of Hip Sockets

Krismer M, Stöckl B, Fischer M, et al (Univ Orthopaedic Hosp, Innsbruck, Austria)

J Bone Joint Surg [Br] 78B:422–426, 1996   2–3

Background.—A major problem in outcome studies of hip replacement is that 10 years of follow-up are needed to obtain reliable information about failure of hip sockets and revision rates. After that length of time, the prosthesis may no longer be available or may have been significantly modified. It would be valuable to predict results of hip replacement early. Studies have shown a higher failure rate of hip sockets that migrate rapidly in the first 2 years than those that do not migrate. The predictive value of socket migration for survival and revision rates was evaluated.

Methods.—In a randomized trial, 120 hip prostheses were implanted in 120 patients with primary or secondary osteoarthritis. Patients were between 50 and 65 years of age. There were 60 Robert Mathys polyethylene cups and 60 Porous-Coated Anatomic cups. Median follow-up was 97 months. Radiologic examination was done annually. Migration was measured with computer-assisted EBRA.

Results.—Threshold migration rates from 1 mm in the first year to 1 mm in 5 years were assessed and related to predetermined revision rates. In 28 cups, a total migration of 1 mm or more in the first 2 years was noted. Thirteen of those 28 cups required revision. Survival curves of cups with and without early migration were very different. Mean survival at 96 months for cups with migration of 1 mm or less in the first 2 years was 0.96. Mean survival at 96 months for cups that showed greater migration was 0.63. Survival rates for the 2 types of cups were similar.

Discussion.—Early migration of hip prostheses is highly predictive of need for later revision. Testing of new hip sockets should be based on studies of early socket migration. Roentgen stereophotogrammetry is the most accurate method of measuring migration. The EBRA method is less accurate, although it is cheaper and simpler.

▶ There have been a number of studies in the past few years in which radiographs accurately measured using radiostereometry have suggested that components which migrate within the first 1–2 years after total hip arthroplasty then have a very high likelihood of subsequent failure. That conclusion that early migration predicts late aseptic failure of hip sockets is confirmed in this study using a computer-assisted measuring method (EBRA).

Accurate radiographic measurement techniques can establish early migration patterns and are valuable predictors of subsequent migration and failure patterns. These powerful techniques should be used in early clinical trials of new prostheses.

R. Poss, M.D.

Osteonecrosis

Core Decompression for Osteonecrosis of the Femoral Head

Markel DC, Miskovsky C, Sculco TP, et al (Wayne State Univ, Southfield, Mich; Cornell Univ, New York)
Clin Orthop 323:226–233, 1996

2–4

Background.—Osteonecrosis is both a biological and biomechanical disease, has clinically and radiographically recognizable patterns, and can be detected at very early stages. Treatment is aimed at preserving the femoral head, preventing disease progression, and restoring function. The best specific treatment for osteonecrosis has not been determined. Results of core decompression for treatment of osteonecrosis of the femoral head were reviewed.

Methods.—The medical records of 45 patients who had simple core decompression of 54 hips during a 10-year period were reviewed. Mean patient age was 38.6 years. Analysis was made of the cause of osteonecrosis, radiographic stage and progression, treatment, function, complications, results, and other data.

Results.—All patients had preoperative pain. A total of 35 hips (30 patients) failed; total hip arthroplasty was done in 26 of those hips. In the other 9 hips (7 patients), function did not improve and patients had virtually no pain relief. At last follow-up, those 7 patients had not undergone total hip arthroplasty. The mean time to hip failure was 11.1 months. A total of 19 hips in 16 patients were successful. At 47.5 months, clinical

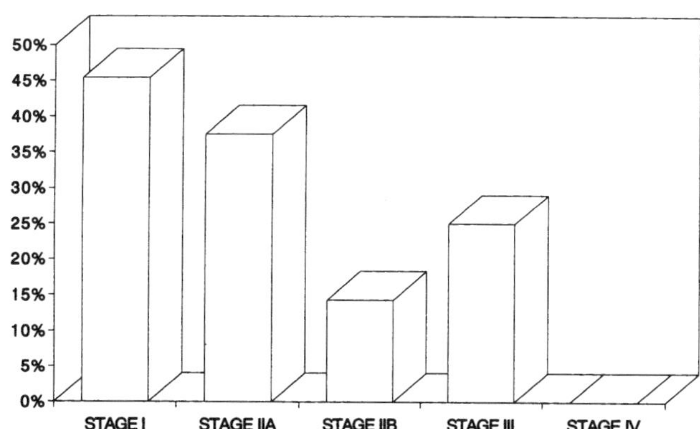

FIGURE 2.—Histogram showing the success rate according to the authors' modification of the Ficat classification. There was a 39.5% success rate in patients with hips staged as Ficat I–IIA. These stages represent 43 of 54 hips, or 76% of the study population. There was a 36% success rate in patients with hips staged as Ficat I–IIB. These stages represent 50 of 54 hips, or 92.5% of the study population. (Courtesy of Markel DC, Miskovsky C, Sculco TP, et al: Core decompression for osteonecrosis of the femoral head. *Clin Orthop* 323:226–233, 1996.)

results were good to excellent in 15 hips and fair in 4 hips. The mean Hospital for Special Surgery hip score was 24.6 points preoperatively (on a scale of 18–38 points), but improved to 34.2 points. Two intertrochanteric femur fractures occurred at about 5.5 weeks postoperatively. The overall success rate of core decompression was 35.2%. The success rate was also determined by the modified Ficat classification (Fig 2).

Discussion.—In these patients, the results of core decompression were poor. The failure rate was 63% and was not attributable to patient selection. Core decompression in this study did not meet the treatment goals of preserving the femoral head, preventing progression, and restoring function. Core decompression had an unpredictable effect on disease progression in these patients.

▶ Thirty of 45 patients who underwent core decompression for osteonecrosis were considered to have had unsatisfactory outcomes after this procedure. The percent of success was greatest in those patients who had idiopathic osteonecrosis when compared to the group as a whole. As with previous reports, the best results were in patients with the earliest stages of osteonecrosis; stage 1 and stage 2A had 45% and approximately 35% of the patients showing improvement. There was a sharp dropoff in success in stage 2B, stage 3, and stage 4. The authors conclude that core decompression is associated with poor results in general and that it has an unpredictable effect on disease progression.

R. Poss, M.D

Femoral Head Reconstruction and Revascularization
Leung PC (Chinese Univ of Hong Kong)
Clin Orthop 323:139–145, 1996   2–5

Background.—Ischemic necrosis of the femoral head has no known idiopathic cause. Spontaneous revascularization can occur, and 30% to 50% of spontaneous recovery is seen in patients with early-stage disease. Evidence of necrotic bone separation indicates failed revascularization and may predict progressive collapse of the femoral head. The early stages of ischemic necrosis are not always diagnosed until there is evidence of collapse of the femoral head. Surgical techniques aimed at saving the femoral joint, such as core decompression, osteotomy, and femoral head reconstruction, have had mixed results. The outcome of a new surgical method of treating ischemic necrosis of the femoral head using a vascular pedicled iliac crest strut graft was analyzed.

Methods.—The technique using a vascular pedicled iliac crest strut graft was performed in 18 consecutive patients and 21 hips. All patients had signs of ischemic necrosis. Mean patient age was 32 years. Follow-up was 4–12 years.

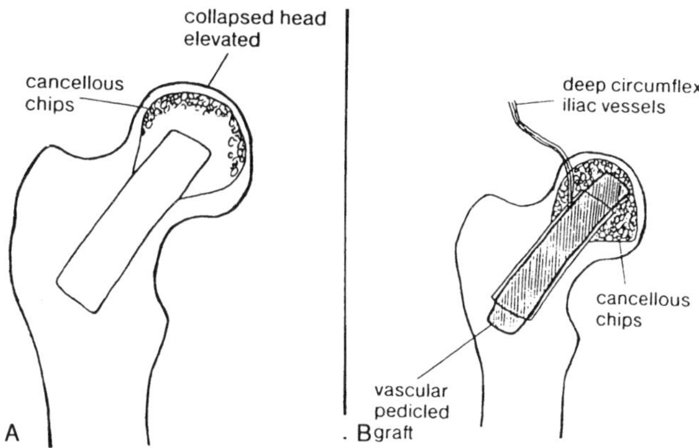

FIGURE 3.—A, an open 1 × 3-cm trough leading from the femoral neck into the femoral head: **B,** the femoral head hollowed from inside via the open trough to leave only a thin shell of subchondral bone and cartilage. (Courtesy of Leung PC: Femoral head reconstruction and revascularization. *Clin Orthop* 323:139–145, 1996.)

Technique.—A bone trough was made in the femoral neck leading into the head. The hard avascular bone and necrotic bone was removed (Fig 3). The cavity in the femoral head was filled with bone that would provide vascularity and strength. The subchondral level was filled with cancellous bone from the ilium, and the remaining space was filled with a tailored piece of iliac crest bone with blood supply intact from the deep circumflex iliac vascular bundle.

Results.—Patients were examined monthly, then every 6 months. Follow-up at 5–12 years showed good results in patients with early involvement. Gait improved significantly, but hip range of motion did not always improve. In the patients with late collapse, pain was controlled, but maintenance of femoral head integrity was unsatisfactory.

Discussion.—This technique is recommended for restoring and maintaining femoral head integrity in patients with ischemic necrosis of the femoral head stage 3 and early stage 4. The long-term results of this technique need further analysis.

▶ The technique to revascularize the femoral head using a vascularized iliac crest bone graft is described. Patients with stage 3 and stage 4 osteonecrotic changes when treated with this method were in the majority of patients to show either good results with maintenance of the height of the femoral head, or late collapse of the femoral head but satisfactory control of pain. The concept of vascularized bone grafting to the femoral head has been associated with overall results of 75% to 80% improvement in patients when vascularized fibular grafts are used.

R. Poss, M.D.

Vascularized Fibular Grafting Compared With Core Decompression in the Treatment of Femoral Head Osteonecrosis

Kane SM, Ward WA, Jordan LC, et al (Carolinas Med Ctr, Charlotte, NC)
Orthopedics 19:869–872, 1996   2–6

Background.—Results of treatment of femoral head osteonecrosis have been mixed. Core decompression and avascular strut grafting have been used in asymptomatic patients with early-stage disease. There have been reports of high failure rates of core decompression in symptomatic patients. Lower revision rates for uncemented total hip arthroplasty have been reported, but the potential life expectancy of joint replacement in younger patients is unknown. Vascularized fibular grafting has been proposed as effective treatment for femoral head osteonecrosis. Results of vascularized fibular grafting were compared with those of core decompression in femoral head osteonecrosis in a prospective, nonrandomized case series.

Methods.—Symptomatic patients with Ficat grade IIA, IIB, or III femoral head osteonecrosis who were treated during a 4-year period were included. There were 39 hips treated in 34 patients. The average patient age was 42 years. Vascularized fibular grafting was done in 20 hips and core decompression was done in 19 hips. Minimum follow-up was 2 years.

Results.—All patients had evidence of disease on plain radiographs or MRI scans and biopsy evidence of avascular bone. The failure rate of vascularized fibular grafting was 20%, with an average time to failure of 17.8 months. The failure rate of core decompression was 58%, with an average time to failure of 15.3 months. Complications in hips that had vascularized fibular grafting included ankle pain and graft vessel thrombosis. There were 2 proximal femur fractures in each group.

Conclusions.—The results of vasculrized fibular grafting were significantly better than results of core decompression in patients with early-stage femoral head osteonecrosis. In some patients, decompressive effects alone may not sufficiently stop disease progression. It may be necessary to use a mechanical strut to compensate for loss of structural support under the subchondral plate at this stage.

▶ Vascularized fibular bone grafting appears superior to cord decompression in Ficat grades 2 and 3 femoral head osteonecrosis.

R. Poss, M.D.

Corrective Osteotomy for Osteonecrosis of the Femoral Head

Mont MA, Fairbank AC, Krackow KA, et al (John Hopkins Univ, Baltimore, Md; Good Samaritan Hosp, Baltimore, Md)
J Bone Joint Surg [Am] 78A:1032–1038, 1996   2–7

Background.—Osteonecrosis is a difficult disease to treat, and the search for procedures that preserve the femoral head continues. Total hip replacement is often the best alternative when patients are first seen after the femoral head has collapsed. Osteonecrosis accounts for about 10% of hip arthroplasties in the United States. The average age of patients in most studies is less than 40 years. Salvage hip replacement often has a high failure rate. Treatment with vascularized or nonvascularized bone grafting, or osteotomy can preserve the femoral head. There have been reports of use of osteotomy for salvage of hips with Ficat and Arlet stage II or III disease. The transtrochanteric osteotomy is a well-known technique in Japan and has had variable success rates. Long-term results of this technique were evaluated.

Methods.—Corrective intertrochanteric osteotomy was performed in 37 hips in 34 patients with Ficat or Arlet stage II and III osteonecrosis of the femoral head. Mean follow-up was 11.5 years. Annual clinical and radiographic examinations were performed. The mean patient age was 32 years.

Results.—Two patients died of causes unrelated to the procedure. Good to excellent results were seen in 28 hips according to the Harris hip scoring system. Seventeen of those hips were in patients who were not taking corticosteroids. Fair to poor results were seen in 9 hips, which later needed total hip arthroplasty. Six of those failed hips were in patients who were taking corticosteroids. Four of them were satisfactory for 5 years or more. Collapse of the femoral head occurred in 5 of 6 hips that had a combined necrotic angle of greater than 200 degrees preoperatively. Good or excellent results were seen in 27 of 31 hips that had a combined necrotic angle of less than 200 degrees preoperatively. There were 3 nonunions and 1 cutout of the compression screw. These were treated and had excellent results. There was 1 case of osteomyelitis that had a poor result.

Discussion.—Corrective intertrochanteric osteotomy for Ficat and Arlet stage II and III osteonecrosis of the femoral head was successful in these patients with small to medium lesions. The success rate was lower in patients who were taking corticosteroids. The success rate in patients not taking corticosteroids was encouraging. Patient selection criteria included age younger than 45 years and a painful hip, stage II or stage III disease, a 20-degree arc of the lateral aspect of the femoral head without necrosis, small to medium lesions, and no continued use of high-dose corticosteroids.

▶ Intertrochanteric osteotomy to deliver the osteonecrotic lesion from the weight-bearing zone was associated with improved clinical outcome in 76% of patients at 11.5 years postoperatively. Patients who had not received corticosteroid treatment had better results than their nonsteroid-treated counterparts. Patient results are similar to those reported for vascularized fibular bone grafting in stage 2 and 3 osteonecrosis.

R. Poss, M.D.

Revision Total Hip Arthroplasty

Revision of the Acetabular Component of a Total Hip Arthroplasty With a Massive Structural Allograft

Garbuz D, Morsi E, Gross AE (Mount Sinai Hosp, Toronto)
J Bone Joint Surg [Am] 78A:693–697, 1996   2–8

Background.—Revision of the acetabular component of total hip arthroplasty is difficult, particularly when there is significant loss of bone stock. A revision procedure on the acetabular side aims to support the cup, approximate normal anatomy, and restore length to the limb. These goals, plus restoration of bone stock, may be accomplished with a structural allograft. Results of revision arthroplasty with a massive allograft on the acetabular side have been varied. Most studies have reported a higher failure rate if more than 50% of the cup is in contact with the structural graft. Results of revision of the acetabular component of total hip arthroplasty with a massive structural acetabular allograft at a minimum follow-up of 5 years were analyzed.

Methods.—Revision of the acetabular component of total hip arthroplasty with a massive structural acetabular allograft was performed in 33 hips in 32 patients. Minimum follow-up was 5 years. The mean patient age was 60 years. All patients had previous hip replacement. Clinical and radiographic follow-up examinations were performed.

Results.—In all patients, the graft supported more than 50% of the cup. No further procedures were needed in 18 hips. In 7 hips, a repeat revision was necessary, but examination showed an intact structural allograft that was used to support the cup at repeat revision. Failure of the prosthesis and allograft occurred in 8 hips. Clinical and radiographic success was based on an increase in hip score of 20 points or more, a stable cup, a united allograft, and no need for further operation. By using these criteria, the success rate was 55%. The method of reconstruction was the only important factor related to outcome. A roof-reinforcement ring and a structural allograft were used in 8 hips, and 7 of those were rated successful at a mean of 7.5 years.

Discussion.—The use of a structural allograft with massive bone loss is supported. The authors use this technique whenever a massive allograft is used on the acetabular side because of the high success rate of acetabular reinforcement rings. These preliminary results are encouraging.

▶ Large structural allografts have been reported to have increasing failure rates with time. In this study, the authors report satisfactory results using large structural allografts, and importantly, even with failure and the need for repeat revision, in a number of cases the allograft provided additional bone stock for subsequent revision. Recently the authors have combined the use of acetabular reinforcement rings to support the allografts and now favor this method of reconstruction. I would agree with this method, and now personally favor the use of acetabular reconstruction rings to protect cancellous allografts as a method of reconstructing segmental defects or even large contained defects in acetabular reconstructions.

R. Poss, M.D.

Acetabular and Femoral Reconstruction With Impacted Graft and Cement

Slooff TJJH, Buma P, Schreurs BW, et al (Univ Hosp Nijmegen, The Netherlands; Medisch Centrum Leeuwarden, The Netherlands)
Clin Orthop 323:108–115, 1996   2–9

Background.—Aseptic loosening is the most common long-term complication of total hip arthroplasty and results in bone destruction, enlargement of the acetabulum, and widening of the femoral medullary cavity. Long-term results of a method of reconstruction of acetabular and femoral defects using a standardized cemented revision procedure with tight impaction of morsellized cancellous autograft or allograft chips were evaluated.

Methods.—Cemented revision hip arthroplasties with impaction grafting and wire meshes, were performed in patients with clinical and radiographic evidence of loosening. The average patient age was 62 years. Follow-up data were collected at an average of 70 months for 88 hips in 80 patients. Ten cemented revision arthroplasties were done with reconstruction of the femoral canal with impacted morsellized allografts and cement. Mean follow-up was 24 months, and the mean patient age was 64 years.

Results.—At an average of 70 months, there were 4 clinical failures and 6 radiologic failures among 88 reconstructions. This gave a 5-year failure rate of 11.4%. The effectiveness of autografts and allografts was similar.

Discussion.—Continued use of this technique in the acetabulum and femur is recommended because of these results and successful results of histologic and biomechanic studies in animals. Impacted morsellized grafts, containment of the graft, and polymethylmethacrylate cement can help replace bone loss, restore normal hip mechanics, and stabilize the hip.

▶ The use of impaction cancellous grafting has gained acceptance in recent years when used in femoral stem revisions. In this paper, a method is described that uses acetabular compaction grafting to restore lost bone in large acetabular defects. The authors report that not only is the method useful in contained acetabular defects, but also where there is a segmental defect. The acetabular rim is reinforced with metal mesh and then compacted cancellous graft is successfully used.

R. Poss, M.D.

Treatment of Femoral Osteolysis With Cementless Total Hip Revision

Hozack WJ, Bicalho PS, Eng K (Jefferson Med College, Philadelphia; Rothman Inst, Philadelphia)

J Arthroplasty 11:668–672, 1996   2–10

Background.—The aim of revision total hip arthroplasty is to relieve pain, stop bone loss, and restore bone stock. It has been shown that in cases of femoral osteolysis, cemented revision arthroplasty cannot restore already deficient bone. Results of the compaction grafting technique of Gie et al. and Ling et al. have been encouraging. The value of cementless revision total hip arthroplasty in restoring deficient femoral bone in patients with osteolytic femoral defects was investigated.

Methods.—In 56 patients, 59 revision total hip arthroplasties with cementless femoral components were performed. The mean patient age was 66.8 years. Revision was done because of aseptic loosening in 55 cases, instability in 1, and infection in 3 cases. Clinical and radiographic examinations were done at 2–5 years.

Results.—Osteolytic defects were classified as stabilized, progressive, regressing, healed, or new. There were no failures and no femoral revisions. Lytic defects did not progress after revision and there were no new defects. Examination revealed 154 preoperative osteolytic defects. Of those, 27 stabilized, 65 regressed, and 62 healed. Revision surgery stopped progression of osteolytic lesions in 100% of patients. A slow remodeling of the lytic lesion seems to occur with a well-fixed, porous, ingrowth prosthesis. There was no additional benefit from cancellous allografting in these patients, although no specifically designed instrumentation was used with the grafting technique. The full potential of grafting may, therefore, not have been achieved.

Discussion.—The type of fixation affects radiographic results. If it is not critical to restore bone stock, then a reasonable choice is cemented femoral components alone. In cases of severe osteolysis, regression of defects can only be achieved with conversion to a cementless femoral component with or without a cancellous allograft.

▶ The authors suggest that with revision surgery that arrests degeneration of particulate debris, osteolytic lesions in the femur do not progress. In this study failed cemented femoral components were removed with complete removal of cemented debris and membrane, and replaced with cementless components. Of interest, there was no significant difference in results when a group that had allograft restoration of the focal defects was compared to a group that underwent cementless arthroplasty with no grafting at all. These results suggest that bone defects are capable of healing once stability has been restored and the source of particulate burden is removed.

R. Poss, M.D.

Revision of the Acetabular Component Without Cement After Total Hip Arthroplasty: A Follow-up Note Regarding Results at Seven to Eleven Years

Silverton CD, Rosenberg AG, Sheinkop MB, et al (Rush-Presbyterian-St Luke's Med Ctr, Chicago)

J Bone Joint Surg Am 78A:1366–1370, 1996   2–11

Objective.—The most common failure mode after total hip arthroplasty is mechanical failure of the acetabular component. Of the 138 revisions (132 patients) of the acetabular component without cement performed at Rush-Presbyterian-St. Luke's Medical Center, Chicago, for aseptic loosening, 7 required repeat revision. Prospective results of an additional 5-year follow-up of these patients were reported.

Methods.—Of the original 132 patients (57 men), aged 20 to 79 years, 111 (115 hips) were available for evaluation after an average of 98 months of follow-up. The condition of the acetabulum and any osteolytic lesions was noted. Failure was defined as loosening or breakage of any component. Implant survival was analyzed statistically, and Harris hip scores were determined.

Results.—The repeat revision rate was 11% (13 hips), which included 6 of the original 7 revisions. There were 6 for infection, 1 for recurrent dislocation, 3 for instability, and 4 for revision of the femoral stem. All cups were stable, and no revisions were performed for aseptic loosening of the acetabular component. Radiographs available for 109 hips (105 patients) commonly showed radiolucent lines, although the total number of zones with radiolucent lines had decreased significantly. Complete radiolucent lines surrounded 5 cups, and partial radiolucent lines were observed in 3 hips. One line was associated with infection, and a radiolucent line was associated with 2 screws in 2 hips. Osteolytic areas were seen in the margin of the acetabular component in 4 hips.

Conclusion.—After a follow-up ranging from 7 to 11 years, there was no increase in the rate of aseptic loosening of the acetabular component without cement after total hip arthroplasty. The repeat revision rate was 11%, and 4 hips showed radiographic evidence of osteolytic lesions.

▶ Revision arthroplasty of the acetabulum using hemispherical porous coated implants have been associated with a high rate of success at 7 to 11 years postoperatively.

R. Poss, M.D.

Revision of a Failed Cemented Total Hip Prosthesis With Insertion of an Acetabular Component Without Cement and A Femoral Component With Cement: A Five to Eight-Year Follow-Up Study

Weber KL, Callaghan JJ, Goetz DD, et al (Iowa Methodist Hosp, Des Moines; Univ of Iowa, Iowa City)

J Bone Joint Surg Am 78A:982–994, 1996　　　　　　　　　　　　　2–12

Background.—The use of "hybrid" fixation—insertion of the acetabular component without cement and the femoral component with cement—has been increasing. One surgeon's experience was reviewed to determine whether the outcomes of revision of failed cemented total hip prostheses could be improved by performing a hybrid fixation.

Methods.—Sixty-one hybrid revision total hip arthroplasties were performed in 55 patients between 1986 and 1988. Mechanical failure of a cemented total hip prosthesis was the indication. The acetabular and femoral components were revised to a porous-coated Harris-Galante acetabular component inserted without cement and an Iowa femoral component inserted with cement. This group of patients was compared with 70 patients who had had revision total hip arthroplasty that used cementing methods for both components.

Findings.—In the first group, the overall prevalence of repeat revision for aseptic loosening was 0% for the acetabular components and 3% for the femoral components. Two percent and 5% of the components, respectively, had radiographic evidence of loosening. In the 43 patients alive at a mean of 74 months after revision, none of the acetabular components and 2% of the femoral components were revised again for aseptic loosening. Another 2% and 6% of the respective components were loose radiographically. Thirty-eight of 41 patients, respectively, were satisfied with the outcome at least 5 years after revision. These results compared favorably with those of the group undergoing revision with cementing techniques.

Conclusion.—The survival of the acetabular component is significantly better after a hybrid revision total hip arthroplasty than after techniques using cement. Hybrid fixation is recommended for most revision hip arthroplasty.

▶ The authors have improved their results in revision arthroplasty by performing hybrid revision total hip replacement compared with their previous practice of performing total hip revision surgery with cemented acetabular femoral components.

R. Poss, M.D.

Complications

Low-Molecular-Weight Heparin (Enoxaparin) as Prophylaxis Against Venous Thromboembolism After Total Hip Replacement

Bergqvist D, Benoni G, Björgell O, et al (Academic Hosp, Uppsala, Sweden; Malmö Univ, Sweden; Rhône-Poulenc Rorer, Paris)
N Engl J Med 335:696–700, 1996   2–13

Objective.—Patients undergoing total hip replacement surgery are at high risk of venous thromboembolism. Anticoagulant prophylaxis can reduce this risk, but it is unclear how long prophylaxis should continue. Two regimens of enoxaparin, a low–molecular-weight heparin, were compared for their ability to prevent venous thromboembolism after total hip replacement: 1 given only during hospitalization and the other continued for 1 month postoperatively.

Methods.—The randomized study included 262 patients undergoing total hip replacement. All received enoxaparin while they were in the hospital. They were then assigned, in blinded fashion, to receive enoxaparin or placebo for 1 month after surgery. About 3 weeks after hospital discharge, the patients underwent bilateral ascending phlebography for evidence of deep vein thrombosis.

Results.—There were 116 evaluable patients in the placebo group and 117 in the enoxaparin group. There were 43 episodes of deep vein thrombosis in the placebo group compared with 21 episodes in the enoxaparin group. Two patients in the placebo group had pulmonary embolism, compared with none in the enoxaparin group. Thus, the total incidence of thromboembolic complications was 39% with placebo and 18% with enoxaparin. Proximal deep vein thrombosis occurred in 24% of the placebo group and 7% of the enoxaparin group (Tables 2 and 3). Hematoma at the injection site was more likely to develop in the enoxaparin group. None of the patients died or experienced major complications.

TABLE 2.—Incidence of Thromboembolic Events in the Patients with Adequate Venography

Event	Placebo (N=116)	Enoxaparin (N=117)	Estimated Odds Ratio (95% CI)	P Value
	no. of patients (%)			
All thromboembolism	45 (39)	21 (18)	2.9 (1.6–5.3)	<0.001
Deep-vein thrombosis				
Proximal	28 (24)	8 (7)	4.3 (1.9–10.0)	<0.001
Indeterminate	2 (2)*	0	—	—
Distal	15 (13)	13 (11)	—	—

*These patients had pulmonary embolism before phlebography was performed. The origin of the thrombi was undetermined.

Abbreviation: CI, confidence interval.

(Reprinted by permission of *The New England Journal of Medicine*, courtesy of Bergqvist D, Benoni G, Björgell O, et al: Low-molecular-weight heparin (enoxaparin) as prophylaxis against venous thromboembolism after total hip replacement. *N Engl J Med* 335:696–700, copyright 1996, Massachusetts Medical Society.)

TABLE 3.—Deep Vein Thrombosis in Patients Who Could Be Evaluated According to Location of Thrombosis

LOCATION OF THROMBOSIS	PLACEBO GROUP (N = 98)			ENOXAPARIN GROUP (N = 96)		
	ALL SITES	PROXAMIL	DISTAL	ALL SITES	PROXIMAL	DISTAL
			no. of patients (%)			
Leg with hip replacement	22 (22)	17 (17)	5 (5)	12 (12)	4 (4)	8 (8)
Contralateral leg	3 (3)	1 (1)	2 (2)	1 (1)	0	1 (1)
Both legs	9 (9)	5 (5)	4 (4)	3 (3)	2 (2)	1 (1)

(Reprinted by permission of *The New England Journal of Medicine*, courtesy of Bergqvist D, Benoni G, Björgell O, et al: Low-molecular-weight heparin (enoxaparin) as prophylaxis against venous thromboembolism after total hip replacement. *N Engl J Med* 335:696–700, copyright 1996, Massachusetts Medical Society.)

Conclusion.—Extending enoxaparin prophylaxis after hospital discharge can significantly reduce the rate of venous thromboembolic complications after total hip replacement. Enoxaparin should be given for a full month after surgery, rather than just during hospitalization. Extended prophylaxis significantly reduces the rates of symptomatic as well as asymptomatic thromboembolism.

▶ There is general consensus that chemical and/or mechanical prophylaxis against venous thromboembolism after total joint replacement is necessary, but there is little agreement as to the optimal duration of treatment—an issue particularly important because of the decreasing length of hospital stays after these procedures In this important paper, 2 groups of patients received 10 to 11 days of low–molecular-weight heparin while in hospital and were then randomly assigned to 1 of 2 groups: 1 group continued to receive an oxyperine for a total treatment time of 1 month, whereas the other group received placebo.

There were significantly fewer venous thromboembolic complications in the group that received prophylaxis for a full month. Importantly, the proximal deep vein thrombosis was significantly different in the 2 groups, whereas the differences in distal thrombosis was not significant. Also of importance, these thromboembolisms occurred in 12 patients during the outpatient phase of the study. Ten of these 12 were in the placebo group. These findings speak strongly to the need for continuing prophylaxis against thromboembolism for an extended period after total hip replacement.

R. Poss, M.D.

Deep Venous Thrombosis After Total Joint Arthroplasty

Garino JP, Lotke PA, Kitziger KJ, et al (Univ of Pennsylvania, Philadelphia)
J Bone Joint Surg Am 78A:1359–1365, 1996   2–14

Objective.—Ascending venography, plethysmography, radioactive fibrinogen uptake, and Doppler testing are techniques for detecting deep vein thrombosis after total joint (hip or knee) arthroplasty. All of these methods have drawbacks such as discomfort, allergy, or lack of accuracy. Screening results for deep vein thrombosis using ultrasonography were compared with results using ascending venography for accuracy and reliability.

Methods.—Phase I involved venograms and ultrasonograms of 121 patients (126 joints), aged 26 to 86 years, who had total joint arthroplasty between September 1989 and February 1991. Phase II included venograms and ultrasonograms of 84 patients (87 joints) who had total joint replacements between April 1992 and October 1992. Venograms and ultrasonograms were independently reviewed and compared for the ability to detect deep vein thromboses.

Results.—In phase I, 3 ultrasonograms were considered to produce positive results. The remaining 123, evaluated as negative, included 7 legs with a clot detected by venography. Venography showed a thrombus in 62 legs. In phase II, 7 ultrasonograms were positive for a thrombus, including 5 wherein venography also confirmed a clot. Venography visualized a thrombus in 43 legs. In phase I, ultrasonography gave false negative results, a sensitivity of 0%, a positive predictive value of 0%, a negative predictive value of 94%, and an accuracy of 92%, primarily as a result of negative readings in 116 legs. Venography had a specificity of 97%. The sensitivity of duplex Doppler ultrasonography was 0%, and the specificity was 98%. In Phase II, the sensitivity of ultrasonography was 100% and the specificity was 98%. The accuracy of ultrasonography was 98%. The development of a clot was not related to the type of arthroplasty nor to the type of anticoagulant therapy. Thrombi distal to the knee were found in 30% of total hip arthroplasties and 71% of total knee arthroplasties. Lack of technical experience is suspected to be the primary reason for false negative ultrasonogram results.

Conclusion.—The expertise of the technician performing ultrasonography determined the accuracy and reliability of detection of deep vein thrombosis after total knee or hip arthroplasty.

▶ Compression ultrasonography is a commonly used procedure for detecting deep venous thrombosis after total joint arthroplasty. The reliability of this technique is shown to be highly dependent upon the experience of the technician.

R. Poss, M.D.

Effect of Intraoperative Blood Loss on the Serum Level of Cefazolin in Patients Managed With Total Hip Arthroplasty: A Prospective, Controlled Study

Meter JJ, Polly DW Jr, Brueckner RP, et al (Walter Reed Army Med Ctr, Washington, DC)
J Bone Joint Surg Am 78A:1201–1205, 1996   2–15

Objective.—Antibiotic prophylaxis has decreased the risk of infection after total joint arthroplasty to less than 1%. Many surgeons increase the frequency of antibiotic administration to maintain adequate serum levels when there is a major blood loss, although there have been no studies to support this practice. Results of a prospective, controlled study of the pharmacokinetic effect of intraoperative blood loss on serum levels of cefazolin in patients with total hip arthroplasty were reported.

Methods.—Preoperative and intraoperative pharmacokinetics of cefazolin were evaluated in 18 patients (5 women), aged 40 to 85 years, who were undergoing total hip arthroplasty. Blood loss, fluid administration, and blood transfusions were monitored. Cefazolin clearance and elimination half-life were calculated for each patient. Preoperative and intraoperative values were compared statistically.

Results.—There were no perioperative complications and no infections during the average 2.4-year follow-up. Patients lost an average of 1,136 mL of blood. The mean creatinine clearance increased significantly from an average preoperative value of 62.06 mL/min to an intraoperative level of 74.02 mL/min. The serum level of cefazolin at 4 hours was 45 µg/mL, which is significantly higher than the minimum inhibitory concentration for *Staphylococcus aureus*. There were no significant differences between mean preoperative and intraoperative values for cefazolin clearance, half-life, or serum concentrations at each time point.

Conclusion.—During the intraoperative period in patients receiving total hip arthroplasty, there was no evidence that intraoperative blood loss significantly affected the serum level of cefazolin during the recommended 4-hour dosing interval.

▶ It is well accepted that prophylactic antibiotics administered IV before skin incision provide a major deterent to infection. The authors address the question of whether maintenance of a minimum inhibitory concentration of cefazolin is compromised when there is increased blood loss. They demonstrate, however, that even when blood loss has approached 2,000 mL, the minimum inhibitory concentration for cefazolin is still exceeded. Therefore, a regimen of cefazolin every 4 hours is adequate for maintaining sufficient blood levels.

R. Poss, M.D.

Aspiration of the Hip Joint Before Revision Total Hip Arthroplasty

Lachiewicz PF, Rogers GD, Thomason HC (Univ of North Carolina, Chapel Hill)
J Bone Joint Surg [Am] 78A:749–754, 1996   2–16

Background.—Authorities continue to disagree about the value of routine hip joint aspiration before hip arthroplasty revision. The outcomes of such aspiration were reviewed to identify clinical or laboratory factors that indicate the presence of infection and thus the need for preoperative aspiration.

Methods and Findings.—Data on 142 hips undergoing presurgical aspiration once or twice were analyzed. Intraoperative culture showed infection in 15% of the hips (although the results in 2 cases were considered false positive). Initial positive aspiration was defined as the presence of organism growth on the solid medium or of grossly purulent fluid. The findings of the initial aspiration were positive for 19 hips. On culture of specimens from 1 hip, *Bacteroides thetaiotaomicron* grew only in the liquid medium. Purulent fluid was obtained from 1 hip, but no organism growth was seen on culture. Fourteen aspirations were repeated, mostly to confirm the presence of an unusual organism. Preoperative aspiration has a sensitivity of 92%, a specificity of 97%, and accuracy of 96%. An abnormally increased erythrocyte-sedimentation rate was associated with infection in 17 of the 19 hips. Although this finding was also noted for 50% of the uninfected hips, the difference was significant. Peripheral leukocyte count was of no benefit for predicting infection. Infection was less likely to occur in hips in which the implants were in place for more than 5 years than in hips with implants in place for 5 years or less. The erythrocyte-sedimentation rate was abnormal in all infected hips in which the implants had been in place for more than 5 years.

Conclusions.—Preoperative hip joint aspiration was very sensitive and specific in predicting infection in the current series. The decision of whether to aspirate can be based on erythrocyte-sedimentation rate and the amount of time that the implant has been in place.

Gram Stain Detection of Infection During Revision Arthroplasty
Chimento GF, Finger S, Barrack RL (Tulane Univ, New Orleans)
J Bone Joint Surg [Br] 78B:838–839, 1996   2–17

Background.—Because infection after revision arthroplasty is disastrous, preoperative assessment must be done to ensure that no infection is present. When infection is suspected clinically but preoperative investigations are not conclusive, intraoperative tests such as Gram staining may demonstrate the presence or absence of infection. The value of Gram-staining performed on swabs obtained during revision hip and knee arthroplasty in patients with known clinical infection was investigated.

Methods and Findings.—One hundred ninety-four revision arthroplasties of the hip and knee were performed during a 10-year period. The findings of intraoperative Gram staining were available for 87%. No evidence of infection was found in 137 joints. Twenty-one knees and 11 hips were infected. However, results of intraoperative Gram staining were negative in all cases. Thus, this technique had a 0% sensitivity for detecting infection.

Conclusions.—Negative Gram-staining results do not reliably indicate the absence of infection. Thus, decisions to proceed with arthroplasty revision should not be based on intraoperative Gram stain findings.

The Reliability of Analysis of Intraoperative Frozen Sections for Identifying Active Infection During Revision Hip or Knee Arthroplasty

Lonner JH, Desai P, Dicesare PE, et al (Hosp for Joint Diseases, New York)
J Bone Joint Surg [Am] 78A:1553–1558, 1996   2–18

Background.—Deciding whether to reimplant at the time of revision arthroplasty can be difficult when the preoperative assessment failed to determine whether infection caused the loosening. Previous retrospective research has suggested that analysis of intraoperative frozen sections reliably identifies active infection during revision hip or knee arthroplasty. A current propsective study determined the reliability of this method.

Methods and Findings.—Data were obtained on 175 consecutive revision total joint arthroplasties. Frozen sections were negative for 152 joints. The remaining 23 had at least 6 polymorphonuclear leukocytes per high-power field and were classified as infected. Frozen-section analysis had an 84% sensitivity for indices of 5 and 10 polymorphonuclear leukocytes per high-power field. Its specificity was 96% and 99% for the 2 indices, respectively. Its positive predictive value increased significantly, from 70% to 89%, when the index was increased from 5 to 10 polymorphonuclear leukocytes per high-power field. For both indices, the negative predictive value of the frozen sections was 98%.

Conclusions.—Obtaining tissue for intraoperative frozen sections during revision hip and knee arthroplasty is of value for detecting infection. Less than 5 polymorphonuclear leukocytes per high-power field reliably indicated the absence of infection, and at least 10 per field reliably predicted infection.

▶ These 3 papers address important questions regarding the reliability of 3 methods that are used to establish whether a wound is infected or not. In Abstract 2–16 the authors address the utility of preoperative aspiration of the hip joint before revision total hip arthroplasty. They find that the accuracy of aspiration is dependent upon the expertise with which a fluid sample can be obtained from the hip joint. On the basis of their findings, they have become more selective in identifying candidates for preoperative aspiration. They believe that aspiration of hips in patients who have had implants in situ for more than 5 years and in patients whose erythrocyte sedimentation rate is normal or only minimally elevated is unlikely to yield evidence of infection. They do recommend preoperative aspiration for all patients that have painful total hip arthroplasties that have been in place for less than 5 years and/or in whom erythrocyte sedimentation is markedly elevated. In Abstract 2–17 the authors assess the utility of intraoperative Gram-staining for the detection of infection. They find that the absence of organisms on intraoperative Gram-staining does not confirm the absence of infection.

In contrast, in Abstract 2–18 the reliability of intraoperative frozen sections for identifying infection is reported. When intraoperative frozen sections reveal 5–10 polymorphonuclear leukocytes per high-power field, there is a high correlation with the presence of infection. The predictive value increases with increasing polymorphonuclear leukocyte count, that is, 10 leukocytes per high-power field provided higher specificity for infection. Quantification of polymorphonuclear leukocytes on intraoperative frozen sections appears to be a valuable method for determining the presence or absence of infection.

R. Poss, M.D.

Factors Affecting the Results of Total Hip Arthroplasty

Early Failure of Acetabular Components Inserted Without Cement After Previous Pelvic Irradiation

Jacobs JJ, Kull LR, Frey GA, et al (Rush-Presbyterian-St Luke's Med Ctr, Chicago)

J Bone Joint Surg Am 77A:1829–1835, 1995   2–19

Objective.—Bone irradiation can result in osteonecrosis. The increased use of noncemented fixation, particularly of the acetabular component, has compelled the examination of the survival of components fixed without cement in patients receiving total hip arthroplasty after periacetabular irradiation.

Methods.—A retrospective analysis of records from a database of 1,319 patients receiving total hip arthroplasty between January 1983 and January 1991 at Rush-Presbyterian-St. Luke's Medical Center in Chicago revealed 8 living patients (9 hips) (1 man), aged 56 to 88 years, with a history of periacetabular irradiation. The type and dose of radiation were determined, and the condition of the component was assessed radiographically. The relationship between irradiation and acetabular component survival was analyzed statistically. Patients were followed for an average of 37 months.

Results.—There were 2 revisions for component failure and 1 additional failure without revision. Failure was the result of acetabular migration in all 3 hips. In 1 patient, the component inserted without cement subsequently failed, and a Girdlestone arthroplasty was performed. The other patient received a cemented component. A fourth patient who was asymptomatic appeared to have a loose component. This patient died of pancreatic cancer. On average, patients were irradiated 31 months before hip symptoms appeared and 77 months before arthroplasty. The time to failure averaged 25 months. Thus, use of noncemented, hemispherical, porous-coated acetabular components without cement was associated with component failure in 4 of 9 irradiated hips.

Conclusion.—Patients receiving pelvic irradiation followed by total hip arthroplasty with noncemented components had a high rate of failure after 25 months. The full effect of irradiation on prosthesis survival will require a study on a larger population of type, dose, and technique of irradiation as well as portals used.

▶ In a recent publication Massin and Duparc[1] describe the difficulties in securing stable acetabular fixation when the pelvis has been previously subjected to radiation therapy. Using cementless fixation, Jacobs et al. in the study abstracted here, found that 4 of 9 acetabular components failed at only 25 months postoperatively, whereas Massin and Duparc report a 52% failure rate at a mean follow-up of 69 months when acetabular components were fixed with cement. They recommended the use of an acetabular reinforcement ring to better stabilize the pelvis but found that even with this method, there was an aseptic acetabular loosening rate of 19%. The patient and surgeon must be aware of the potential complications when contemplating total hip arthroplasty in a previously irradiated pelvis.

R. Poss, M.D

Reference

1.   Massin P, Duparc J: Total hip replacement in irradiated hips. *J Bone Joint Surg Br* 77B:847–852, 1995.

▶ The next 2 papers address the subject of variations in the diameter of prosthetic femoral heads and the possible consequences of articulation "mismatch" and degeneration of polyethylene wear products. In Abstract 2–20, the authors compare the range of prosthetic femoral head diameters from 9 manufacturers. They found that with 28-mm and 32-mm heads, the measurements were within narrowed tolerances, but with 22-mm heads, there were 2 distinct populations of sizes. They conclude that it is probably acceptable to exchange 28-mm or 32-mm heads of different manufacturers, but that the exchange of 22-mm heads may be accompanied by significant variation in head dimensions.

R. Poss, M.D.

Femoral Head Size: Variation Among Manufacturers

Ritter MA, Meding JB, Faris PM, et al (Ctr for Hip and Knee Surgery, Mooresville, Ind)
Orthopedics 19:877–878, 1996   2–20

Background.—In some patients with loosening of a total hip replacement component, the acetabular or femoral component, but not both, may need revision. It is unclear whether the loose component of one manufacturer's prosthesis can be replaced with that of another manufacturer with confidence that the diameter specifications are similar. The outside diameters of most available femoral heads were compared.

Methods and Findings.—Nine manufacturers were asked for the specific femoral head diameters of their 22-mm, 28-mm, and 32-mm femoral components. The 22-mm heads averaged 0.869 inch. All were within 1 SD, although the SD was great. The 28-mm heads averaged 1.101 inches. Eighty-nine percent of these were within 1 SD. The 32-mm heads averaged 1.258 inches. Seventy-eight percent were within 1 SD.

Conclusions.—Different manufacturers' femoral and acetabular components can apparently be used together when a 28-mm or 32-mm femoral head is used. However, when a 22-mm femoral head is needed, the surgeon should check with the manufacturer of the prosthesis previously placed, as the variation among these prostheses is wide.

Adaptive Finite Element Modeling of Long-term Polyethylene Wear in Total Hip Arthroplasty
Maxian TA, Brown TD, Pedersen DR, et al (Univ of Iowa, Iowa City)
J Orthop Res 14:668–675, 1996   2–21

Background.—Polyethylene wear debris and the resulting aseptic loosening are a major cause of the abrupt decline in total hip component survivorship after 10 years. Ideally, all new constructs would be assessed for their long-term effects before implantation. To date, methods of assessing wear have been problematic. A new adaptive remeshing formulation was developed and used to investigate the evolution of wear fronts and long-term wear in total hip replacements.

Methods and Findings.—Loads and femoral head excursions were obtained from a physically validated gait analysis model of a patient with an instrumented total hip replacement. Otherwise identical 22-, 28-, and 32-mm components were used. The least volumetric wear but most linear wear occurred for the 22-mm head. The polyethylene thickness in a 22-mm component was then decreased to the same as that in a 32-mm component. The volumetric wear rate for the smaller component continued to be much less than that for the larger component. This showed that sliding distance rather than polyethylene linear thickness was mainly responsible for the difference in rates. In a 28-mm series, for which head sizes were varied across the range of currently accepted industrial tolerances, long-term volumetric wear was almost the same regardless of initial clearance, although wear rates were greatest for the least congruent articulations (Fig 6).

Conclusions.—The sliding-distance-coupled finite element formulation is useful for design-oriented parametric studies. It is clearly better than inferring wear from contact stress alone. Although the differences in predictions of the postoperative wear rate in the different head sizes persisted during long-term simulation, marked differences in predicted postoperative wear rates in the conformity series converged rapidly to similar wear behaviors.

▶ Using finite element modeling to address questions of polyethylene wear in total hip arthroplasty, the authors confirm previous findings that the most linear wear occurs with 22-mm heads but the most volumetric wear occurs wih 32-mm heads. Even when polyethylene thickness was reduced in the 22-mm head simulation to equal that of the 32-mm component, the volumetric wear rate was still significantly less in a 22-mm head

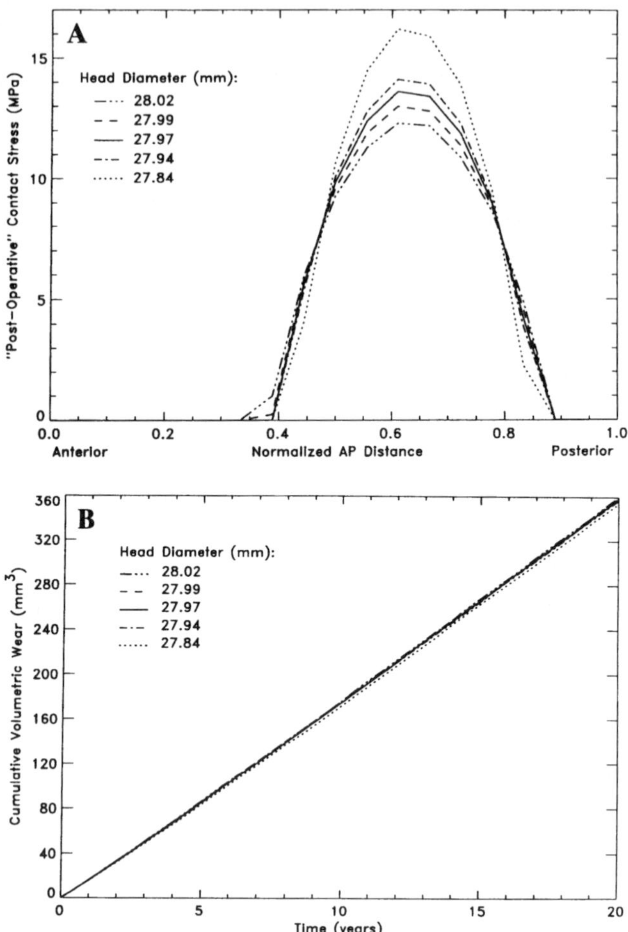

FIGURE 6.—A, initial contact stress distributions for the congruency series. The stress distribution from the peak gait load is plotted from anterior to posterior across a set of nodes passing through the peak loading region. As the head size decreased, the peak contact stress increased. B, cumulative volumetric wear for the head size tolerance series. The cumulative wear volumes are virtually the same across the series for the range of time studied. *Abbreviation: AP,* anterior-posterior. (Courtesy of Maxian TA, Brown TD, Pedersen DR, et al: Adaptive finite element modeling of long-term polyethylene wear in total hip arthroplasty. *J Orthop Res* 14:668–675, 1996.)

construct. Addressing the question of the possible deleterious effect of a mismatched articulation because of slight variations of head sizes attributable to industrial tolerances, the authors conclude that although initial wear rates were high (wear in), evaluation of the long-term volumetric wear showed negligible differences across the range of sizes tested. Thus, slight variations in diameter within the industrial tolerance limits are of less significance to the ultimate performance of the articulation and the generation of particulate debris than the initial choice by the surgeon of the diameter of the femoral head articulation.

R. Poss, M.D.

The Effect of Superior Placement of the Acetabular Component on the Rate of Loosening After Total Hip Arthroplasty: Long-term Results in Patients Who Have Crowe Type-II Congenital Dysplasia of the Hip
Pagnano MW, Hanssen AD, Lewallen DG, et al (Mayo Clinic and Mayo Found, Rochester, Minn)
J Bone Joint Surg Am 78A:1004–1014, 1996   2–22

Introduction.—The proper position of the acetabular component in patients with congenital dysplasia of the hip has not been defined. The long-term results of total hip arthroplasty with cement in 117 patients (145 hips) with Crowe type-II congenital dysplasia of the hip were analyzed to determine the effect of the initial position of the acetabular cup on the long-term durability of the femoral and acetabular components.

Methods.—Patient records were reviewed retrospectively for measurement of preoperative and postoperative radiographs and functional evaluations. The position of the acetabular cup outside of the true acetabular region was determined preoperatively. A 7-zone system was used to assess the position of the acetabular component postoperatively. The effect of the initial position of the acetabular component on eventual loosening of the acetabular and femoral components was determined. The mean patient age was 51 years and the mean duration of follow-up was 14 years.

Results.—Significant correlations were observed between revision of the femoral components and the initial position of the acetabular cup outside of the true acetabular region and outside of zone 1 (inferior and medial). Increased rates of loosening and revision of the femoral and acetabular components were significantly correlated with cups that were initially more than 15 mm superior to the approximate femoral head center, without lateral displacement.

Conclusion.—Superior positioning of the acetabular component, even in the absence of lateral displacement, is associated with increased rates of loosening of the femoral and acetabular components. Findings indicate that the acetabular component should be positioned in or near the true acetabular region.

▶ Proponents of a high hip center state that it poses no biomechanical disadvantages as long as the hip is not lateralized. In this paper, the authors refute that proposition and find that superior positioning of the acetabular component, even without lateral displacement, was associated with increased rates of loosening of both femoral and acetabular components. The authors advocate attempting to place the acetabular component in the anatomical position.

R. Poss, M.D.

Congenital Hip Disease in Adults

Hartofilakidis G, Stamos K, Karachalios T, et al (Athens Univ, Greece)
J Bone Joint Surg [Am] 78A:683–692, 1996   2–23

Background.—Early attempts at treating congenital hip disease in adults with total hip arthroplasty often failed because the true acetabulum could not be identified at the time of surgery, resulting in incorrect placement of the acetabular component and inadequate component coverage and containment. This failure prompted a study of the pathoanatomy of the acetabulum associated with congenital hip disease in adults and the development of a classification system. The classification of acetabular deficiencies and operative treatment with acetabuloplasty combined with total hip arthroplasty were presented.

Classification.—Three distinct types of congenital hip disease in adults have been identified: dysplasia, in which the femoral head is contained in the original true acetabulum; low dislocation, in which the femoral head articulates with a false acetabulum, the inferior lip contacting or overlapping the superior lip of the true acetabulum, giving the appearance of 2 overlapping acetabula; and high dislocation, in which the femoral head has migrated superposteriorly, with no contact between the true and false acetabulum.

Treatment and Outcomes.—In some patients, the anterior, posterior, and superior aspects of the acetabular component cannot be covered during a total hip arthroplasty because of a deficient acetabulum. In such patients, an acetabuloplasty technique termed *cotyloplasty* can be performed. This procedure involves medial advancement of the acetabular floor by creating a controlled comminuted fracture of its medial wall, autogenous bone grafting, and the implantation of a small acetabular component with cement. The outcomes of this technique were satisfactory after 2- to 15-year follow-up in 49 hips with high dislocation, 31 with low dislocation, and 6 with dysplasia. Only 2 acetabular components required revision for aseptic loosening. The cumulative success rate for the acetabular components at 5 years was 100% and at 10 years was 93.2%.

Conclusions.—A common terminology is needed to describe the different types of congenital hip disease in adults for better treatment planning and outcome evaluation. The use of the terms dysplasia, low dislocation, and high dislocation is proposed.

▶ Some of the most difficult total hip reconstructions are in patients who have degenerative changes secondary to congenital hip disease. This paper describes the acetabular abnormalities and resulting bony acetabular deficiencies encountered in this group of patients and also describes the surgical techniques by which they obtain adequate bone coverage.

R. Poss, M.D.

The Porous-coated Anatomic Total Hip Prosthesis: Failure of the Metal-backed Acetabular Component

Astion DJ, Saluan P, Stulberg BN, et al (Hosp for Special Surgery, New York; Case Western Reserve Univ, Cleveland, Ohio; Cleveland Ctr for Joint Reconstruction, Ohio; et al)

J Bone Joint Surg [Am] 78A:755–766, 1996   2–24

Background.—Porous-coated anatomical acetabular components have been reported to have a high rate of failure. Implants retrieved at revision were analyzed to determine the reasons for clinical failures associated with this component.

Methods.—One hundred seventy-three patients were implanted with the original porous-coated anatomical prosthesis in a total of 199 procedures between 1983 and 1987. The component was a preassembled, metal-backed polyethylene device. Beads were sintered to the metal backing to permit bone ingrowth. Two pegs were used for initial fixation. Twenty-three components (12%) failed because of migration or severe osteolysis, and 13 hips were revised at a mean 69.5 months after the initial procedure.

Findings.—Extensive polyethylene damage was discovered on the articular and back surfaces of the liners. Commonly, the polyethylene rim of the liner was cracked, and the antirotation notch in the polyethylene rime was deformed. Polyethylene density was greater than expected. There was less particle fusion with surrounding polyethylene than was anticipated.

Conclusions.—Factors related to both the design and material of the porous-coated anatomical acetabular component appear to contribute to the failure of these devices. Patients implanted with this type of prosthesis should be monitored closely for the onset of pain and for the development of osteolytic lesions or component migration. Such findings signal the impending failure of the component.

▶ The original acetabular component of the porous-coated anatomical hip prosthesis (PCA) was composed of a preassembled metal-backed polyethylene liner. The authors report a 12% failure rate because of migration or osteolysis. The incidence of osteolysis increased with the duration that the implant had been in place, and osteolysis was also more prevalent in hips in which the polyethylene thickness was 8.5 mm or less. Patients who have this first generation PCA acetabulum in place should be observed closely and for an indefinite period to assess the status of these components.

R. Poss, M.D.

Primary Total Hip Replacement With Insertion of an Acetabular Component Without Cement and a Femoral Component With Cement

Woolson ST, Haber DF (Stanford Univ, Calif)
J Bone Joint Surg [Am] 78A:698–705, 1996   2–25

Background.—The "hybrid fixation"—insertion of an acetabular prosthesis without cement along with a femoral prosthesis with cement—has been done in total hip replacement since the early 1980s. However, few intermediate and no long-term follow-up studies have been reported. One group of patients undergoing hybrid fixation between 1985 and 1989 was studied retrospectively.

Methods.—Clinical data on 114 patients with 125 affected hips were analyzed. Radiographic data were also available for 110 of these patients. Minimum follow-up was 56 months, with a mean of 72 months.

Findings.—The mean Harris hip score increased from 47 to 91 points. Three percent of the hips needed revision for aseptic loosening of the femoral component at an average of 55 months after surgery. Two femoral components were definitely loose radiographically. Eight percent of the hips had endosteal lysis of the femur. Overall, 5% of the femoral components were revised for loosening or had definite radiographic evidence of loosening. None of the acetabular components had loosened. Clinical outcomes were excellent in 115 hips.

Conclusions.—Hybrid fixation for primary total hip replacement has yielded excellent intermediate outcomes in this series of patients. Surgeons are encouraged to use this technique in all elderly patients and young patients in whom femoral fixation without cement is not appropriate because of femoral osteoporosis. An adequate mantle of cement is needed in the proximal part of the femur with the use of a rasp that enables enough space for cement and possibly with the use of a proximal cement-spacer.

▶ In this 6-year follow-up of the results of so-called hybrid fixation, the authors find excellent clinical and radiographic results of the acetabular fixation, a finding consistent with other reports. In contrast, the cemented femoral components using third-generation cementing techniques demonstrated a 5% incidence of aseptic loosening. The authors attribute these failures to an inadequate cement mantle, possibly caused by a rasp envelope that was not sufficiently oversized to allow for a minimum 2-mm-thick cement mantle proximally. Two stems fractured, probably by the same mechanism of good distal fixation but poor proximal fixation.

Hybrid total hip replacement has been reported as being satisfactory by most authors, but its success is highly dependent on good surgical and cement technique.

R. Poss, M.D.

The Bone-Implant Interface of Femoral Stems With Non-circumferential Porous Coating
Urban RM, Jacobs JJ, Sumner DR, et al (Rush Presbyterian St Luke's Med Ctr, Chicago)
J Bone Joint Surg [Am] 78A:1068–1081, 1996   2–26

Background.—Porous-coated femoral stems implanted without acrylic cement, used widely in hip arthroplasty in younger patients, have yielded disappointing short-term clinical outcomes. The prevalence and amount of bone ingrowth are reportedly far less than initially reported in animal studies. Currently, neither the basic design parameters of the location and extent of the porous coating nor the amount of bone ingrowth needed to maintain a biologically stable interface have been established. The bone-implant interface of 15 titanium-alloy femoral stems with porous coating limited to 3 proximal areas not covering the full circumference of the device was studied histologically.

Methods.—Specimens were obtained at autopsy from 10 patients who had received the implant a mean 46 months earlier. Histomorphometric techniques were used to determine the volume fraction of bone in the porous spaces and extent of bone ingrowth.

Findings.—Eleven of the 15 stems had bone in the porous coating in continuity with the surrounding medullary bone. In these specimens, the mean volume fraction of bone ingrowth was 26.9%. The mean extent of bone ingrowth was 64.3%. Both parameters increased with time. In the 4 remaining stems, the bone did not show continuity with the surrounding trabecular bed. Two had a limited amount of bone in the porous coating, and 2 (from 1 patient) showed no bone ingrowth. The uncoated surfaces of the stems were covered by periprosthetic membranes surrounded by a shell of trabecular bone. The membranes of implants that had been in place for at least 8 months showed polyethylene wear debris and other particles at the level of the joint within histiocytes throughout the length of the femoral stem.

Conclusions.—The ingrowth of bone into the porous surface was of greater magnitude in these femoral stems retrieved at autopsy than in previously described failed prostheses. In addition, bone ingrowth progressively increased with time. Interruptions in the circumferential extent of the porous surface are associated with periprosthetic membrane development, which provides a pathway for migration of particulate wear and corrosion products to the distal part of the stem. A circumferential coating may hinder particle access, thus reducing the possibility of diaphyseal osteolysis.

▶ The bone-implant interface of femoral stems with noncircumferential porous coating was investigated in an autopsy retrieval study. Although there was reasonably good bone ingrowth in the areas that had porous coating, the uncoated surfaces of the stems were surrounded by a membrane and this membrane demonstrated the presence of polyethylene wear debris. The authors conclude that a larger area of the stem, preferably circumferential, should contain ingrowth material for at least 2 reasons: (1), to eliminate the possibility of a periprosthetic membrane, which may provide a pathway for migration of particulate wear debris; and (2) to provide a larger surface area to achieve bone ingrowth stability of the implant and thus lessen the likelihood of fatigue fracture of the supporting trabeculae.

R. Poss, M.D.

Incidence of Thigh Pain After Uncemented Total Hip Arthroplasty as a Function of Femoral Stem Size

Vresilovic EJ, Hozack WJ, Rothman RH (Univ of Pennsylvania, Philadelphia; Jefferson Med College, Philadelphia; Rothman Inst, Philadelphia)
J Arthroplasty 11:304–311, 1996   2–27

Background.—The incidence of mechanical thigh pain in uncemented femoral components ranges from 10% to 20%. Proposed mechanisms for this pain include an indequate fit or fixation of the femoral component in the femoral canal and excessive stress concentration in the femur resulting from changes in the femoral flexural and torsional rigidity caused by the stem in the femoral canal. The incidence of thigh pain for an uncemented femoral component as a function of femoral stem size was determined.

Methods.—Two hundred seventy-one patients undergoing a total of 297 primary total hip arthroplasties were assessed for thigh pain 2 years postoperatively. The femoral components used were the same wedge-shaped geometry but were different sizes.

Findings.—Radiographically, all components were stable. In a regression analysis, the presence of thigh pain was associated directly with increasing stem size. Proximal and distal component moments of inertia for bending in the mediolateral plane were even more strongly positively correlated with thigh pain (Table 2).

Conclusions.—Femoral stem size significantly influences the incidence of thigh pain associated with uncemented femoral components. Thus one

TABLE 2.—Incidence of Thigh Pain as a Function of Stem Size

Femoral Size (mm)	Thigh Pain Yes (%)	No	Total
5	0 (0)	6	6
7.5	6 (15)	34	40
10	2 (3)	69	71
12.5	11 (12)	78	89
15	9 (15)	51	60
17.5	6 (23)	20	26
20	2 (40)	3	5
Total	36 (12)	261	297

(Courtesy of Vresilovic EJ, Hozack WJ, Rothman RJ: Incidence of thigh pain after uncemented total hip arthroplasty as a function of femoral stem size. *J Arthroplasty* 11:304–311, 1996.)

source of thigh pain may be changes in bone mechanical stress from the femoral component. Designing more flexible components, either through material modifications or structural modification such as slots or hollow components, may help avoid the problem of size-related thigh pain. Another possibility may be to use cemented stems.

▶ The authors report that thigh pain after use of uncemented femoral stems in total hip arthroplasty is highly correlated with the stiffness of the prosthesis. Femoral stems of larger diameters, thereby having a larger stem to host femur stiffness mismatch, were more likely to be associated with thigh pain.

R. Poss, M.D.

The Elevated-rim Acetabular Liner in Total Hip Arthroplasty: Relationship to Postoperative Dislocation
Cobb TK, Morrey BF, Ilstrup DM (Mayo Clinic, Rochester, Minn)
J Bone Joint Surg [Am] 78A:80–86, 1996   2–28

Background.—The postoperative stability of a total hip prosthesis is thought to be improved by an acetabular component with an elevated rim. However, the clinical value of this has not been established. The effect of an augmented acetabular component on the cumulative probablity of dislocation after total hip arthroplasty was investigated.

Methods and Findings.—The outcomes of 5,167 total hip arthroplasties performed at 1 center between 1985 and 1991 were reviewed. There were 2,469 acetabular components with an elevated-rim liner and 2,698 with a standard liner. Forty-eight hips with an elevated-rim acetabular liner dislocated within 2 years, compared to 101 with the standard acetabular liner. The 2-year probability of dislocation was 2.19% and 3.85%, respectively. The trend at 5 years was similar. The hips with an elevated-rim liner also had increased stability at 2 years when hips were analyzed according to the surgical approach, mode of fixation, sex of the patient, and type of total hip arthroplasty.

Conclusions.—Although stability after total hip arthroplasty is improved when an elevated liner is used, especially in hips at greater risk for prosthesis dislocation, the long-term effect of this elevated liner on wear and loosening is unknown. Further study is needed to address this concern.

▶ There are theoretical advantages and disadvantages to the use of an elevated-rim acetabular liner. One purported advantage is that an elevated liner should protect against total hip dislocation. The authors have reviewed a large cohort of patients and find that an elevated-rim liner does confer a small, but significant, increased protection against posterior hip dislocation, but they caution that the long-term effect of an elevated liner on wear and loosening remains an area of concern. Prevention of total hip dislocation requires exacting surgical technique and proper placement of the components to achieve an impingement-free range of motion. When these criteria are met, it is this author's opinion that an elevated-rim liner adds little to the stability of the hip.

R. Poss, M.D.

The Influence of Clinical Factors on Periprosthetic Bone Remodeling

Sychterz CJ, Engh CA (Anderson Orthopaedic Research Inst, Arlington, Va)
Clin Orthop 322:285–292, 1996   2–29

Background.—Mechanically induced bone remodeling after femoral prosthesis implantation is difficult to quantify. Changes in bone mineral content resulting from bone remodeling were quantitated by analyzing femurs retrieved at autopsy from patients with unilateral total hip replacements to determine the importance of patient age and weight, implant size, implantation duration, and bone mineral quality on the remodeling process.

Methods.—Femurs were obtained from 11 patients who had had well-functioning unilateral hip replacements before they died. Dual energy x-ray absorptiometry was performed to analyze periprosthetic bone remodeling. The porous-coated endoprostheses had remained in place for a mean 5.9 years. A matching prosthesis was implanted in vitro in the contralateral femur to serve as a control.

Findings.—The in vivo implanted femurs had a mean bone mineral content decrease of 22.6%. Women had significantly greater mean bone loss than men, with percentages of 31.2% and 12.3%, respectively. In a longitudinal analysis, the mean reduction in bone mineral content was found to be 42.1% proximally, 23% in the midsection, and 5.5% distally. Percent reductions in total bone mineral content were associated with patient weight and age, implant diameter, duration of implantation, and contralateral femoral bone mineral content. Bone mineral content of the contralateral femur was the only variable with strong predictive value, bone loss being greater in femurs with low bone mineral content than in those with high bone mineral content. Bone loss was unassociated with patient weight or age, implant diameter, and implantation duration.

Conclusions.—In this study, the single variable predicting bone loss was the total bone mineral content of the control femur. This suggests the intriguing possibility that the most important factor in bone remodeling after uncemented total hip arthroplasty is the mechanical and biological state of the femur at arthroplasty rather than the mechanical properties of the stem.

▶ Although implant material of fabrication and diameter (the relative prosthesis–bone stiffness mismatch has been implicated as a major contributor to stress shielding), the authors find in a series of 11 autopsy-retrieved specimens that the most predictive indicator of bone loss was the bone mineral content of the contralateral femur. Thus, patients who have osteopenia at the time of initial total hip arthroplasty are most likely to experience the greatest loss of periprosthetic bone.

R. Poss, M.D.

Porosity Reduction in Bone Cement at the Cement-Stem Interface
Bishop NE, Ferguson S, Tepic S (AO/ASIF Research Inst, Davos, Switzerland)
J Bone Joint Surg [Br] 78B:349–356, 1996   2–30

Background.—Fatigue failure of bone cement results in stem loosening and is probably one reason why cemented total hip replacements fail. Strong evidence suggests that cracks in the cement begin at voids that act as stress risers, especially at the cement-stem interface. The preferential development of voids at this site is caused by shrinkage during polymerization and the initiation of this process at the warmer cement-bone interface, which causes bone cement to shrink away from the stem. Reversing the direction of polymerization would shrink the cement on the stem and decrease or eliminate void formation at this interface. The transient temperature distribution in the stem-cement-bone system was modeled to find the best temperature at which the stem should be implanted.

Methods and Findings.—Hip prostheses at room temperature or preheated to 44°C were implanted into human cadaver femora kept at 37°C. Hand-mixed or vacuum-mixed bone cement was used before implantation. Preheating the stem markedly decreased the area of porosity at the cement-stem interface. The preheating temperature of 44°C determined by computer analysis of transient heat transfer was the minimum needed to induce initial polymerization at the cement-stem interface. Temperatures determined during these experiments showed that stem preheating caused a negligible increase in bone temperature (Fig 2).

Conclusions.—Moderate preheating of the stem practically eliminates shrinkage-induced porosity at the cement-stem interface. This was observed with normal and low-viscosity cements mixed by hand and under vacuum. The minor increase in temperature at the cement-bone interface will probably not significantly damage the bone.

▶ Because of evidence that voids and cement fracture are initiated at the cement-stem interface, the authors developed a method to avoid the shrinkage of the cement mantle from the metallic stem during prepolymerization. By preheating the hip implant, the areas of porosity at the cement-stem interface were reduced. It will be of great interest to find out whether this technique, which may result in an improved cement-stem interface, confers an increased longevity on cemented implants. Centralization of femoral components is currently viewed as an essential part of proper surgical technique because the goal of cemented implants is to have a symmetric and complete cement mantle of at least 2 mm in all areas. In this study, the effect of 5 different designs on the cement mantle was evaluated. There was greater porosity in the specimens containing centralizers than in con-

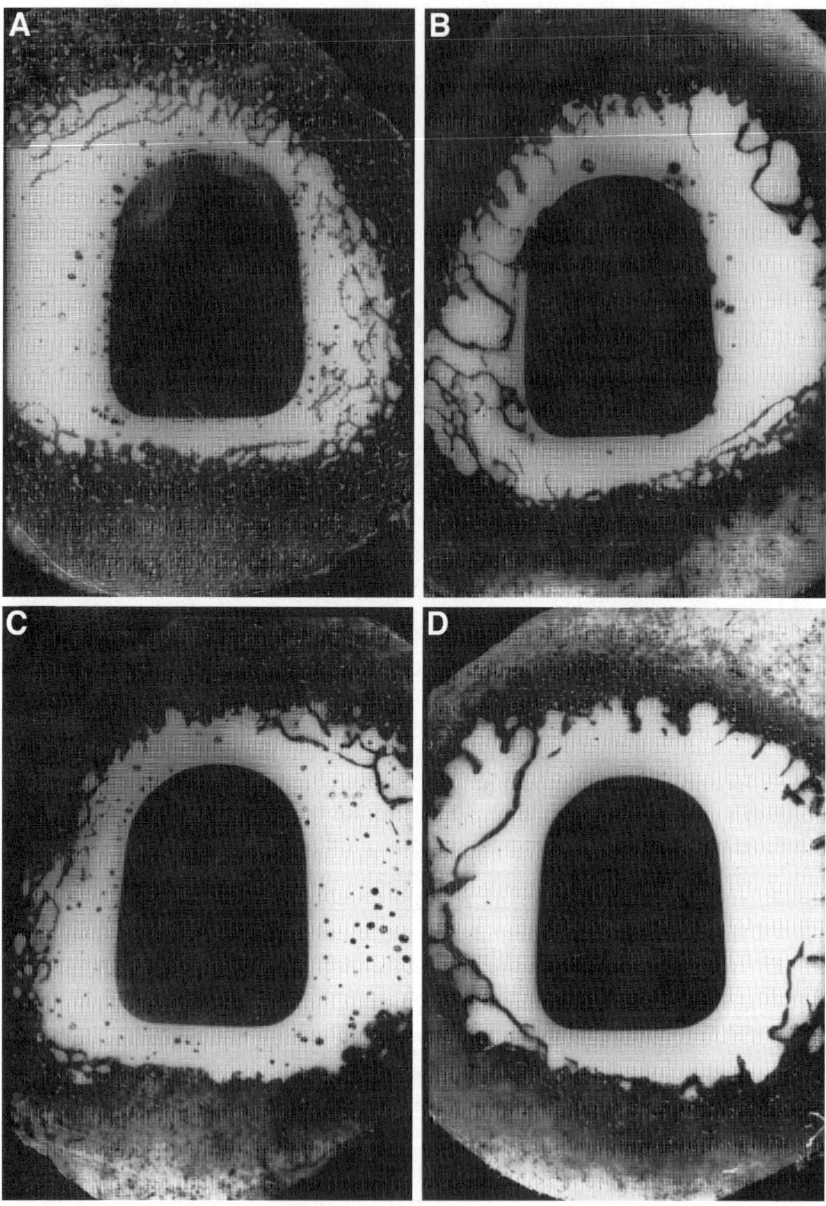

FIGURE 2.—Cross-sections at the junction of the middle and distal thirds of the prosthesis, implanted in Sulfix 60 bone cement. The black lines in the cement are cross-sections of bony trabeculae. **A,** hand-mixed cement implanted with a stem at 23°C. There are a number of pores at and around the cement-stem interface. **B,** vacuum-mixed cement implanted with a stem of 23°C. All the pores result from cement shrinkage, because all others have been removed by the vacuum mixing. The pores are at and around the stem. **C,** hand-mixed cement implanted with a stem at 44°C. There are no pores at the cement-stem interface. **D,** vacuum-mixed cement implanted with a stem at 44°C. There are very few pores in the cement. (Courtesy of Bishop NE, Ferguson S, Tepic S: Porosity reduction in bone cement at the cement-stem interface. *J Bone Joint Surg [Br]* 78B:349–356, 1996.)

trols and different designs of centralizers induced varying degrees of porosity. Centralization is an important feature of total hip arthroplasty, but optimum use of centralizers under design awaits further study.

R. Poss, M.D.

Effects of Distal Femoral Centralizers on Bone-Cement in Total Hip Arthroplasty: An Experimental Analysis of Cement-Centralizer Bonding, Cement Void Formation, and Crack Propagation
Smith SG, Kabo JM, Kilgus DJ (Univ of California, Los Angeles School of Medicine; VA Med Ctr, Los Angeles)
J Arthroplasty 11:687–692, 1996   2–31

Background.—Manufacturers of total hip prostheses have begun providing methacrylate cement spacers that insert into the distal tip of femoral stems to facilitate centralization of cemented femoral stem components in the intrameduallary canal. The use of these centralizers is believed to be a simple, effective way of achieving a uniform cement mantle around total hip arthroplasty femoral stems. However, it is not known whether their use adversely affects the long-term durability of polymethyl methacrylate cement. Whether distal femoral centralizers increase the risk of cement crack formation as a result of incomplete bonding of the prepolymerized spacer to the cement or by increasing cement porosity as a result of changes in cement flow in the region of the centralizer was determined.

Methods.—Five different types of distal femoral centralizers were inserted into model femoral stems and cemented into closed-ended tubes simulating a proximal femoral canal. Cyclic loads from 50 to 500 lb were applied for 0–10 million cycles.

Findings.—Analysis of each specimen revealed no cement cracks or lack of bonding at the interface between the cement and the centralizers. Specimens containing centralizers had more porosity than the control specimens without centralizers. The cement surrounding 2 of the centralizer designs had a significantly smaller amount of porosity than that surrounding the other 3 types. Neither centralizer use, centralizer type, nor cycling duration affected the number of cracks that occurred. Failure to plug the centralizer receptacle hole in the stem tip adequately resulted in very large cement voids in the control specimens.

Conclusions.—These data indicate that centralizer use is an effective way of producing an even cement mantle around femoral stems. All designs tested in this model were equally effective.

▶ Does osteolysis cause loosening or does loosening cause osteolysis? In a rat model, the authors conclude that mechanical loosening is of primary importance and that the events initiated by loosening are later accelerated by the reaction to particulate debris.

R. Poss, M.D.

Periprosthetic Bone Resorption

Aspenberg P, Herbertsson P (Lund Univ, Sweden)
J Bone Joint Surg [Br] 78B:641–646, 1996   2–32

Background.—Lack of initial stability and the presence of particulate debris appear to be important factors in the cause of prosthetic loosening. A model that can differentiate between particles and movement as a cause of bone resorption at an established bone-titanium interface was used to determine whether particles induce bone resorption in the absence of arthritis, whether a fibrous membrane develops at a bone-metal interface because of the presence of particles and/or movement, and whether these particles have a detrimental effect after the formation of a fibrous membrane.

Methods.—A bone-to-titanium interface was created in rats. Phagocytosable high-density polyethylene particles were applied between the bone and implant initially or after the interface matured. No fibrous membrane nor bone resorption occurred.

Findings.—Fibrous membrane developed when sliding movements were begun at the interface after 2 weeks. Additional application of particles did not change membrane thickness. Only minor qualitative changes were noted. Creating a membrane by movement followed by cessation of movement and application of particles caused the membrane to persist. In a particle-free control group, bone-to-metal contact was re-established.

Conclusions.—Mechanical stimuli are of major importance in prosthetic loosening. Particles may modulate the later stages of the loosening process.

Surgical Experience Related to Dislocations After Total Hip Arthroplasty

Hedlundh U, Ahnfelt L, Hybbinette C-H, et al (Univ Hosp, Malmö, Sweden; NÄL County Hosp, Trolhättan, Sweden; Kalmar County Hosp, Kalmar, Sweden)
J Bone Joint Surg Br 78B:206–209, 1996   2–33

Objective.—Whether increased surgical experience decreases the rate of hip dislocation has not been determined. The rate of dislocation after primary total hip arthroplasty (THA) over a period of 8 to 11 years was examined in relation to surgeon experience in 3 Swedish hospitals.

Methods.—Of the 4,230 primary THAs performed, there were 129 primary dislocations. Each surgeon had performed at least 50 THAs using a standardized posterior approach. Patients with and without dislocation were compared statistically.

Results.—The rate of dislocation was significantly higher for the first 15 THAs performed by a surgeon during the first year of experience. Experienced surgeons performed more THAs on patients with rheumatoid arthritis or other problem diagnoses. Regardless of the surgeon or the age of the patient, the rate of dislocation was significantly higher for patients with nonunion fractures of the hip (relative risk, 2.6) than for patients with osteoarthritis and significantly higher for patients with rheumatoid arthritis (relative risk, 2.6). Whereas patient age and surgeon experience were not correlated, there was an increased risk of dislocation with an increase in age of 10 years. The dislocation rate decreased after approximately 30 surgeries, significantly declining 1.5 times for every 10 THAs/year performed.

Conclusion.—The rate of dislocation after THA is related to the number of surgeries performed, leveling off at about 30 operations. The risk of dislocation decreases by a factor of 1.5 for every 10 THAs performed/year. Patients with nonunion fractures have a higher risk of dislocation.

▶ Prevention of total hip dislocation requires precise surgical technique, particularly concerning the position in which the components are implanted. To what degree does surgical experience influence the incidence of dislocation? The authors have found that the incidence of dislocation after THA was twice as high when inexperienced surgeons performed the operation. The frequent performance of a surgical procedure is likely to be associated with fewer technical complications.

R. Poss, M.D.

Bilateral Total Hip Arthroplasty: One Stage Versus Two Stage Procedure
Eggli S, Huckell CB, Ganz R (Univ of Bern, Switzerland; Johns Hopkins Hosp, Baltimore, Md)
Clin Orthop 328:108–118, 1996   2–34

Introduction.—Earlier reports suggest an increased incidence of pulmonary embolism, less improvement in motion capacity, and more heterotropic bone formation in patients who undergo simultaneous bilateral total hip arthroplasty (THA), compared with patients who undergo 2-stage procedures. A prospective, multicenter trial was conducted to evaluate differences in the early complication rate, short-term clinical outcome, and length of hospital stay between patients with 1-stage and 2-stage procedures.

Methods.—Clinical data from 255 patients (510 hips) from 19 clinics were collected between 1982 and 1992. Patients were assigned to 1 of 3 groups: group A (1-stage procedure)—simultaneous bilateral hip arthroplasty performed under 1 anesthesia; group B (2-stage procedure)—surgeries performed less than 6 weeks apart (126 hips); and group C—(2-stage procedure)—surgeries performed between 6 weeks and 6 months apart (256 hips). Patients in group B underwent the second surgery within the same hospital stay. The average follow-up was 1.5 years.

Results.—Patients with 1-stage procedures were significantly younger than 2-stage patients. There were no between-group differences in perioperative complications. The incidences of pulmonary embolism and deep vein thrombosis were similar for all 3 groups. One-stage procedure patients with a preoperative total hip range of motion of less than 50 degrees gained significantly more motion, compared with 2-stage patients. Group B patients with a preoperative total range of motion greater than 50 degrees had greater improvement than group A or group C patients. The degree of postoperative pain was similar in all 3 groups. One-stage procedure patients had a significantly better capacity for walking after surgery, compared with 2-stage patients. A 5- to 6-day shorter hospital stay and a single visit to the operating room resulted in a 30% reduction in overall hospital cost for 1-stage patients, compared with 2-stage patients.

Conclusion.—Patients with 1-stage bilateral THA were significantly more likely than 2-stage patients to be younger, have bilaterally stiff hips preoperatively, and have decreased hospital costs. One-stage patients had similar complication rates and pain reduction but better walking capacity than 2-stage patients.

▶ The authors commend bilateral simultaneous THA as being efficatious and cost effective. They particularly recommend its use in a patient group in which there is marked limited motion of the hips. The incidence of complications was no higher in the simultaneous group than it was in the control groups of staged procedures.

R. Poss, M.D.

New Issues

The Use of Erythropoietin in the Management of Jehovah's Witnesses Who Have Revision Total Hip Arthroplasty
Sparling EA, Nelson CL, Lavender R, et al (Univ of Arkansas for Medical Sciences, Little Rock)
J Bone Joint Surg Am 78A:1548–1552, 1996   2–35

Purpose.—Jehovah's Witnesses will not accept blood or blood products by transfusion. This can limit their therapeutic options in some cases, especially during orthopedic procedures associated with substantial blood loss. The glycoprotein hormone erythropoietin regulates erythrocyte production. Recombinant human erythropoietin has been used to treat both medically and operatively induced anemia. Its use in the management of Jehovah's Witnesses undergoing revision total hip arthroplasty was reported.

Methods.—The experience included 5 Jehovah's Witnesses undergoing revision total hip arthroplasty. There were 4 women and 1 man (average age, 66 years). All received preoperative recombinant human erythropoietin in an attempt to optimize their hematocrit for surgery. The erythropoietin dose started at 100 IU/kg given subcutaneously 3 times per week. The duration of preoperative treatment depended on the patient's hematocrit at presentation and ranged from 2 weeks for patients with an initial hematocrit of 0.40 to 0.449 to 4 weeks for those with an initial hematocrit of 0.30 to 0.36. Weekly hematocrit monitoring determined the dose up to the time of surgery. If the hematocrit rose above 0.45, erythropoietin treatment was stopped. The hematocrit and hemoglobin levels recorded from presentation to discharge were analyzed.

Results.—All 5 operations were successfully carried out without blood transfusion. There were no complications caused by excessive blood loss or low hematocrit. The average hematocrit rose from 0.395 at presentation to 0.476 at admission to the hospital. The patients received erythropoietin for an average of 26 days before surgery and 4 days afterward. The hematocrit averaged 0.368 immediately after surgery and 0.308 at discharge. There were no problems with deep venous thrombosis.

Conclusion.—Preoperative erythropoietin treatment can optimize the hematocrit in patients scheduled for surgery. This adjunct can safely achieve a relatively high hematocrit of 0.45 to 0.50, providing some margin of safety during a procedure involving substantial intraoperative blood loss. Flexibility of timing makes preoperative erythropoietin replacement especially well suited to joint replacement and revision surgery. Larger studies with longer follow-up are needed to determine the ultimate place of preoperative erythropoietin therapy.

▶ Erythropoietin has been shown to be effective in elevating the hematocrit level preoperatively. One obvious application of this technique is in patients such as Jehovah's Witnesses in whom alternative methods of blood banking are unacceptable.

R. Poss, M.D.

Effect of Preoperative Donation of Autologous Blood on Deep-vein Thrombosis Following Total Joint Arthroplasty of the Hip or Knee
Anders MJ, Lifeso RM, Landis M, et al (Univ of Buffalo, NY)
J Bone Joint Surg Am 78A:574–580, 1996   2–36

Background.—Without prophylaxis, deep vein thrombosis after elective total joint arthroplasty can occur in as many as 84% of patients. Many prophylactic strategies have been described in an attempt to reduce the prevalence of potentially fatal pulmonary embolism. Preoperative donation of autologous blood has been routine since the mid-1980s. The effect of preoperative autologous blood donation on postoperative deep vein thrombosis was investigated.

Methods and Findings.—Two hundred thirty-seven men at high risk for deep vein thrombosis undergoing elective total hip or knee arthroplasty for noninflammatory degenerative joint disease were included. In 54 patients, venography showed evidence of deep vein thrombosis of the lower extremity. Most of these patients had asymptomatic clots distal to the knee. Deep vein thrombosis occurred in 16% of 116 patients after total hip arthroplasty and in 29% of 121 patients after total knee arthroplasty. This complication developed in 17% of the 161 patients who had donated blood before surgery and in 34% of the 76 patients who had not. Logistic regression analysis indicated that autologous blood donation significantly reduced the development of postoperative deep vein thrombosis for patients undergoing total knee arthroplasty but not in those have total hip arthroplasty. In an additional neural network analysis, autologous blood donation was the most important prognostic factor in predicting the absence of postoperative deep vein thrombosis.

Conclusion.—Although autologous blood donation alone is not sufficient prophylaxis against deep vein thrombosis after total joint arthroplasty, it appears to protect against this complication after total knee arthroplasty in this high-risk population. Thus, this is an added benefit of preoperative donation of autologous blood, which also reduces the need for homologous blood transfusion.

▶ The authors report that in addition to the well-recognized advantages of autologous blood donation, such as avoiding the need for homologous transfusion, autologous blood donation may offer protection against postoperative deep vein thrombosis after total knee arthroplasty.

R. Poss, M.D.

Preoperative Irradiation for Prevention of Heterotopic Ossification Following Total Hip Arthroplasty

Pellegrini VD Jr, Gregoritch SJ (Univ of Rochester, NY)
J Bone Joint Surg Am 78A:870–881, 1996   2–37

Introduction.—Heterotopic ossification occurs frequently in patients who have undergone total hip arthroplasty (THA) and can cause functional impairment. If preoperative irradiation is as effective as postoperative irradiation in preventing heterotopic ossification, it could be used to avoid the transport discomfort associated with postoperative irradiation. The efficacy of a single 800-cGy dose of limited field radiation administered preoperatively was compared with the same dose given postoperatively in 85 patients (86 hips) considered at high risk for heterotopic ossification after THA.

Methods.—Patients were randomized to receive a single 800-cGy dose of limited field radiation administered either preoperatively (group I) or postoperatively (group II). The most common risk factor for heterotopic ossification in both groups was radiographic evidence of hypertophic osteoarthritis or diffuse idiopathic skeletal hyperostosis. Minimum follow-up was 6 months.

Results.—Group I and II patients were irradiated within 6.1 hours preoperatively or within 51.3 hours postoperatively. Thirty-seven of 49 group I hips (76%) treated with preoperative irradiation exhibited no new heterotopic ossification; 11 progressed to grade I or grade II ossification, and there was 1 progression from grade II to grade III in a patient with Paget disease. Twenty-seven of 37 group II hips treated with postoperative irradiation showed no new heterotopic ossification; 9 progressed from grade 0 to grade I ossification; and 1 progressed from grade III to grade IV. The last was a patient with Parkinson's disease. Extra-field ossification was observed in 12 hips (24%) irradiated preoperatively and 3 hips (8%) irradiated postoperatively. There was no association between extra-field ossification and symptoms of bursitis of the greater trochanter. Three hips treated with preoperative irradiation and none treated with postoperative irradiation required revision of the trochanter for nonunion.

Conclusion.—Preoperative irradiation was as effective as postoperative irradiation in preventing heterotopic ossification. Preoperative irradiation may be used to avoid the discomfort and morbidity associated with conventional postoperative treatment.

▶ The effectiveness of irradiation to protect against heterotopic ossification has been well demonstrated. Current protocols use a single dose of approximately 700 cGy delivered within the first 72 hours after surgery. In this study, the authors found that preoperative irradiation with a single 800-cGy dose confers similar protection. Patients who are candidates for irradiation may find that its administration preoperatively is associated with less discomfort and morbidity.

R. Poss, M.D.

Intercalary Replacement of Canine Femora Using a New Bioactive Bone Cement

Senaha Y, Nakamura T, Tamura J, et al (Kyoto Univ, Japan)
J Bone Joint Surg Br 78B:26–31, 1996   2–38

Introduction.—The problems associated with polymethylmethacrylate (PMMA) have prompted an ongoing search for more efficient bonding materials. A bioactive bone (BA) cement consisting of bioactive glass powder and bis–glycidyl methacrylate resin was developed. It has a low curing temperature and bonds directly to bone with high strength. A comparison of BA and PMMA cement for strength of fixation of metallic prostheses to bone was reported.

Methods.—Eighteen femora of 9 mongrel dogs underwent operation for intercalary replacement of part of the bone by a metal prosthesis. All dogs underwent operation of both legs, 1 bonded with PMMA and the other with BA cement. Three dogs were sacrificed at 4, 12, and 26 weeks after surgery. Fixation strength was evaluated by means of a push-out test. Histologic examination was performed using Giemsa surface staining and scanning electron microscopy.

Results.—Both cements allowed weight-bearing and running without limping during outside exercise. Histologic examination showed fibrous tissue intervening between bone and PMMA cement. The BA cement had bonded directly to bone at 12- and 26-week evaluation. The mean PMMA cement fixation strengths at 4, 12, and 26 weeks were 46.8, 50.0, and 58.2

kgf, respectively, compared with means of 56.8, 67.2, and 72.8 kgf, respectively, for BA cement. Fixation strengths were significantly stronger at 26 weeks, compared with 4 weeks. The fixation strength was greater for BA cement than for PMMA cement at 12 weeks after surgery.

Conclusion.—Findings indicate that BA cement may be useful in providing long-lasting fixation of implants to bone under weight-bearing conditions and may reduce the incidence of aseptic loosening.

▶ By mixing bioactive glass powder into bone cement, pores in the cement are created that, through either osteoinduction or osteoconduction, permit direct bonding of the cement to bone. The authors demonstrate this finding and, importantly, show that there is no loss of mechanical strength of the cement with this admixture. Fibrous tissue present at 4 weeks at the cement-bone interface was still present in longer-term studies in the PMMA animals but was replaced by direct bonding to bone in the bioactive cement cohort. This exciting new use of cement, if confirmed, provides the optimal type of fixation with initial immediate mechanical fixation supplemented subsequently by biological fixation.

R. Poss, M.D.

Rabbit Articular Cartilage Defects Treated With Autologous Cultured Chondrocytes

Brittberg M, Nilsson A, Lindahl A, et al (Univ of Göteborg, Sweden)
Clin Orthop 326:270–283, 1996   2–39

Introduction.—Cartilage defects have been treated by widely differing techniques with widely differing results. Results of cartilage defects treated with chondrocyte transplantation in New Zealand White rabbits were reported.

Methods.—After patellar dislocation, a 3-mm full–cartilage-thickness patellar chondral lesion was created that extended down to the calcified zone. Samples from the defect and a non–weight-bearing area were collected for cell isolation. These trypsin-treated chondrocytes were allowed to grow in culture for 2 weeks. At 2 weeks, the operative site was reoperated and a free periosteal flap from the medial proximal tibia was sutured to the defect. The patella defects were harvested and transplanted into 1 knee of 10 rabbit recipients. Mechanically harvested chondrocytes were transplanted in the other side. Some defects were covered with periosteum but no cells, and other defects were left untreated without cells or periosteum (control group). In other knees, carbon fiber pads seeded with chondrocytes were used as scaffolds. Scaffolds without seeds were placed in some knees. The rabbits were euthanized and healing was assessed at 8, 12, and 52 weeks.

Results.—The amount of newly formed repair tissue was significantly increased in knees with chondrocyte transplantation, compared with control knees. There was a significant increase in repair at 12 and 52 weeks in chondrocyte-seeded knees vs. knees with scaffolds with no chondrocytes. All knees treated with chondrocytes had significantly better histologic quality scores for repair tissue than knees treated with periosteum alone. There was a tendency for the repair tissue to make an incomplete bond to adjacent cartilage.

Conclusion.—Findings indicate that isolated autologous articular chondrocytes that have been expanded for 2 weeks in vitro can stimulate the healing phase of chondral lesions. A gradual maturation of the hyaline-like repair with a more pronounced columnarization was observed as late as 1 year after surgery.

▶ In this experimental study in rabbits performed by the originators of the carticel technique, chondrocyte transplantation into patellar defects produced significantly better healing when the chondrocytes were implanted as part of a carbon fiber scaffold. These findings suggest that a truly effective and long-lasting repair of articular cartilage defects will occur not when hyaline cartilage is produced, but when an organized tissue, articular cartilage, is produced. Remodeling of the initial hyaline cartilage transplantation into a tissue that can successfully transmit load and can bond to the articular cartilage boundaries of the defect and to the bony subchondral bed, remains a goal, not a reality.

R. Poss, M.D.

Repair of Partial-Thickness Defects in Articular Cartilage: Cell Recruitment From the Synovial Membrane
Hunziker EB, Rosenberg LC (Univ of Bern, Switzerland)
J Bone Joint Surg Am 78A:721–733, 1996   2–40

Introduction.—It is not known why partial-thickness defects in articular cartilage do not heal spontaneously. It has been suggested that these defects do not heal because they are walled off from marrow and have no access to macrophages, endothelial cells, and mesenchymal cells. Factors that prevent healing in partial-thickness defects were evaluated.

Methods.—Defects were created in the articular cartilage of New Zealand White rabbits and Yucatan minipigs. Rabbits were placed in 1 of 5 treatment groups: I—control (defect untreated), II—treatment with chondroitinase ABC, III—application of growth factors after chondroitinase ABC, IV—defects filled with fibrin after chondroitinase ABC treatment, and V—treatment with mitogenic growth factor after chondroitinase ABC treatment. Minipigs were treated according to protocols for groups I, IV, and V.

Results.—Light microscopic examination showed sporadic patches of mesenchymal cells along the surface of the defect in control animals. Treatment with chondroitinase ABC caused an increased coverage of the defect surface with mesenchymal cells. The combination of chondroitinase ABC and the local application of a mitogenic growth factor caused more extensive coverage, but mesenchymal cells did not extend into and fill the defect completely. Treatment with chondroitinase ABC and fibrin clot caused a migration of cells within the fibrin matrix, but at a low population density, and proliferation of cells throughout the defect. The deposited fibrin matrix was remodeled by the mesenchymal cells, then replaced by a loose fibrous connective tissue. Addition of a mitogenic growth factor to chondroitinase ABC caused mesenchymal cells to fill the entire cavity of the defect. Cell density was greatly increased when transforming growth factor-$\beta 1$ was used. Cartilage did not form in any experiments in which a growth factor was added to the growth matrix. At 48-week evaluation, the bulk of the repair tissue was a fibrous connective tissue without differentiation into hyaline cartilage.

Conclusion.—The treatment protocol used did not result in the production of cartilage, but findings indicate that the failure of partial-thickness defects to heal is not completely caused by a lack of access to mesenchymal cells.

▶ The authors have shown that in partial-thickness defects in articular cartilage in rabbits, mesenchymal cells can be recruited from the local area to populate these defects. It may be possible, therefore, to induce these mesenchymal cells to modulate into chondrocytes by further adjustment of the local environment.

R. Poss, M.D.

Effects of Fluid-Induced Shear on Articular Chondrocyte Morphology and Metabolism *In Vitro*
Smith RL, Donlon BS, Gupta MK, et al (Veterans Affairs Med Ctr, Palo Alto, Calif; Stanford Univ, Calif; Merck, Sharp and Dohme Research Labs, Rahway, NJ)
J Orthop Res 13:824–831, 1995   2–41

Introduction.—High contact pressures in joints cause fluid to be exuded and imbibed cyclically, with most fluid exchanges occurring at the superficial layers where flattened chondrocytes are most common. A potential for physical damage to the matrix exists below the superficial layers where there is less fluid exchange. The effects of fluid-induced shear on human and bovin articular chondrocytes were evaluated in vitro using a cone viscometer.

Methods.—Samples of normal human adult knee articular cartilage were obtained at autopsy within 24 hours after death. The human and bovine cartilages were dissected and exposed to continuous laminar fluid-induced shear using a cone viscometer for periods of 24, 48, and 72 hours. A phase distribution analysis was used to ascertain the extent to which the cells realigned in response to fluid-induced shear.

Results.—Fluid-induced shear caused individual chondrocytes to elongate and align tangential to the direction of cone rotation at 48 and 72 hours but not 24 hours. There was a twofold increase in glycosaminoglycan synthesis in response to fluid-induced shear. The length of newly synthesized proteoglycans was increased by fluid-induced shear. The hydrodynamic size of newly synthesized proteoglycans was increased in human, but not in bovine, cultures. Prostaglandin E_2 release was increased 10- to 20-fold after 48 hours. Compared with controls, the messenger RNA (mRNA) signal levels for tissue inhibitor of metalloproteinase increased ninefold in human chondrocytes. Major changes were not detected in mRNA signal levels for the neutral metalloproteinases, collagenase, stromelysin, or 72-KD gelatinase.

Conclusion.—Fluid-induced shear changed the alignment of the cells with respect to one another, resulting in an axial polarization tangential to the direction of rotation of the cone viscometer. Articular chondrocyte metabolism responded directly to physical stimulation in vitro. It may be that mechanical loading directly influences cartilage homeostasis in vivo.

▶ Articular cartilage is a tissue that must respond to physical stresses. In this study, the authors demonstate that the metabolism of articular chondrocytes responds directly to physical stimulation and that its loading environment influences its physiologic responses.

R. Poss, M.D.

Correlation of Patient Questionnaire Responses and Physician History in Grading Clinical Outcome Following Hip and Knee Arthroplasty: A Prospective Study of 201 Joint Arthroplasties

McGrory BJ, Morrey BF, Rand JA, et al (Mayo Clinic and Found, Rochester, Minn)

J Arthroplasty 11:47–57, 1996   2–42

Introduction.—Questionnaires are commonly used to help determine outcome in orthopedic trials. Their validity has not been evaluated systematically. The emphasis on minimizing health care costs and comparison of interinstitution results has underscored the need for quantification of clinical outcomes. Patient questionnaire responses were correlated with physician interviews to determine clinical outcome after total hip arthroplasty (THA) and total knee arthroplasty (TKA).

Methods,—Ninety-two and 83 patients, respectively, who underwent THA and TKA (a total of 201 surgeries) were asked to return a standardized questionnaire by mail before their first scheduled routine appointment for evaluation of their arthroplasty. Responses recorded by physicians during the clinical visit were reviewed and patients were assigned to 1 of 4 treatment outcome categories: excellent, good, fair, and poor.

Results.—A comparison of patient and physician responses indicated that 71.6% of responses were the same and 97.3% were within 1 grade for all patients. Physician and patient responses were similar for clinical hip scores, but physicians gave significantly higher knee scores than patients for both short- and long-term follow-up. Physicians were 8.5% more likely than patients to give a higher clinical score when good-excellent and fair-poor categories were considered.

Conclusion.—Findings suggest that clinical scores may be reliably estimated by means of a single questionnaire in patients who have undergone THA and TKA. However, accurate differentiation between excellent, good, fair, and poor outcomes was not possible, even in the presence of highly correlated physician and patient scores.

▶ Questionnaires will undoubtedly become a necessary instrument by which outcomes are assessed. In this study, there was a high degree of agreement between scores calculated from patient responses on the questionnaire and those elicited from patients during a visit to the physician when evaluating the results of hip and knee arthroplasty. The authors caution, however, that questionnaires alone provide poor differentiation between excellent, good, fair, and poor outcomes.

R. Poss, M.D.

Differences Between Patients' and Physicians' Evaluations of Outcome After Total Hip Arthroplasty
Lieberman JR, Dorey F, Shekelle P, et al (Univ of California, Los Angeles; West Los Angeles VA Ctr)
J Bone Joint Surg Am 78A:835–838, 1996   2–43

Introduction.—The success of total hip arthroplasty is typically determined by the physician's assessment of pain and the functional ability of the patient. The assumption is that patients concur with their physician's assessment. Physician and patient assessments of results of total hip arthroplasty were compared in a series of 147 consecutive patients.

Methods.—Patients and physicians independently evaluated pain and over-all satisfaction with the outcome of hip arthroplasty using a visual analogue scale with a scoring system of 0 to 10 cm. Questionnaires were also completed by both groups.

Results.—Patients' perceptions were as follows: 118 (80%) thought their health was good, very good, or excellent; 128 (87%) reported their 2 most important expectations had been met; 105 (71%) thought surgery substantially improved their quality of life; and 110 (75%) thought they were somewhat or substantially more independent than before surgery. The mean analogue ratings for overall satisfaction were 8.6 cm and 8.8 cm for patients and physicians, respectively. The mean analogue ratings for pain were assessed as 1.7 and 1.0 cm, respectively, by patients and physicians. As patients' analogue ratings for pain increased and/or satisfaction decreased, the contrast between patient and physician scores widened. Thirty patients assessed their pain experience as more than 4.0 cm. Their mean pain score was 6.8 cm, compared with a mean of 3.6 cm assessed by their physicians. Nineteen patients rating their satisfaction as less than 7.0

cm had a mean rating of 3.8 cm, compared with a mean physician rating of 6.5 cm. Physicians gave better ratings than patients regarding general health, walking ability, pain in the thigh, and improvements in quality of life.

Conclusion.—Patient and physician scores were similar when patients had little or no pain and were satisfied with operative results. The disparity between rating scores widened as patients' pain ratings increased and satisfaction decreased.

Clinical Significance.—Traditionally, assessments of the outcome of total hip arthroplasty are based on physicians' assessment of pain and functional status. Findings indicate that patients and physicians may evaluate success differently, particularly when patients are not completely satisfied with the result. Patient rating may be an important component of determining the success of total hip arthroplasty.

▶ Patients' and physicians' evaluations of the results of total hip arthroplasty differ, and the discrepancy increases when the patient is dissatisfied with the result. The authors—correctly, in my view—advocate a continuation of traditional physician-generated assessment instruments in addition to patient-derived information to better assess the results and outcomes of these procedures.

R. Poss, M.D.

3 Orthopedic Oncology

Introduction

The major advances seen during the 1980s in adjuvant treatment for patients with musculoskeletal tumors have proved to be of significant benefit. More patients are surviving and more limbs are saved. No new dramatic adjuvant treatments have been found recently, but we are learning more about the long-term results of patients treated with limb salvage techniques and the side effects of some of our treatments.

As more patients with Ewing's sarcoma survive, we are discovering that their risk of complications from local treatment is significant. Although no prospective studies have been done, nor is it likely that they will be done, surgical treatment seems to be better than irradiation for the primary tumor.

Better understanding of how to do surgical resections and how to reconstruct the extremity after a limb salvage operation are being developed as more patients are monitored for longer periods of time. Our experience with significant numbers of patients is getting large enough that we can collect data rather than just speculate as we have done in the past. We will now begin to see how well we can reconstruct our failures from prior reconstructions. In all likelihood, future decisions about how best to do the original reconstruction will be influenced by how well we can do the second reconstruction.

We should begin to reconsider amputation as a means of treating some patients who are having limb salvage procedures. We have abandoned amputation as a primary treatment for all but the largest tumors, but the amputee has the least complicated treatment and is usually the most active of all patients surviving a malignant tumor of a major long bone.

Dempsey S. Springfield, M.D.

Surgery

Limb Salvage for Neoplasms of the Shoulder Girdle: Intermediate Reconstructive and Functional Results

O'Connor MI, Sim FH, Chao EYS (Mayo Clinic Jacksonville, Fla; Mayo Clinic and Mayo Found, Rochester, Minn)
J Bone Joint Surg (Am) 78A:1872–1888, 1996

3–1

Objective.—Although limb-sparing curative resections for malignant or destructive benign tumors of the shoulder girdle are possible, reconstruction is a problem because of inadequate compensation by prosthetic devices. The functional results of various reconstruction techniques are reviewed.

Methods.—Between January 1980 and May 1990, 57 patients (25 females) aged 5–71 years, were operated on for primary sarcoma of bone ($n = 53$) or extensive benign giant cell tumor of the shoulder girdle ($n = 4$). Resections were classified by the system of the Musculoskeletal Tumor Society. Patients were followed up for an average of 4.6 years. There were 17 tumors of the scapula and 40 of the proximal humerus; 4 were chondrosarcomas, 20 were osteosarcomas, 6 were Ewing sarcomas, 1 was a fibrosarcoma, and 4 were giant-cell tumors. Reconstructive procedures used were resection of the scapular blade with the abductor mechanism intact (SIA); resection of the glenoid cavity with the abductor mechanism disrupted (S2B); resection of the entire scapula with the abductor mechanism disrupted (S12B); resection of the entire scapula and the proximal humeral epiphysis and metaphysis with the abductor mechanism disrupted (s1234B); resection of the glenoid cavity and proximal humeral epiphysis and metaphysis with the abductor mechanism disrupted (S123B); resection of the glenoid cavity and the proximal humeral epiphysis, metaphysis, and diaphysis with the abductor mechanism disrupted (S2345B); resection of the proximal humeral epiphysis and metaphysis with the abductor mechanism intact (S34A) or disrupted (S34B); and resection of the proximal humeral epiphysis, metaphysis, and diaphysis with the abductor mechanism intact (S345A) or disrupted (S345B).

Results.—Forty patients had a wide resection, and 13 had a marginal resection. Four patients, including 1 with a giant-cell tumor, had a local recurrence. Ten patients died an average of 1.8 years after surgery, 8 of their disease. The 43 survivors were followed up for an average of 5.3 years. S1234B resection with a functional spacer gave a poor functional result. S234B and S2345B resections gave good functional results with the osseous arthrodesis method of reconstruction but not with the functional spacer or prosthetic arthrodesis methods of reconstruction. The preferred method, using an osteoarticular allograft, resulted in osseous union in 8 patients but later failed in 3 patients when the articular and subchondral regions of the allograft fractured. All results were satisfactory with respect to pain, emotional acceptance, and functionality.

Conclusion.—Postoperative satisfaction with shoulder reconstruction after tumor removal is dependent on selecting the procedure that is appropriate for the patient and counseling the patient about what to expect after surgery.

▶ Limb salvage surgery for sarcomas around the shoulder girdle have been done longer and more often than for any other site. The importance of the hand and the relatively limited importance of reconstructing the shoulder are the 2 most important reasons for the frequency of limb salvage surgery for shoulder girdle tumors. Fortunately, the neurovascular bundle is usually not involved in the tumors that arise in the shoulder girdle, so it is oncologically safe in most cases to do a limb-sparing resection. O'Connor and associates have reviewed their experience with limb salvage resections in the shoulder girdle.

Their results suggest that, for most patients, a limb salvage resection is safe. They had 5 patients (9%) with a local recurrence. This is a little higher than ideal but is acceptable. They used a variety of reconstructions, and the reconstructions were selected by the surgeon and the patient without a protocol, so it is impossible to compare reconstructions; however, some understanding of the expected outcome can be gained. There are 3 large functional groups: essentially normal function; able to abduct and flex the humerus away from the body; and a flail shoulder. The most important variable is the amount of functioning muscle left after the resection. The second most important variable is the reconstruction used.

When the rotator cuff and deltoid can be spared, the patient's shoulder can be reconstructed with a prosthesis or osteoarticular allograft; almost normal motion and strength can then be expected in the shoulder. When the deltoid is resected but a normal rotator cuff is spared, an articulating reconstruction can be done; most patients will have almost normal function, but when the deltoid and rotator cuff is removed, an articulating reconstruction will function as a flail shoulder. An arthrodesis is probably the best reconstruction for the patient who wants or needs a strong upper extremity and who must use the hand in space. The range of motion is better than it seems it can be, and most patients find the function to be excellent. The position of the extremity is important and can be difficult to determine at the time of the operation. A prebent plate is useful. The patient should be able to rest the upper arm on the side of the body and should be warned of the loss of rotation. A flail shoulder is often the best choice when the patient does not need to use the hand in space and particularly when the patient is frail. The flail shoulder reconstruction is the least difficult, and there is little need for extensive immobilization or physical therapy after surgery. The less active patient will find the flail shoulder functional, and as long as the remaining humerus is suspended from the remaining scapula, clavicle, or rib, it is a comfortable extremity.

These resections and reconstructions are difficult and not for most surgeons. The patient should be prepared for a long operation and lengthy rehabilitation, especially if a reconstruction with an articulating shoulder or arthrodesis is done.

D.S. Springfield, M.D.

Surgical Resection of Primary Soft-Tissue Sarcoma: Incidence of Residual Tumour in 95 Patients Needing Re-excision after Local Resection
Goodlad JR, Fletcher CDM, Smith MA (St Thomas' Hosp, London)
J Bone Joint Surg Br 78B:658–661, 1996   3–2

Background.—Soft-tissue sarcomas are rare. Treatment involves surgical removal of the primary tumor with a wide margin of normal tissue. Effective treatment relies on accurate preoperative diagnosis and assessment of tumor extent, which are best achieved by a multidisciplinary team of specialists. One experience with the treatment of these rare tumors was reported.

Patients and Findings.—Two hundred thirty-six consecutive patients have been seen at a soft-tissue sarcoma clinic since its inception in 1987. Ninety-five patients had a primary soft-tissue sarcoma excised elsewhere but with inadequate margins. These patients required a secondary, wider re-excision. Tissue removed at re-excision was assessed histologically. Definite tumor tissue was detected in 29 of 66 lower limb specimens, in 16 of 25 upper limb specimens, in 7 of 10 trunk specimens, and in 4 of 5 head and neck specimens. Some residual tumor was evident macroscopically in 31 cases. In 59% of the 95 patients, primary tumor had been excised incompletely.

Conclusion.—Surgical assessment of the adequacy of excision in patients with soft-tissue sarcomas appears to be very inaccurate. Most local recurrences are the result of inadequate primary surgery. A coordinated multidisciplinary approach to the management of patients with soft-tissue sarcoma is essential.

▶ One of the more frustrating situations for a surgical oncologist is the patient who has had a soft-tissue sarcoma removed but with inadequate margins. If the surgeon and pathologist agree that there is tumor left in the patient, it is not difficult for the patient to understand the need for another operation, but if, as is most often the case, the initial surgeon believes all the tumor has been removed, it is often difficult for the patient to understand the need for re-excision. In addition, after a soft-tissue sarcoma has been removed, it is almost impossible to determine the original extent of the tumor. The most common situation in which soft-tissue sarcomas are removed with inadequate margins is when the lesion is thought to be benign and is removed with little or no determination of its exact extent.

In the experience of Goodlad and associates, 40% of the patients they saw with soft-tissue sarcomas (95 of 236) were referred after an inadequate resection. As others have advised, Goodlad and associates re-excised the tumor bed and, as others have shown, residual tumor was more often than not found (59%). Almost surely, some of the resected specimens in which tumor was not found contained tumor but in such small amounts that the pathologist was unable to see it.

In my experience, the incidence of local recurrence is high in patients who have had inadequate surgical resection (usually excisions of a soft-tissue lesion thought by the surgeon to be benign), even if they receive postoperative irradiation. Re-excision is the standard recommendation for all patients who have had an inadequate resection of a soft-tissue sarcoma. Most of us will also use adjuvant irradiation, either before or after re-excision, for high-grade lesions but perhaps not for low-grade soft tissue sarcomas.

D.S. Springfield, M.D.

The Surgical Treatment and Outcome of Pathological Fractures in Localised Osteosarcoma

Abudu A, Sferopoulos NK, Tillman RM, et al (Royal Orthopaedic Hosp, Birmingham, England)
J Bone Joint Surg Br 78B:694–698, 1996   3–3

Background.—Osteosarcoma is the most common primary malignant bone tumor in children and young adults. The incidence of pathologic fractures in patients with high-grade disease ranges from 5% to 10%. Such fractures occur spontaneously or after minimal trauma because of high cellularity, poor differentiation, and loss of matrix. The influence of fractures on the survival and preservation of the limb was studied in 1 group of patients.

Methods.—Forty patients with pathologic fractures from localized osteosarcoma of the long bones were treated at 1 center between 1975 and 1994. Age at diagnosis ranged from 2 to 46 years. The median follow-up was 55 months.

Findings.—Limbs were salvaged in 27 patients. In 13, amputation was needed. Resection margins were radical in 5 patients, wide in 26, marginal in 6, wide but contaminated in 2, and intralesional in 1. Nineteen percent of patients undergoing limb salvage and none having amputation had local recurrence. Overall, the cumulative 5-year survival rate was 57%. The survival rate was 64% among those treated by limb salvage and 47% among those needing amputation.

Conclusion.—In many patients with pathologic fractures from primary osteosarcoma, limb-sparing surgery with adequte margins can be performed without compromising survival. However, the risk of local recurrence with such treatment is significant.

▶ Limb salvage surgery as the treatment of primary osteosarcoma of bone has become the standard of care. I believe there has been an increase in the frequency of pathologic fractures among patients with osteosarcoma, mainly because of the tumor being left in the patient while adjuvant chemotherapy is being given. Once the decision has been made to save a limb, it is difficult to change that decision, and even after a pathologic fracture has occurred, there is usually considerable desire to save the limb. Therefore, whether it is safe to do limb salvage resection for osteosarcoma after a pathologic fracture is important.

All pathologic fractures are not the same. The authors do not classify the pathologic fractures. How many were displaced? How many patients had swelling or other evidence of a hematoma in the extremity away from the bone? The authors say that only those patients who had involvement of a joint were offered an amputation. We do not know how many met this criterion. Other amputations were done based on intraoperative findings. Of the 40 patients, 13 had a primary amputation. These 13 were selected from the 40 and were probably not similar to the 27 who had limb salvage.

Despite the dissimilarity between the groups, we can learn something from these data. Local recurrence was higher in those patients who had a limb salvage. Survival, on the other hand, was not significantly different between the groups. This finding is similar to that of a study done by the Musculoskeletal Tumor Society and reported by Simon et al. in 1986.[1] In that article, local recurrence was found to be more frequent in patients who had had limb salvage or above knee amputation compared with a hip distarticulation for an osteosarcoma in the distal femur, but there was not a significantly higher incidence of metastatic disease.

As one would expect, the incidence of local recurrence was related to the surgical margin. When the tumor was violated during the operation, local recurrence was frequent. When a wide margin was obtained, local recurrence was not frequent. Another interesting finding was that no patient with an amputation had a local recurrence, but this did not reduce their risk of the development of metastatic disease.

It seems safe to say that limb salvage for an osteosarcoma can be safely done after a pathologic fracture, but it remains important to obtain a wide margin and not to contaminate the operative field during the resection by cutting into the tumor. It is likely that patients with displaced fractures that occur before the patient has received chemotherapy are more likely to have distant spread of disease and an increased risk of local recurrence, compared with a patient who sustains a minimally displaced fracture while receiving chemotherapy.

D.S. Springfield, M.D.

Reference

1. Simon MA, Aschiliman MA, Thomas N, et al: Limb-salvage treatment versus amputation for osteosarcoma of the distal end of the femur. *J Bone Joint Surg Am* 68:1331–1337, 1986.

Aseptic Loosening in Cemented Custom-made Prosthetic Replacements for Bone Tumours of the Lower Limb

Unwin PS, Cannon SR, Grimer RJ, et al (Royal Natl Orthopaedic Hosp Trust, Stanmore, England; Royal Orthopaedic Hosp, Birmingham, England)
J Bone Joint Surg Br 78B:5–13, 1996   3–4

Background.—Recent studies have shown that aseptic loosening is surpassing infection as the principal mode of prosthetic failure. The risk from aseptic loosening in 3 types of lower limb replacement used most commonly for tumor resection, in relation to patient age at limb salvage and percentage of bone replaced, was studied.

Methods.—A total of 1,001 custom-made prostheses implanted after surgery for bone tumors were analyzed retrospectively. Four hundred ninety-three were distal femoral prostheses, 263 were proximal femoral, and 245 were proximal tibial. The main mode of implant failure was aseptic loosening. Seventy-one patients underwent revision for aseptic loosening of a cemented intramedullary stem.

Findings.—The probability of a patient surviving aseptic loosening for 120 months was 93.8% among those with proximal femoral replacements, 67.4% among those with distal femoral prostheses, and 58% among those with a proximal tibial implant. Patient age at surgery and the percentage of bone resected were associated with the risk of aseptic loosening in patients with distal femoral replacements. The prognosis for prosthetic survival without aseptic loosening was poorest for young patients with distal femoral prostheses in whom a high percentage of the femur had been replaced. Percentage of bone removed significantly affected the proximal tibial replacement group, but patient age did not. Neither age nor percentage of bone removed affected proximal femoral replacement (Fig 3).

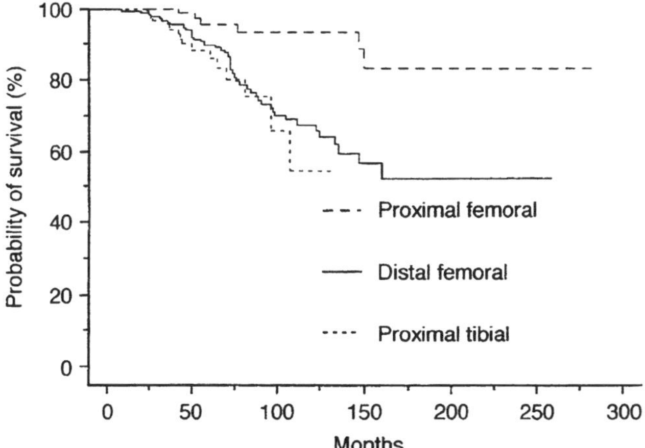

FIGURE 3.—The probability of surviving aseptic loosening with respect to the site of the implant. (Courtesy of Unwin PS, Cannon SR, Grimer RJ, et al: Aseptic loosening in cemented custom-made prosthestic replacements for bone tumors of the lower limb. *J Bone Joint Surg Br* 78B:5–13, 1996.)

Conclusion.—In this series, the main cause of failure of cemented massive prostheses in the leg after bone tumor resection was aseptic loosening, a complication that may not be detected in studies of short-term outcomes. Anatomical location, percentage of bone resected, and patient age significantly affected the incidence of aseptic loosening.

▶ Limb salvage surgery is now accepted as the usual treatment of malignant and some locally aggressive benign bone tumors. Amputation is rarely needed as a means of controlling the local tumor. This trend started in the mid-1970s but did not reach complete acceptance until almost a decade later. As the number of survivors increases they live longer, more is learned about the quality of the reconstructions done after the limb salvage operation.

The 2 institutions that have combined their follow-up results and the surgeon and engineers who have authored this paper have been leaders in the field of limb salvage and endoprosthetic replacements. This retrospective examination of 1,001 patients with lower extremity, cemented, custom-made prosthesis provides us with valuable information about what to expect from an endoprosthetic replacement and what to tell a patient who is deciding what reconstruction to elect, as well as its use as a means of comparison with other methods of reconstruction (i.e., autogenous, allograft, and allograft-endoprosthetic). It also suggests that amputation is not as bad in comparison as one might expect.

The data presented represents the best we can expect. Although the average follow-up was 45.7 months, 186 of the 1,001 patients were followed for less than 3 months. In addition, with an average age of 29.9 years, the patients who survive want a reconstruction that will last 40 years more than 10 times the average follow-up of these patients. As can be seen in Figure 3, there tends to be continued failure of protheses with time, especially those replacements of the distal femur or proximal tibia. Less than half of the patients (38.5%) have had no problems with their reconstruction. It is likely that many, if not most, of these (the authors do not tell us how many) are patients in their early postoperative period.

These data are as good as have been reported, and the authors probably have been honest. Limb salvage surgery can be done and local disease controlled (5.4% of local recurrence reported by these authors is acceptable and close to what would be achieved with amputation) but the reconstructions need to be improved. Some patients will be better off with an amputation and a conventional prosthesis.

D.S. Springfield, M.D.

Tumor Survival Assessment

Thallium-201 Scintigraphy to Assess Effect of Chemotherapy in Osteosarcoma

Ohtomo K, Terui S, Yokoyama R, et al (Natl Cancer Ctr Hosp, Tokyo; Japanese Orthopaedic Assoc, Tokyo)
J Nucl Med 37:1444–1448, 1996   3–5

Objective.—Intensive chemotherapy has improved the survival rate of patients with high-grade osteosarcoma of the extremities. There is evidence that the degree of necrosis after preoperative chemotherapy is predictive of outcome. Correlations among [201]T1-chloride scintigraphic appearance before and after preoperative chemotherapy, histologic degree of tumor necrosis, and prognosis are discussed.

Methods.—[201]T1 scintigraphy was performed before and after preoperative chemotherapy in 30 patients with high-grade osteosarcoma of the extremities. Tumor-to-background count ratio (TBR) was classified as group 1 for a ratio less than 0%, grade 2 for a ratio of 0% to 99%, and grade 3 for a ratio greater than 100%. Twenty patients had limb-sparing surgeries, and 10 had wide or radical amputations. The area of tumor necrosis found at pathologic examination was categorized as grade 1, necrosis less than 60%; grade 2, necrosis 60% to 89%; and grade 3, necrosis greater than 90%. Survival data were analyzed using the Kaplan–Meier test, and groups were compared using the Kruskal–Wallis test.

Results.—Before chemotherapy, tumor uptake was much higher than background. After chemotherapy, tumor uptake had increased significantly in 10 patients, was peripheral in 5, showed invasion into the epiphysis in 3, and was unchanged in 3. Tumor (volume and uptake had decreased in 17 patients. Ten patients in group 1 and 1 in group 2 had a grade 1 response. Nine group 2 patients had a grade 2 response. Two group 2 patients and 8 group 3 patients had a grade 3 response. The differences between grades were significant. Fourteen patients are disease free, and 1 died from an unrelated cause. Fifteen patients have had metastases, and 5 are alive and disease free after treatment. The 5-year disease-free survival rate was 48.9%. The grade 1 response was 27.3%, the grade 2 response was 51.9%, and the grade 3 response was 75.0%. The differences in responses and disease-free survival rates between groups were significant.

Conclusion.—T1-scintigraphy provides an accurate assessment of the effect of chemotherapy in patients with high-grade osteosarcoma.

▶ Since it was recognized that the percent of necrosis of an osteosarcoma after preoperative chemotherapy was predictive of the patient's outcome, there has been a search for methods of predicting the percent of necrosis before an operative resection. Numerous reports have shown that there needs to be more than 90% necrosis for there to be a statistically significant improvement in survival rates, and predicting with sufficient accuracy has been difficult. Recently, it has been suggested that the patient who has more than 90% necrosis can have a limited resection with no increased risk of local recurrence. This has heightened interest in being able to predict the percent of necrosis before an operation so that the operation may be adjusted based on the degree of necrosis. Thallium scanning has been suggested as a means of determining the percent of necrosis of an osteosarcoma after preoperative chemotherapy, but limited studies have been done. Ohtomo and associates have added to the body of data, and their study supports the use of thallium-201 as a means of predicting necrosis.

Even though it is likely that the patient with 85% necrosis has a better chance of surviving than the patient with 50% necrosis, this has not been shown. Only if the percent of necrosis is greater than 90% do the data support a better survival rate. Therefore, to be useful, the preoperative examination needs to discriminate between the patient with more than 90% necrosis and those with less. Ohtomo and associates graded the thallium scans based on the visual appearance and by an alteration ratio. The visual inspection of the scan was not useful except for the fact that it did predict a poor response for those patients whose thallium scans had increased activity after preoperative chemotherapy. There were 17 of 30 patients whose scans improved, but 7, or almost half, had less than 90% necrosis. The alteration ratio was more predictive. Only 1 patient whose alteration ratio was more than 90% had less than 90% necrosis, and that patient has not had a metastasis. No patient with less than 90% necrosis had an alteration ratio of less than 90%. More patients need to be studied, but this is strongly suggestive that thallium-201 scanning is predictive of the percent of necrosis of an osteosarcoma treated with preoperative chemotherapy.

D.S. Springfield, M.D.

Benign Versus Malignant Intraosseous Lesions: Discrimination by Means of PET With 2-[F-18]Fluoro-2-Deoxy-D-Glucose
Dehdasht F, Siegel BA, Griffeth LK, et al (Mallinckrodt Inst of Radiology, St Louis, Mo; Washington Univ, St Louis, Mo)
Radiology 200:243–247, 1996   3–6

Background.—The ability of CT, MRI, and bone scintigraphy to differentiate benign from malignant intraosseous lesions is limited, often necessitating invasive methods for making a definitive diagnosis. The efficacy of positron emission tomography (PET) with 2-[fluorine-18]fluoro-2-deoxy-D-glucose (FDG) in distinguishing benign from malignant intraosseous lesions was investigated.

Methods.—Twenty patients with strictly intraosseous lesions underwent FDG PET. In all patients, histologic assessment confirmed the final diagnosis. Uptake of FDG in each lesion was assessed qualitatively and semiquantitatively by determining standard uptake value (SUV).

Findings.—Assessment of FDG accumulation in osseous lesions with SUV was better than subjective visual analysis for discriminating between benign and malignant lesions. By using a 2.0 cutoff value for SUV, 14 of 15 malignant lesions were classified correctly, compared with 12 of 15 classified correctly by subjective image evaluation. Four of 5 benign lesions were categorized correctly with both methods.

Conclusion.—The feasibility and clinical potential of FDG PET in differentiating benign from malignant intraosseous lesions large enough to be assessed without major partial volume averaging were demonstrated in this study. Quantitative SUV analysis appears to be more accurate than subjective image interpretation.

▶ On plain radiographs, malignant bone tumors are usually separated from benign bone tumors based on the degree of aggressive behavior seen. Infiltration of bone, destruction of cortex without a complete periosteal containment, multiple layers of periosteal reaction (onion skinning), bone formation perpendicular to the cortex (sunburst reaction), and poor marginalization between the tumor and adjacent unaffected bone (broad border of transition) are the hallmarks of an aggressive—and, therefore, assumed to be malignant—bone tumor. Most bone lesions can be recognized as either inactive or minimally active (therefore, assumed to be benign) or aggressive (therefore assumed to be malignant), but there are some whose plain radiographic appearance is not sufficient to make that distinction. In addition, some malignant bone tumors can have the plain radiographic presentation of an inactive or minimally active bone tumor and some benign bone tumors can have an aggressive radiographic appearance. Osteomyelitis can do either.

Diagnostic radiologists and orthopedists have been looking for a radiographic tool that can distinguish malignant from benign tumors in all cases. These authors have investigated whether PET scanning has that capability. It does not.

As the authors state, PET scans measure the uptake of whatever radioactive material is used and the uptake is determined by the metabolic activity of the tissue. Because malignant bone tumors almost always have higher metabolic activity compared with benign bone tumors, PET is an excellent candidate for a test that would be able to distinguish benign from malignant tumors. Unfortunately, even though PET is reasonably accurate, it is not perfectly accurate and, unless it is perfectly accurate or very nearly so, it still means that some lesions will need to be submitted to biopsy before a final decision can be made.

The authors examined only 20 cases and all but 5 were malignant. The most common setting in which it is critical to distinguish a benign from a malignant bone tumor is in a patient with a diagnosed malignancy who has a solitary bone lesion without other evidence of metastatic disease. If the physician is not able to distinguish a metastatic focus from a benign bone lesion with a PET scan in almost every case and if it not possible to know when the results are unreliable, PET scanning is of little use.

D.S. Springfield, M.D.

Langerhans Cell Histiocytosis

Langerhans' Cell Histiocytosis (Histiocytosis X) of Bone: A Clinicopathologic Analysis of 263 Pediatric and Adult Cases
Kilpatrick SE, Wenger DE, Gilchrist GS, et al (Mayo Clinic, Rochester, Minn)
Cancer 76:2471–2484, 1995   3–7

Introduction.—A group of histologically similar disorders is encompassed by Langerhans' cell histiocytosis, or histiocytosis X. These disorders include Hand-Schuller-Christian disease, eosinophilic granuloma, and Letterer-Siwe syndrome. These disorders have variable and often unpredictable behavior, and the biological behavior is poorly understood, although the findings provide ample evidence for a neoplastic origin. The clinical and pathologic features of patients with this disorder were comprehensively reviewed to provide insights into the natural history of Langerhans' cell histiocytosis of bone.

Methods.—There were 172 children and 91 adults with biopsy-proven Langerhans' cell histiocytosis who ranged in age from 2 months to 71 years at presentation; This study evaluated the clinical and pathologic features of these patients during an 80-year period. Clinical follow-up ranged from 3 months to 50 years and was available for 245 patients. To determine associations between age, sex, visceral disease, extent of osseous involvement, and pathologic features, chi-square tests were conducted. Univariate and multivariate Cox regression methods were used to perform survival analyses.

Results.—Pain was the most common presenting complaint, which was often worse at night. The most frequent osseous site in children and adults was the skull. In 40 patients, diabetes insipidus was documented. Skeletal recurrence or new bone lesions or both occurred in 44 children, and 19 of these children had diabetes insipidus. Radiologic findings found that 69% of the lesions were in the flat bones of the axial skeleton and that 31% were in the long tubular bones. Langerhans' cell histiocytosis was responsible for the direct or indirect death of 14 children and 3 adults, and all but 2 children were 3 years or younger at presentation. All 9 children with thrombocytopenia and all 7 children with hepatosplenomegaly died. There were 3 or more bone lesions among 9 of the 14 children who died. Systemic amyloidosis occurred in 1 adult patient. No patients with isolated skeletal disease died of Langerhans' cell histiocytosis.

Conclusion.—A poor prognosis is associated with hepatosplenomegaly, young age at diagnosis, polyostotic disease with 3 or more bones involved, and thrombocytopenia. The presence of diabetes insipidus was strongly correlated with recrudescence in children but not in adults. The course of this disorder when it was fatal, progressed to death within 3 years of presentation. A favorable prognostic indicator was significant eosinophilia, according to the results of 2 additional studies.

Langerhans Cell (Eosinophilic) Granulomatosis: A Clinicopathologic Study Encompassing 50 Years
Lieberman PH, Jones CR, Steinman RM, et al (Mem Sloan Kettering Cancer Ctr, New York; Rockefeller Univ, New York)
Am J Surg Pathol 20:519–552, 1996   3–8

Introduction.—The term histiocytosis X was applied to 3 conditions, including Letterer-Siwe disease, Hand-Schuller-Christian disease, and eosinophilic granuloma of bone. Other terms are histiocytosis h and Langerhans' cell histiocytosis. The concept that these disorders had a single nosologic entity was challenged by a review of the literature. The most appropriate term would be Langerhans' cell granulomatosis to avoid confusion with the concept of histiocytosis X because there is evidence that Langerhans' cells are not a member of the mononuclear phagocyte system and are not a tissue macrophage. The pathologic course of the disease is reviewed.

Methods.—The study was based on 238 patients ranging in age from 1 month to 66 years with Langerhans' cell granulomatosis, designated either as Langerhans' cell granulomatosis or eosinophilic granuloma. Of these patients, 198 were followed up for a median of 10.5 years. The pathologic course of the disease was reviewed using electron microscopy, histology, and immunolabeling.

Results.—Unless overtreated, the patients did well, and no deaths were attributed to the disorder itself. Except for occasional residual orthopedic problems of residual diabetes insipidus, all patients recovered completely. Although the granulomas occur primarily in bone, they also occur in the lung, skin, and lymph nodes. The accumulation of Langerhans' cells is the hallmark of the disease. The major associated cells are mature eosinophils rather than T cells. Most patients had the disease within the first 15 years of life. Unifocal Langerhans' cell granulomatosis was found in 153 patients (64.3%) and most involved the skull (16%), femur (15%), pelvic bones (13.2%), ribs (12.4%), vertebrae (10%), jaw (7.2%), humerus (6.5%), clavicle (3.3%), or other bones (7.2%).

Conclusion.—Langerhans' cell granulomatosis is a reactive process, analogous to sarcoidosis. The underlying process may be clonal. It has been helpful to consider unifocal vs. multifocal disease as a staging tool. Factors involved in treating the disease include the histology of the lesions; the distribution of the disease; determination and elimination of triggering antigens, such as tobacco, marijuana, perfumes, coal smoke, wood smoke, sandblasting, fiberglass, paint fumes, welding fumes, animal saliva, and bird droppings; the history of trauma; and evidence of untreated endocrinopathy.

▶ It is likely that we have overtreated many of the patients with isolated Langerhans' cell histiocytosis (eosinophilic granuloma). Observation is probably all that is needed for the majority of the patients, and it is uncommon for a patient with only 1 lesion to have any problems. On the other hand, when the patient has any involvement with an organ system, we do not know who needs treatment and who does not. We have systemic drugs that are effective, but we have yet to completely understand when to use them.

These are both reviews of patients seen over many years. Langerhans' cell histiocytosis continues to be poorly understood, and these reviews help us know what to expect in patients with this disorder. Once it was thought that eosinophilic granuloma, Hand-Schuller-Christian disease, and Letterer-Siwe were 3 separate disorders. In the 1940s, it was speculated that they were a spectrum, and now it seems clear that they are all a disorder of the Langerhans' histiocyte. The separation of the disease into 3 syndromes is probably inappropriate; thus, the term *Langerhans' cell histiocytosis* or *Langerhans' cell granulomatosis* is better.

Kilpatrick and associates (Abstract 3–7) reviewed cases from the records of the Mayo Clinic. Lieberman and associates (Abstract 3–8) reviewed cases from the records of Memorial Sloan-Kettering Cancer Center. Both groups reviewed enough cases to give us an understanding of this disorder. Both groups believe that there is enough evidence to establish Langerhans' cell histiocytosis as a neoplastic disorder of the Langerhans' histiocyte and not just a reactive inflammatory disorder. They also tell us that many of the patients are adults before the disease is diagnosed, and both groups had patients in their 8th decade of life when first given diagnoses. Langerhans' cell histiocytosis is not just a disease of the pediatric age group. At least two thirds of the patients had solitary lesions, and these patients did very well. Patients with isolated lesions need to be followed up for at least 2 years (more than 90% who develop more lesions will do so within 2 years) but need little, if any, treatment for their lesions. No patients with a solitary lesion or even with lesions isolated to bone died of their disease. They had no systemic sequelae or sequelae caused by local structural abnormalities.

Patients with involvement of soft tissues, particularly the liver and the spleen, probably need systemic treatment, although it is difficult to document that treatment improves the course of the disease. Irradiation has been used and is effective for local sites. Small doses, usually around 1,000 cGy (1,000 rad) is sufficient. Radiation is probably most indicated for the patient with spinal cord compression from soft-tissue extension from a vertebral involvement. Prednisone, methotrexate, and vinblastine are the drugs of choice. Usually a single drug regimen will be sufficient. Overtreatment is a problem, and less is often better than more.

D.S. Springfield, M.D.

Ewing's Sarcoma

▶ Ewing's sarcoma is an uncommon malignant tumor of bone that is seen almost exclusively in patients between the ages of 8 or 9 and 25 years of age. Before the advent of adjuvant chemotherapy in the late 1960s, almost every patient died of their disease. Since the use of multidrug chemotherapy protocols, the survival rate has dramatically improved. Now we expect at least 55% of the patients to be continuously disease free at 5 years, and we, therefore, believe them to be cured. Since the original description of the disease, there has been controversy as to how to treat the primary site; however, because of the infrequent occurrence and the poor survival rate until recent years, the issue of primary site management has been of minor importance. Surgical resection is clearly the best means of eradicating the disease, but, until recently, it was thought that major morbidity from surgery was not acceptable and that irradiation was the treatment of choice if surgical resection would cause a significant functional impairment. There is a considerable amount of data, although collected retrospectively, suggesting that surgical resection improves the overall survival rate, and it is common now for the recommended treatment of the primary site to be a resection, even if there are functional consequences.

The next 7 articles are related to this issue. Prospective studies to address the management of the primary site have not been done, and there probably will not be because of the limited number of patients and the difficulty of doing prospective surgical studies. We will have to rely on retrospective data with all of their limitations.

D.S. Springfield, M.D.

Ewing's Sarcoma of the Proximal Femur

Damron TA, Sim FH, O'Connor MI, et al (Mayo Clinic and Mayo Found, Rochester, Minn; Mayo Clinic Jacksonville, Fla)
Clin Orthop 322:232–244, 1996   3–9

Introduction.—The evolution in the treatment of Ewing's sarcoma continues. Surgical resection has been reserved for expendable bones, and traditional treatment has consisted of radiotherapy and chemotherapy. With the improved rate of survival and local control after surgery, there is an increase in surgical management. Treatment of Ewing's sarcoma of the proximal femur during the era of multiagent chemotherapy was reviewed, as were the structural problems encountered, including the incidence, prognosis for healing, time of presentation, and a management scheme.

Methods.—The cases of 16 patients with Ewing's sarcoma of the proximal femur were reviewed. Chemotherapy and radiotherapy were the initial treatment for 14 of 16 patients. Wide local resection was performed after chemotherapy and radiotherapy for 1 patient. Amputation followed by chemotherapy was performed for 1 patient. The follow-up averaged 6.3 years.

Results.—There were 2 patients with a local recurrence. The pathologic fracture rate was 79%, excluding the 2 patients whose femurs were fixed prophylactically. The pathologic fracture rate was 92% by additionally excluding the 2 patients who died before any fracture occurred. In 5 of the 7 pathologic fractures not treated by resection (71%), nonunion occurred. Five additional surgical procedures were required for these fractures to obtain union. No evidence of disease was found at follow-up. Five had died of the disease, and 1 with the disease was alive.

Conclusion.—The most common site of long bone involvement by Ewing's sarcoma is the femur. After completion of chemotherapy with or without radiotherapy, primary resection and reconstruction or prophylactic internal fixation should be considered as the options for management. Prevention strategies include earlier diagnosis, greater awareness of the possibility, appropriate biopsy techniques, patient education about weight-bearing restrictions, and prophylactic fixation vs. resection–reconstruction.

▶ This report is from the group at the Mayo Clinic. They were one of the first groups to report improved survival rates with surgical resections. The purpose of this review of 16 patients with Ewing's sarcoma of the proximal femur treated since the acceptance of adjuvant chemotherapy is to demonstrate the difficulty of management of these patients. The proximal femur is a common site of involvement, and the local complications are significant. Most of these patients were treated with chemotherapy and irradiation. The incidence of pathologic fractures was 92% among those patients who survived and were not treated prophylactically with internal fixation. The authors discuss the difficulty of reconstructing the proximal femur in the young patient, and they conclude that they do not know what is the best treatment.

I believe the treatment should be individualized. The patient who has completed growth and who has a large primary tumor is probably better treated with a surgical resection and replacement of the proximal femur with either an allograft or prosthesis. The patient with a small lesion, especially if it responds well to preoperative chemotherapy, may have the primary site successfully treated with irradiation. Irradiation usually arrests the local growth plate; unfortunately, the risk of later irradiation-associated sarcomas is real, but the functional consequences of resecting and reconstructing the proximal femur are significant.

D.S. Springfield, M.D.

Treatment of Femoral Ewing's Sarcoma
Terek RM, Brien EW, Marcove RC, et al (Brown Univ, Providence, RI; Orthopaedic Hosp, Los Angeles; Mem Sloan-Kettering Cancer Ctr, New York; et al)
Cancer 78:70–78, 1996   3–10

Introduction.—Treatment for Ewing's sarcoma, a small round-cell tumor of the bone, includes chemotherapy for local and systemic disease; however, only about 15% of patients were long-term survivors with only radiotherapy. With the introduction of multiagent chemotherapy, radiotherapy, and surgical resection, survival rates increased to 60% for 5 years. Results of treatment of patients with Ewing's sarcoma of the femur are described. The contribution of surgery and radiation to the multimodality treatment of this disease is also evaluated.

Methods.—The study included 32 patients with Ewing's sarcoma of the femur who were retrospectively reviewed. Patients were categorized into 3 treatment groups: 10 received chemotherapy and radiotherapy (5,320 cGy of radiation); 9 received surgery and chemotherapy; and 13 received surgery, chemotherapy, and radiotherapy (3,590 cGy of radiation). All patients received multiagent cyclophosphamide–doxorubicin-based chemotherapy. Wide resection or amputation was used for surgery. Surviving patients had a minimum follow-up of 45 months.

Results.—A higher risk of local recurrence was found in patients in the chemotherapy and radiotherapy group than in the other 2 groups. For 7 of the 10 patients in the group receiving chemotherapy and radiotherapy, surgery was needed because of the combination of local recurrences and treatment complications. There were 1 of 9 in the chemotherapy and surgery group and 4 of 13 in the chemotherapy, radiotherapy, and surgery group who had a combination of local recurrences and treatment complications that necessitated surgery. For all patients, the median survival rate was 39 months. In the chemotherapy and radiotherapy group, the 5-year survival rate consisted of 1 of 10 patients; in the chemotherapy and surgery group, the 5-year survival rate was 2 of 9; and in the chemotherapy, radiotherapy, and surgery group, the 5-year survival rate was 7 of 13. Among the 3 survival curves, there were no statistically significant differences. A significant prognostic variable was tumor location within the femur with a distal femoral location having a survival advantage compared with mid-femur or proximal locations.

Conclusion.—A poor prognosis is associated with femoral Ewing's sarcoma. There is a high rate of local recurrence and complications with radiation alone for local treatment. Surgery in all and adjuvant radiotherapy in many of the patients is the current local treatment strategy for femoral Ewing's sarcoma. For high-risk Ewing's sarcoma, more effective treatments are needed. A multi-institutional trial is necessary to determine optimal timing and the sequence of surgery and radiotherapy.

▶ This is another retrospective analysis of a group of patients with Ewing's sarcoma. This group of patients were treated at Memorial Sloan-Kettering Cancer Center. These authors reviewed the experience at their institution with patients who had a Ewing's sarcoma of the femur. As was shown in the group from Mayo Clinic previously discussed (Abstract 3–9), these patients have a worse overall prognosis compared with other patients with Ewing's sarcoma. This is probably a result of the larger size of their tumors. These authors suggest that resection is a better treatment for the patient, although their retrospective review does not demonstrate an improved survival rate.

As mentioned in the discussion of the paper from the Mayo Clinic, specific treatment for these patients needs to be individualized. When a surgical resection can be done with limited functional consequences, it is the treatment of choice. When a surgical resection will result in a major loss of function, the consequences of irradiation should be considered. For the patient with a small lesion that has responded well to chemotherapy, irradiation may be the better local treatment.

D.S. Springfield, M.D.

Local Control and Functional Results After Twice-Daily Radiotherapy for Ewing's Sarcoma of the Extremities
Bolek TW, Marcus RB Jr, Mendenhall NP, et al (Univ of Florida, Gainesville)
Int J Radiat Oncol Biol Phys 35:687–692, 1996   3–11

Introduction.—The predominant local treatment for Ewing's sarcoma of the bone has been radiotherapy. Surgery was considered too radical for a disease in which less than 10% of patients survived before chemotherapy became available. The issue of local control has become even more important with the improved prognosis of patients. The differences in local control and functional outcome were compared with once-daily vs. twice-daily radiotherapy for patients with Ewing's sarcoma of the bone occurring in the extremities.

Methods.—There were 37 patients who had nonmetastatic Ewing's sarcoma of the bone with a primary lesion in an extremity in a 19-year period. Three patients had amputation, and 34 were treated with radiotherapy. Of these, 3 had a combination of radiotherapy and local excision, and 31 had radiotherapy alone. Once daily radiotherapy was given to 14 patients (47–61 Gy at 1.8–2 Gy per fraction), whereas twice-daily radiotherapy was given to 17 patients (50.4–60 Gy at 1.2 Gy per fraction). Total body irradiation was also given to some patients in the twice-daily group before their marrow-ablative therapy with stem cell rescue.

Results.—For patients treated twice daily, the actuarial local control rate at 5 years was 81%, whereas for patients treated once daily, the rate was 77%. In patients treated twice daily, no posttreatment pathologic fractures occurred, whereas in those treated once daily, there were 5 fractures. In the twice-daily group, there was less loss in range of motion (15 degrees vs. 28 degrees of loss), and a lesser degree of muscle atrophy (8% vs. 21% loss in muscle circumference) when compared with the once-daily group. In patients treated twice a day, there was a trend toward less local alopecia and less fibrosis. A higher Musculoskeletal Tumor Society functional rating was given to patients treated twice daily than to those treated once daily.

Conclusion.—In the 2 groups, local control rates were similar (77% for once daily vs. 81% for twice daily); however, in the group treated twice daily, functional results were superior. Excellent functional results can be obtained with radiotherapy in patients with Ewing's sarcoma of an extremity.

▶ The group at the University of Florida prefers irradiation for the treatment of Ewing's sarcoma. They reviewed 37 patients but concentrated on 31 who had irradiation as the treatment of their primary tumor. They were most interested in whether treating the patient twice a day with 2 smaller doses was better than treating them once a day with the total dose. They had a local recurrence incidence in both groups that is probably unacceptable. They had a total of 6 local recurrences in the 31 patients treated with chemotherapy and irradiation. That is an incidence of almost 20%. On the other hand, they demonstrate little functional impairment as a consequence of irradiation. When evaluated using the Musculoskeletal Tumor Society functional scoring system, both groups did well, and most had minimal functional deficits. The twice daily treated patients did a little better, but both were acceptable.

Once again, this is a retrospective analysis, and the number of patients is small. On the other hand, the incidence of local recurrence is high. Local recurrence after surgical resection has been much less than 20%, and, although showing that this results in a higher survival rate has been difficult, most agree that local recurrence is not good. I think this article supports using surgical resection whenever possible.

D.S. Springfield, M.D.

Ewing's Sarcoma of Bone: Oncologic and Functional Results
Renard AJS, Veth RPH, Pruszczynski M, et al (Univ of Nijmegen, The Netherlands; Univ Hosp of Groningen, The Netherlands)
J Surg Oncol 60:250–256, 1995   3–12

Background.—In the past decade, the limitations of radiotherapy alone for Ewing's sarcoma (ES) have become apparent. High rates of local failure and secondary tumors have been reported, together with poorer functional outcomes compared with surgery in selected patients. Thus, surgical treatment of ES has been re-evaluated. Treatment outcomes in 1 series of patients were analyzed.

Methods and Findings.—Twenty-nine patients with ES of the bone were treated with chemotherapy plus surgery and/or radiotherapy at 1 center between 1975 and 1990. In 24% of the patients, osteomyelitis was the primary diagnosis. Five of the 9 patients receiving radiotherapy alone died of disease. None of the 12 patients undergoing wide excision had evidence of disease. All 3 patients undergoing radical disarticulation died of disease. Disease-free survival at 1.5 years was 66%, and at 5 years, it was 55%.

Conclusion.—Wide excision of tumors in expendable bone is the preferred treatment for optimum oncologic and functional outcomes. This is also true for femoral and radial tumors, with implantation of resection mega-endoprosthesis or bone grafting, respectively. None of these patients had local recurrence, including those who had not had radiotherapy.

▶ These authors retrospectively examined the results of treatment of 29 patients with ES. Only 9 patients had their primary disease treated with irradiation alone. The remainder had surgery alone or surgery and irradiation. Of the 9 treated with irradiation, 5 died and 1 of the remaining 4 had a local recurrence. The patients who had a resection with negative margins are alive without disease. Three patients had hip disarticulation; all 3 died. It is clear that there is a selection bias among these patients and it is not possible to know what role the surgery played in the patient's outcome.

Functional results are interesting. Sixty percent of the patients seen with localized disease alone were alive at 5 years. Only 3 of them underwent reconstruction with mega-endoprostheses, whereas the others treated with a resection did not need a reconstruction, were reconstructed with an arthrodesis, or had an amputation. As is too often the case, function is not closely followed. Only 11 of the 29 patients had a functional evaluation. The patients with amputations were rated as fair. We tend to downgrade the function of an amputee unfairly. Most amputees are as active as they want to be and are allowed unrestricted activities, which is not the case for most limb-salvage patients. Most limb-salvage patients have to limit their physical activities to protect their reconstruction. There were only 3 patients treated with irradiation in the functional analysis group. Two were rated fair and I was rated poor. There were not enough patients followed after irradiation to know the functional consequences, but the results of these 3 patients reminds us that irradiation is not without functional consequences.

This article does not give us much information about how to treat patients except to reinforce the impression gained from other retrospective studies that individualized management is indicated. Local irradiation for extremity disease has a slightly higher risk of local recurrence and not necessarily better function. On the other hand, many of the patients treated with surgery in this series have lesions in a rib, fibula, clavicle, or small bone of the hand, all of which can be resected with limited functional deficit.

D.S. Springfield, M.D.

Significance of Surgical Margin on the Prognosis of Patients With Ewing's Sarcoma: A Report From the Cooperative Ewing's Sarcoma Study
Ozaki T, Hillmann A, Hoffmann C, et al (Westfälische Wilhelms-Univ, Münster, Germany; Martin Luther Univ Halle-Wittenberg, Germany)
Cancer 78:892–900, 1996   3–13

Background.—Few data are available on adequate surgical margins for local control of Ewing's sarcoma (ES). The influence of surgery and surgical margins on local control and overall survival in patients with ES was investigated.

Methods.—Two hundred forty-four patients with ES undergoing surgery were included. Ninety-four had definitive surgery alone, 131 had postoperative irradiation, and 19 had preoperative irradiation. The surgical margins were radical in 29 patients, wide in 148, marginal in 39, and intralesional in 28.

Findings.—The local or combined relapse rate after surgery with or without irradiation was significantly reduced compared with that after definitive irradiation; the rates were 7% and 31%, respectively. The local or combined relapse rate after complete resection with or without irradiation was lower than that after incomplete resection with or without irradiation (5% and 12%, respectively). Radiation treatment after incomplete surgery did not greatly reduce the local or combined relapse rate. In groups with good or poor histologic response, the difference in systemic or combined relapse rate between patients undergoing complete and incomplete surgery was nonsignificant. At 10 years, the survival rate for patients with radical margins was 58%; for those with wide margins it was 65%; for those with marginal margins, it was 61%; and for those with intralesional margins it was 71%.

Conclusion.—In patients with ES, surgical treatment increases the safety of local control. With the current intensive chemotherapy and radiation therapy regimen, complete tumor resection appears to reduce the risk of local recurrence.

▶ The European oncologists have cooperated to study ES. The group, whose study is called the Cooperative Ewing's Sarcoma Study, have combined their efforts to study different aspects of the treatment of ES. Numerous reports have been presented and published based on these data. This article is a review of 244 patients with ES treated by members of the cooperative group. The local disease was treated with irradiation alone, surgery alone, or a combination of the 2. The treatment of the primary disease was determined jointly by the surgeon and the patient. The idea was to resect all lesions that could be resected with limited morbidity of functional deficity while others were irradiated.

This is a retrospective study, and the selection of treatment of the primary tumor was not controlled but, as with other studies, surgical resection was associated with a better overall survival. Local control was much better when the primary tumor could be resected but distant metastases were more frequent in those patients who had a resection, compared with those who were treated with irradiation. The increased incidence of pulmonary metastasis in patients having surgery may be the result of physical manipulation or may be just coincidence. No other reports have made this observation. The answer remains unknown, but the increased incidence of local recurrence more than offset the less frequent distant metastasis among the patients who had irradiation, so the overall survival was better among patients who had surgery. The surgical margin did not seem to affect the outcome, but this may result from the use of postoperative irradiation for patients with positive margins.

These data suggest that for patients who can have a wide surgical margin resection, surgery alone is the treatment of choice. For those who will have a marginal or intralesional resection, preoperative irradiation (with or without postoperative irradiation) is advised. All patients should have preoperative chemotherapy. This treatment rationale seems to make the most sense, based on the information we have available, but it is still not proven.

D.S. Springfield, M.D.

Second Malignancies After Ewing's Sarcoma: Radiation Dose-Dependency of Secondary Sarcomas

Kuttesch JF Jr, Wexler LH, Marcus RB, et al (St Jude Children's Reseach Hosp, Memphis, Tenn; Univ of Tennessee, Memphis; Univ of Florida, Gainesville; et al)
J Clin Oncol 14:2818–2825, 1996   3–14

Background.—Survivors of childhood Ewing's sarcoma (ES) have an increased risk of second malignancies. A multicenter database was used to reassess this risk and identify possible reasons for it.

Methods and Findings.—The database included 266 survivors of ES. During a median follow-up of 9.5 years, second malignancies developed in 16 patients. Ten were sarcomas and 6 were other malignancies. The median time to the diagnosis of the second malignancy was 7.6 years. The 20-year estimated cumulative incidence rate for any second malignancy was 9.2% and for secondary sarcoma, 6.5%. This cumulative incidence rate was radiation dose dependent. None of the patients given less than 48 Gy had secondary sarcomas. Among those receiving 60 Gy or more, the absolute risk of secondary sarcoma was 130 per 10,000 person-years of observation.

Conclusion.—The overall risk of second malignancies after ES is comparable with that associated with the treatment of other childhood malignancies. Reductions in radiation doses appear warranted.

Radiotherapy, Alkylating Agents, and Risk of Bone Cancer After Childhood Cancer

Hawkins MM, Kinnier Wilson LM, Burton HS, et al (Univ of Oxford, England; Royal Manchester Children's Hosp, Pendlebury, England; Univ of Texas, Houston)
J Natl Cancer Inst 88:270–278, 1996   3–15

Background.—The risk of bone cancer is greater than that of any other type of second primary cancer in persons who had childhood cancer. The incidence and etiology of second primary bone cancer after childhood cancer were investigated in a cohort and case-control study.

Methods.—Data were obtained from the population-based National Registry of Childhood Tumours in Britain. The cohort study included 13,175 three-year survivors of childhood cancers diagnosed between 1940 and 1983. Fifty-five bone cancers subsequently developed in this cohort. The nested case-control study included 59 patients with second primary bone cancers and 220 control patients matched for sex, type of first cancer, age at first cancer, and interval between the diagnosis of the first cancer and subsequent bone cancer.

Findings.—The proportion of 3-year survivors who had bone cancer within 20 years was 0.9% or less in most patient groups. Exceptions were those with heritable retinoblastoma, with 7.2% developing bone cancer;

those with Ewing's sarcoma (ES), 5.4%; and those with other malignant bone tumors, 2.4%. The risk of bone cancer rose markedly with increased cumulative radiation dose to the bone, although at the highest exposure levels, this risk seemed to decline somewhat. At worst, a dose of less than 10 Gy was associated with a small increased relative risk of bone cancer. The risk of bone cancer increased linearly with increases in the cumulative dose of alkylating drugs.

Conclusion.—Most survivors of childhood cancer can be assured that their risk of bone cancer developing within 20 years of 3-year survival does not exceed 0.9%. The relative risks associated with certain radiation dose levels should be considered in decision making regarding future treatment protocols.

▶ Secondary sarcomas associated with irradiation have been one of the reasons surgeons have wanted to reduce the number of patients with ES who are treated with irradiation. The risk is difficult to determine. The number of survivors has been few and the time between the irradiation and their associated sarcoma is long, so it has been difficult to accurately calculate the risk. As more patients survive, the significance of the risk increases. It has been suggested that children are at greater risk compared with adults and that alkylating agents in combination with irradiation increase the risk. Kuttesch et al. (Abstract 3–14) have tried to find out the risk of a secondary sarcoma developing. They found 16 (6%) in 266 survivors. This is probably the best incidence figure currently available. Remember, though, that the risk remains present forever; 6% is the lowest incidence and it will increase with longer follow up. The authors remind us that this is a smaller risk than has been reported.

Hawkins and associates (Abstract 3–15) reviewed the incidence of secondary bone tumors in patients who had a childhood malignancy and survived at least 3 years. This review confirmed the increased risk among patients with ES. The authors also found that increased doses of irradiation increased the incidence of a secondary bone tumor. The incidence increases with higher doses of irradiation (more than 6,000 cGy or 6,000 rads). Their conclusion is probably true, but an incidence of 6% is too high, especially when the risk does not decrease after a few years but actually increases. The authors are correct is stating that continued work needs to be done on strategies to reduce the dose required. As a surgeon, I suggest that a total surgical resection is the best method for reducing the incidence of irradiation-associated sarcomas.

D.S. Springfield, M.D.

Miscellaneous

Cytoxicity of Phenol to Musculoskeletal Tumours
Quint U, Vanhöfer U, Harstrick A, et al (Univ of Essen, Germany)
J Bone Joint Surg Br 78B:984–985, 1996   3–16

Background.—Local treatment with phenol is commonly used after intralesional excision of chondroblastomas and giant-cell tumors of bone.

Such treatment has been shown to decrease recurrence rates. The best concentration of phenol has not been established. Because of its high absorption rate and toxicity, determining the best concentration is important.

Methods and Findings.—The efficacy of various concentrations of phenol was tested on standard sarcoma cell lines. After 3 cycles of incubation for 1 minute with 5% phenol solution, the cell count showed a survival fraction of 7%. Concentrations of 7.5% and 10% in vitro resulted in only minimal gains in antitumor activity, to 6.5% and 3.8%, respectively.

Conclusion.—A 5% solution of phenol is effective against dispersed single cells. Higher concentrations are not more effective and are associated with problems in homogeneous mixing, temperature, and safety.

► Many, in fact most, benign bone tumors can be successfully treated with observation or simple curettage. Only a few benign tumors have a significant enough incidence of local recurrence to warrant more aggressive treatment. Giant cell tumor (GCT) of bone is the most common benign bone tumor that needs more treatment than a simple curettage. Even with aggressive curettage, the incidence of local recurrence for GCT of bone is at least 20%. A variety of adjuvants have been and are being used. More radical surgery has been used with the en bloc method (wide surgical margins) being done for some patients' GCTs. This works but usually leaves the patient with significant functional loss. Cryosurgery is used and does reduce the frequency of local recurrence but with damage to adjacent tissue. Polymethylmethacrylate is thought by some to be an adjuvant, but this has not been proven. Phenol has been used as an adjuvant for many years. Its origins are not clear, but its effects on tumor cells have rarely been been reported.

Quint and associates have made an effort to examine the effect of phenol on tumor cells. They used a monolayer of cultured human sarcoma cells and exposed these cells to different concentrations of phenol. The lowest concentration of phenol studied (5%) was effective in killing almost all of the cells, even with the shortest time of exposure (1 minute times 3). It may be that even less concentration for less time is effective. The use of 5% phenol is probably safe although this was not studied.

It should be pointed out that the concentration of phenol, although reported as a percent, is probably grams percent. Therefore, 5% means 5 g of phenol in 100 mL of water. As mentioned by the authors, phenol and water do not mix well, and it is difficult to have very concentrated solutions of phenol.

The time of exposure to phenol may be important. We have done some work with phenol's effect on cell viability of fresh GCT of bone (C. Jennings et al., unpublished data) and found that constant contact for 10 minutes produced more cell death than did shorter time periods.

More work needs to be done on the effects and safety of phenol. If it is a useful adjuvant with acceptable or no side effects, it should be used for all locally aggressive benign tumors. It would be important to know how much of the phenol is absorbed and what, if any, is the risk of systemic effect.

D.S. Springfield, M.D.

Isolated Limb Perfusion With High-dose Tumor Necrosis Factor-α in Combination With Interferon-γ and Melphalan for Nonresectable Extremity Soft Tissue Sarcomas: A Multicenter Trial
Eggermont AMM, Koops HS, Liénard D, et al (Univ Hosp Rotterdam-Daniel den Hoed Cancer Ctr, The Netherlands; Univ Hosp, Groningen, The Netherlands; Netherlands Cancer Inst, Amsterdam; et al)
J Clin Oncol 14:2653–2665, 1996   3–17

Background.—About 60% of soft_tissue sarcomas occur in the extremities and are often large when initially diagnosed. Amputation or exarticulation may be done for locally advanced extremity soft-tissue sarcomas. If at all possible, limb-sparing procedures are extensive and are usually followed by high-dose radiation therapy, which may mutilate and markedly compromise limb function. An investigation was conducted of the efficacy of isolated limb perfusion (ILP) with tumor necrosis factor (TNF) -α combined with interferon (IFN)-γ and melphalan as induction treatment to make tumors resectable in an attempt to avoid amputation in patients with nonresectable extremity soft-tissue sarcomas.

Methods.—Fifty-five patients underwent subcutaneous IFN administration for 2 days before ILP with TNF, IFN, and melphalan. Delayed marginal resection of the tumor remnant was usually done 2 to 3 months after ILP. Thirty patients had primary tumors, and 25 had recurrent sarcoma. Forty-eight sarcomas were high grade.

Findings.—Eighty-seven percent of the patients had a major tumor response, and resection was possible in most. Eighteen percent had complete responses, 64%, had partial responses, and 18% had no response. Eighty-four percent had limb-salvaging procedures. In 39 patients, resection of the tumor remnant (single or multiple) was done after ILP was performed. Local recurrence developed in 13% of these patients. Local recurrences were frequent when no resection was performed. However, limb salvage was often achieved but patients died of systemic disease. Regional toxicity was limited. Systemic toxicity was minimal to moderate, causing no deaths.

Conclusion.—This induction biochemotherapy regimen effectively and safely enables limb salvage in patients with nonresectable extremity soft-tissue sarcoma. In the setting of ILP, TNF is an active anticancer drug.

▶ Limb salvage for soft-tissue sarcomas has become the expected management. Some soft-tissue sarcomas can be safely treated with surgery alone, but most do not lend themselves to an adequate surgical margin (at least a "wide" surgical margin) and in order to salvage a limb, an adjuvant to the surgery is needed. Irradiation has been used as the adjuvant almost exclusively in North America to allow a less than "wide" surgical resection. Intra-arterial infusions are used by some, either with or without irradiation. Limb perfusion is not often used as an adjuvant for limb salvage of soft-tissue sarcoma, but it is used in the management of some patients with melanoma.

Eggermont and associates have used adjuvant limb perfusion as a method of assisting in limb salvage. The theoretical advantage of infusional chemotherapy over irradiation is the ability of the normal tissues in the extremity to recover from chemotherapy better than from irradiation. This needs to be proven. Another unproven, theoretic advantage is less risk of a treatment-related malignancy. These are uncommon, but they are a risk with irradiation. The major disadvantages of infusional chemotherapy are the technical difficulties of administering this type of treatment and the limitations of anatomical locations that can be treated. Infusional chemotherapy requires careful arterial access, complete venous occlusion of all veins not cannulated by the infusional system, and monitoring of the patient during treatment. Many soft-tissue sarcomas and most of the large ones are proximal to thigh, buttock, and low pelvis. These anatomical areas are difficult or impossible to access with infusional treatment.

Infusional chemotherapy for soft-tissue sarcomas has some advantages and needs additional study. Whether it will be indicated sufficiently often for any centers to become comfortable in its use is uncertain.

D.S. Springfield, M.D.

4 Spinal Disorders

Introduction

A balanced set of articles were reviewed this year. No particular area was heavily emphasized. Besides diagnostics and therapeutics, articles include complications, infections, and tumors.

I have continued to look for good outcome studies addressing the use of instrumentation in degenerative conditions of the lumbar spine. There are a number of studies, but none really conclusive. This is the most controversial area in spine surgery today, and hopefully we will have answers in the near future.

Finally, the evaluation of bone morphogenic protein for fusions continues. It will probably be investigated in humans within the next year. Hopefully this will provide an alternative to autograft with a more predictable rate of union.

Sam W. Wiesel, M.D.

Imaging

Clinical Impact of Contrast-enhanced MR Imaging Reports in Patients With Previous Lumbar Disk Surgery

Milette PC, Fontaine S, Lepanto L, et al (Hôpital Saint Luc, Montreal)
AJR Am J Roentgenol 167:217–223, 1996   4–1

Background.—Symptoms that suggest a recurrent lumbar disk herniation may occur in patients after successful lumbar disk surgery, sometimes after intervals of many years. Magnetic resonance imaging has been shown to have excellent accuracy in the evaluation of the postoperative lumbar spine. The cost of MRI demands, however, that it not only be accurate but have benefit for patients. The clinical usefulness of MRI for the evaluation of patients who had previous lumbar disk surgery was assessed by determining the influence of MR examinations on the decision to have repeat surgery and by evaluating the outcome of these repeat surgeries.

Methods.—Magnetic resonance imaging studies were performed in 257 patients. The patients' status was then followed to determine their treatment and outcome. The studies were interpreted by 4 experienced radiologists. Relationships between their reports and the decision to undergo

"

surgery were analyzed. The 6-month postoperative outcomes of patients who underwent repeat surgery were determined.

Results.—Of the 257 patients, 52 underwent repeat surgery after the MR examination. When positive MRI test results were defined as reports of a probable or definite single herniation at the level of the previous surgery, repeat surgery was performed in 32% of patients who had positive test results and in 14% of those who had negative results. When positive MRI test results were defined as reports of 1 or more herniations at any level, repeat surgery was performed in 29% of patients who had positive test results and in 9% of those who had negative results. Repeat surgery of all types, and particularly the frequency of disk exploration, was significantly associated with positive test results of either definition and with the reported size of the main herniation. Poor surgical outcome was significantly associated with younger age and with Worker's Compensation status. At 1 year after surgery, a 50% symptomatic improvement was reported by 8% of patients who had Worker's Compensation and by 23% of those who did not.

Conclusions.—Although enhanced MRI has high accuracy in detecting disk herniation and significantly influences the decision to undergo repeat lumbar disk surgery, it has little patient benefit, because the repeat surgery has poor efficacy in relieving symptoms. More well-designed outcome research is therefore needed to determine selection criteria for repeat surgery and to define a clinically useful role of MRI in patients who have undergone previous lumbar disk surgery.

▶ Currently, contrast-enhanced MRI is the diagnostic study of choice to differentiate scar tissue from a recurrent herniated disk in a patient who has had multiple back operations. This study demonstrates that the clinical outcome is not as good as we would like to achieve. I definitely agree with the conclusion that further work and a better diagnostic test are probably necessary for us to get better surgical results in this challenging group of patients. I suspect that there will be other contrast agents to use with MRI in the near future.

S.W. Wiesel, M.D.

Value of SPECT Imaging of the Thoracolumbar Spine in Cancer Patients
Delpassand ES, Garcia JR, Bhadkamkar V, et al (Univ of Texas, Houston)
Clin Nucl Med 20:1047–1051, 1995   4–2

Background.—It is difficult to determine the exact anatomical site of vertebral abnormalities with planar bone scintigraphy and to differentiate between benign and malignant vertebral lesions. The exact location of bone abnormalities can be detected, however, with single-photon emission CT (SPECT). The usefulness of SPECT bone imaging in defining the precise location of vertebral lesions and in determining whether the abnormality is benign or malignant was evaluated prospectively.

Methods.—Fifty patients who had different cancers and no known skeletal metastases and had abnormalities on planar images of the thoracolumbar spine were included. The patients all underwent SPECT imaging of either the thoracic spine (25 patients) or the lumbar spine (25 patients), as directed by the planar bone scintiscan findings. The SPECT images were interpreted by 2 blinded physicians to determine the exact location of the vertebral lesions. These findings were correlated with other diagnostic studies and with at least 6 months of clinical follow-up, which revealed whether the lesions were benign or malignant.

Results.—The SPECT images revealed 53 thoracic spine abnormalities in 25 patients and 57 lumbar spine abnormalities in 25 patients. Of the 53 thoracic spine abnormalities, 23 were metastases, as were 12 of the 57 lumbar spine abnormalities. Abnormalities of the vertebral body that extended into posterior elements were metastatic in 93% of thoracic cases and in 100% of lumbar cases. All abnormalities confined to the disk space, the articular process, and the anterior vertebral body were benign, whereas 26% of the abnormalities confined to the vertebral body and 25% of the abnormalities confined to the spinous process were malignant.

Conclusions.—Single-photon emission CT has clinical utility in determining the exact anatomical location of vertebral abnormalities. These locations are useful in determining the likelihood that the lesion is benign or malignant. Because of its costliness, however, SPECT imaging should be reserved for patients with cancer whose bone scans reveal abnormalities limited to the thoracolumbar spine, who have back pain but no abnormalities on planar bone scans, or whose planar bone scans reveal a new thoracolumbar spine abnormality but no typical skeletal metastatic pattern.

▶ It is sometimes difficult to isolate the precise location of a lesion in the spine and to differentiate whether it is a metastatic or benign process. Single-photon emission CT imaging is a new technique, and this article nicely demonstrates that it is quite helpful in achieving both goals. It can differentiate the location of a particular lesion better than our traditional studies. In addition, SPECT imaging gives information as to whether an abnormality is a metastatic process or a benign lesion.

S.W. Wiesel, M.D.

Fat Suppressed Contrast Enhanced MR Imaging in the Assessment of Sacroiliitis

Wittram C, Whitehouse GH, Bucknall RC (Univ of Liverpool, England)
Clin Radiol 51:554–558, 1996   4–3

Background.—Magnetic resonance imaging can be useful in reaching a diagnosis for patients with a clinical suspicion of sacroiliitis. The role of fat-suppressed gadolinium-diethylenetriamine-pentaacetic acid (Gd-DTPA) enhancement of T1-weighted with fat suppression (T1FS) MRI

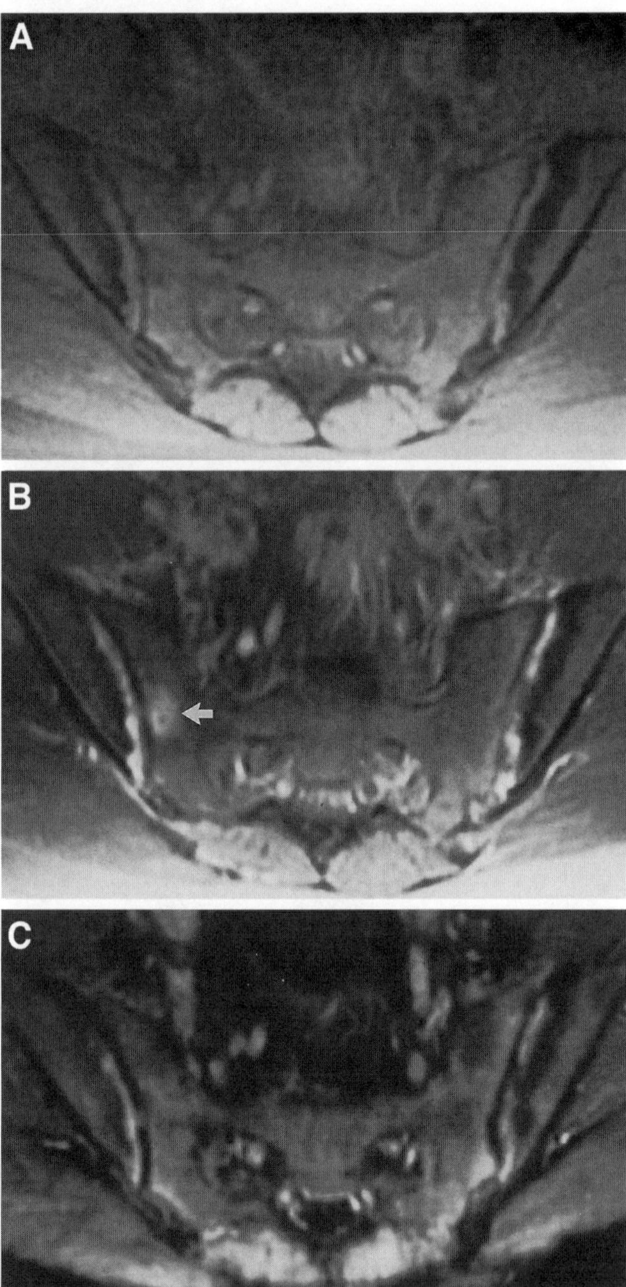

FIGURE 1.—Images of a woman, aged 26 years, with definite sacroiliitis with a symptom rating score of 9/10. **A,** T1-weighted with fat suppression (*T1FS*) (500/19) image shows widening of the synovial compartment of the sacroiliac joint, cortical erosions, and subchondral sclerosis particularly affecting the iliac bones. **B,** T1FS (500/19) contrast-enhanced image at approximately the same level as 1A shows abnormal enhancement of the synovial compartment of the sacroiliac joint and the subchondral marrow (*arrows*). **C,** fast STIR (3000/16EF inversion time 160 msec with an echotrain of 8) at approximately the same level as Fig 1B, shows abnormal high signal in the synovial compartment and abnormal patchy increase in signal in the adjacent subchondral marrow, indicating active inflammation. (Courtesy of Wittram C, Whitehouse GH, Bucknall RC: Fat suppressed contrast enhanced MR imaging in the assessment of sacroiliitis. *Clin Radiol* 51:554–558, 1996.)

images in reaching a diagnosis for patients with a clinical suspicion of sacroiliitis was studied.

Methods.—The study group consisted of 25 participants: 5 controls, 15 with confirmed sacroiliitis and 5 with a clinical diagnosis of sacroiliitis and abnormal high signal on Fast STIR images, but who had negative results from CT. The enhancement factor was calculated for T1FS images.

Findings.—Abnormal Gd-DTPA enhancement of the sacroiliac joints or adjacent subchondral marrow was detected in 14 out of 15 patients with sacroiliitis and in 1 of 5 patients with a clinical suspicion of sacroiliitis. The regions of abnormal enhancement on the T1FS images corresponded to the regions of abnormal high signal on the Fast STIR images in the subchondral marrow (Fig 1).

Conclusions.—When active inflammation is revealed by the distribution of abnormal high signal on Fast STIR images, there is no need to administer Gd-DTPA. When Fast STIR images are inconclusive, Gd-DTPA enhancement may provide additional evidence for a diagnosis of sacroiliitis.

▶ The diagnosis of sacroiliitis can be difficult to make—especially early in its course. This article describes the technique using a Gd-DTPA MRI with fat suppression. It seems to work well. This article is worth noting in that one has to be able to ask the neuroradiologist for this type of study if the diagnosis of sacroiliitis is suspected.

S.W. Wiesel, M.D.

Discographic Pain Report: Influence of Psychological Factors
Block AR, Vanharanta H, Ohnmeiss DD, et al (Texas Back Inst Research Found, Plano)
Spine 21:334–338, 1996   4–4

Background.—Typically, injection into disrupted disks is painful, whereas injection into nondisrupted disks is not. However, sometimes results are discordant, which makes diagnosis difficult. The current study determined whether patients with increased scores on the Minnesota Multiphasic Personality Inventory (MMPI) scale were more likely to report pain on injection of a nondisrupted disk than patients without increased scores.

Methods and Findings.—Seventy-two patients underwent CT/diskography at the 3 lowest lumbar levels and completed the MMPI. Patients reporting pain on injection into a nondisrupted disk had significantly higher scores on the hypochondriasis and hysteria scales than those not reporting pain. Scores on the depression scale showed a similar trend. These findings persisted after adjustment for the possible confounding effects of age, symptom duration, and sex in a multivariate analysis.

Conclusion.—Diskographic pain reports are influenced by personality, as reflected by MMPI scores, as well as anatomical abnormalities. Patients with increased scores on the hypochondriasis, hysteria, and depression-scales of the MMPI may report pain during injection into nondisrupted disks.

▶ Diskography is somewhat controversial as a diagnostic test for invasive therapeutics at this moment. Everyone agrees that for a diskogram to be positive, it has to reproduce the patient's pain. This is a nice paper regarding the psychological factors that can influence that pain interpretation. I think that one must carefully appreciate the subjective nature of a positive diskogram because it does involve a patient's subjective response.

S.W. Wiesel, M.D.

Magnetic Resonance Imaging for the Evaluation of Patients With Occult Cervical Spine Injury
Benzel EC, Hart BL, Ball PA, et al (Univ of New Mexico, Albuquerque; Dartmouth-Hitchcock Med Ctr, Lebanon, NH)
J Neurosurg 85:824–829, 1996   4–5

Objective.—Routine x-ray films, tomography, and CT may miss occult soft-tissue damage in acute cervical spine injuries. Magnetic resonance imaging has proved useful for assessing soft-tissue injury in knee, shoulder, and other extremities. The utility of MRI in visualizing extradural soft-tissue injury after surgical spine trauma was examined in a 42-month study at the University of New Mexico School of Medicine.

Methods.—T1- and T2-weighted sagittal MR images were obtained in all 174 post-trauma patients, aged 15 months to 91 years, within 72 hours of injury; axial images were obtained in those with suspected disk herniation. Injuries were catalogued as ventral soft-tissue, dorsal soft-tissue, or disk interspace disruption.

Results.—Soft-tissue injuries, all clinically significant, were found in 62 patients. T2-weighted sagittal images were the most instructive in demonstrating soft-tissue injuries. There were disk interspace disruptions in 27 patients, 4 with ventral and dorsal ligamentous injuries, 3 with ventral ligamentous injuries, 18 with dorsal ligamentous injuries, and 2 with no dorsal or ventral injuries (Fig 2). There were isolated ligamentous injuries in 35 patients, 8 with ventral and dorsal ligamentous injuries, 5 with ventral ligamentous injuries, and 22 with dorsal ligamentous injuries. There were 50 patients with no soft-tissue injuries but with loss of lordosis in 37, serious degenerative changes in 11, and congenital abnormalities in 2. One patient had a dorsal fusion with foraminotomy. The patients were treated with a semirigid cervical collar (35 patients), including the surgery patient, or a thermoplastic Minerva jacket (27 patients). All patients recovered with no spinal or neurologic deficits.

Conclusion.—T2-weighted sagittal images were the most useful in providing information about acute soft-tissue injuries. Disk herniations and ligamentous injuries were common. Additional studies are needed to de-

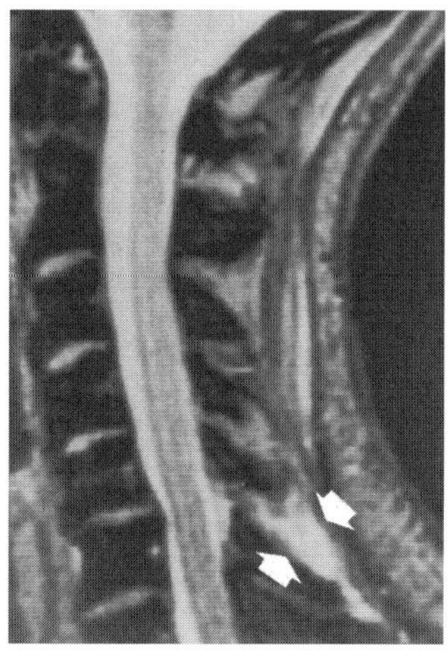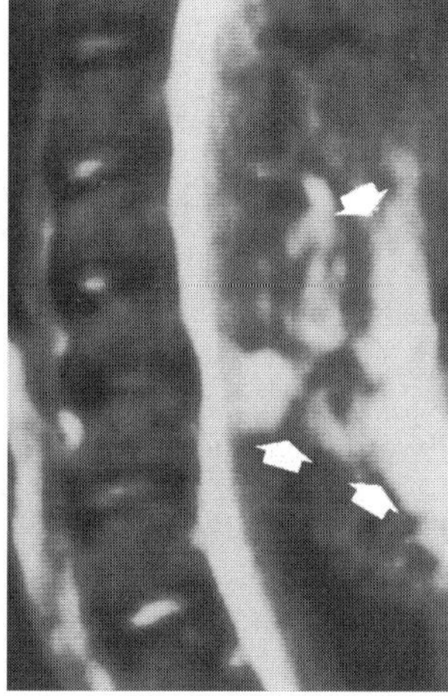

FIGURE 2.—A high-field (1.5-T) sagittal T2-weighted MR image (**left**) and a low-field (0.064-T) sagittal T2-weighted MR image (**right**) obtained on the same day in a patient with a cervical spine injury. Note that the abnormal signal intensity in the soft tissues (*arrows*) is much more striking on the low-field than on the high-field image. However, also note that the anatomical resolution is much better with the high-field image. (Courtesy of Benzel EC, Hart BL, Ball PA, et al: Magnetic resonance imaging for the evaluation of patients with occult cervical spine injury. *J Neurosurg* 85:824–829, 1996).

termine whether this modality is cost effective in assessing acute cervical spine trauma.

► Traditionally, it has been assumed that if x-ray films do not give one all the diagnostic information required, CT scans should be the next step. This article shows eloquently that with the sophistication of today's MRI, it is perhaps the diagnostic modality of choice. It certainly picks up soft-tissue injuries that otherwise would not be appreciated on either plain x-ray films or CT scans.

S.W. Wiesel, M.D.

Complications

Meningitis Complicating Spinal Surgery

Twyman RS, Robertson P, Thomas MG (Auckland Hosp, New Zealand)
Spine 21:763–765, 1996   4–6

Purpose.—Meningitis is rare as a complication of spinal surgery; no case series has been reported nor have incidence statistics been published. The incidence and clinical features of this illness were described.

Methods.—The records of all patients in Auckland, New Zealand, who showed bacterial meningitis after spinal surgery in 1990 through 1992 were reviewed retrospectively. A total of 2,180 spinal operations (excluding those involving planned durotomy) were performed during this period. Postsurgical bacterial meningitis developed in 4 of these patients, for an overall incidence rate of 0.18%.

Case Report 1.—Woman, 78, underwent elective decompression and fusion from L4 to the sacrum for severe spinal stenosis. A small hematoma discharged from the wound 10 days after surgery. Fourteen days after surgery, she showed clinical signs of meningitis. *Escherichia coli* was isolated from the aspirated hematoma, and deep wound infection with associated bacterial meningitis was diagnosed.

Case Report 2.—Man, 27, underwent elective decompression of the L5 and S1 nerve roots for persistent right-sided radicular pain. Clinical signs of meningitis appeared within 7 days after surgery. *Staphylococcus aureus* was isolated from pus near the wound.

Case Report 3.—Woman, 69, underwent elective laminectomy and bilateral foraminotomy from C5 to C7 for treatment of cervical spondylosis and radicular compression. Clinical signs of meningitis appeared on the sixth postsurgical day. *S. aureus* and *Staphylococcus epidermidis* were cultured from wound pus.

Case Report 4.—Man, 53, experienced accidental durotomy during a second elective L4–L5 diskectomy and showed a persistent leak of CSF. A redivac drain was placed on day 11 and removed on day 15; on day 16, the patient showed clinical signs of meningitis. *Streptococcus faecalis* was isolated from aspirated CSF.

Discussion.—These data indicate that the incidence of meningitis is ten-fold less than the recognized incidence of post–spinal surgery wound infection. All patients recovered with appropriate antibiotic therapy. A CSF leak was found in only 1 patient. Meningitis after spinal surgery occurred in association with deep wound infection. Prophylactic antibiotics might reduce the incidence of meningitis after spinal surgery. Outcome for these patients was good; factors that may improve prognosis include early diagnosis, prompt drainage and lavage of the wound, intensive care support, and advice on optimal antimicrobial therapy from infectious disease physicians.

▶ Infection after spinal surgery is an unfortunate complication. True meningitis is often talked about as 1 type of infection. This article demonstrates that the actual incidence is small, and then describes a practical approach to handling the problem that is useful.

S.W. Wiesel, M.D.

Deep Vein Thrombosis After Major Reconstructive Spinal Surgery
Rokito SE, Schwartz MC, Neuwirth MG (Orthopaedic Inst, New York)
Spine 21:853–859, 1996   4–7

Background.—Deep venous thrombosis (DVT) is a serious complication of major surgery, but its incidence and prophylaxis in association with spinal surgery have not been thoroughly investigated. Reported incidences of thrombotic complications after spinal surgery have ranged from 0.9% to 14%. To determine better the incidence of DVT after major spinal surgery in adults and to evaluate modes of prophylaxis, patients undergoing major reconstructive spinal surgery were evaluated prospectively.

Methods.—Of the 329 patients evaluated, 110 were randomly allocated to receive 1 of 3 different forms of DVT prophylaxis and to undergo duplex Doppler scanning between the fifth and seventh postoperative days. Forms of prophylaxis included bilateral thigh-high thrombosis embolic deterrent (TED) depression stockings, TED stockings and thigh-length cuffs that provided sequential pneumatic compression to the calf and thigh, or TED stockings and low-dose coumadin. The remaining 219 patients received DVT prophylaxis according to the preference of their surgeon. Patients were monitored for clinical signs and symptoms of DVT; total duration of clinical follow-up was at least 1 year.

Results.—Duplex scans performed in patients who received randomized prophylaxis were normal in 109; the remaining scan was initially indeterminate, but the results of a follow-up venogram were negative. All these patients were clinically asymptomatic. Excessive blood loss was experienced by 2 patients who received low-dose coumadin (5.7%). One clinically detectable proximal DVT (confirmed by duplex ultrasonography) was detected in a patient from the nonrandomized group. The only perioperative form of prophylaxis used by this patient was graduated compression stockings worn during hospitalization. Overall incidence of DVT among these 329 patients was 0.3%.

Conclusions.—The incidence of DVT in adult reconstructive spinal surgery patients appears low; hence, routine screening for asymptomatic thrombi may be unwarranted. Mechanical prophylaxis with graduated compression stockings and pneumatic compression boots appears preferable to anticoagulation therapy.

▶ The complication of phlebitis with subsequent pulmonary embolus is an ever-present problem in orthopedic surgery. In spinal surgery, the prophylactic treatment of DVT can lead to complications, such as an epidural hematoma, in and of itself. This study demonstrated that the incidence (0.3%) is so low that prophylaxis with medication in most cases is probably not indicated. Mechanical prophylaxis, such as compression stockings or pneumatic compression boots, has little to no downside risk and is appropriate.

S.W. Wiesel, M.D.

Superior Gluteal Artery Injury During Iliac Bone Grafting for Spinal Fusion

Lim EVA, Lavadia WT, Roberts JM (Univ of Cincinnati, Ohio; Cincinnati Orthopaedic and Spine Inst, Ohio)
Spine 21:2376–2378, 1996   4–8

Background.—A few cases of damage through the superior gluteal artery during bone graft harvesting have been reported in the literature. Direct vessel ligation is performed to manage this complication. A patient sustained injury to the superior gluteal artery during iliac bone grafting for spinal fusion.

Case Report.—Woman, 33, was treated for degenerative, end-stage collapse of the L4–L5 disk space associated with foraminal stenosis and nerve root entrapment. Surgery was performed through a posterior midline approach. After decompression, trans-pedicular screws and instrumentation were inserted from L4 to S1. The iliac crest was easily palpated through the same midline incision and approached subcutaneously. The corticocancellous iliac crest bone graft was readily obtained. When bone graft harvesting was completed, a great deal of bleeding was noted. Although the source could not be pinpointed, it appeared to be coming from the sciatic notch. Because the patient was obese, the consulting vascular surgeon thought that neither a posterior nor anterior approach to the vessel was appropriate. The wound was closed superficially with packing in place, and the patient was taken to the angiography suite. The catheter was advanced into the superior gluteal vessel through the contralateral femoral artery, and dye extravasated readily. An arteriovenous fistula indicated the presence of a traumatic injury to the superior gluteal vein. After selective coil emobilization of the superior gluteal artery, repeat angiography showed rapid cessation of bleeding and no additional dye extravasation. The next day, the initial procedure could be completed. Subsequently the patient recovered with no complications. A solid fusion was obtained.

Conclusions.—Injury to the superior gluteal artery during elective bone graft surgery is avoidable. In the current patient, therapeutic arterial embolization successfully controlled hemorrhage. Radiographically guided arterial embolization of the lacerated vessel was a fast and effective treatment of this potentially fatal complication.

▶ Harvesting of bone graft, whether anteriorly or posteriorly, is not an innocuous procedure. This article calls attention to the fact that significant complications can occur and presents an interesting way of handling an injury to the superior gluteal artery. I thought this was innovative. One should keep this article's advice in one's armamentarium.

S.W. Wiesel, M.D.

Perioperative Complications of Anterior Procedures on the Spine
McDonnell MF, Glassman SD, Dimar JR II, et al (Univ of Louisville, Ky)
J Bone Joint Surg Am 78A:839–847, 1996   4–9

Introduction.—Anterior procedures on the spine are thought to involve risk in certain patient populations, but no previous study has focused on the perioperative complications of these procedures. The operative and hospital records of 447 patients were reviewed to determine the prevalence and types of complications associated with anterior procedures on the spine for deformity, fracture, tumor, or infection.

Methods.—Patients underwent procedures on the thoracic, thoracolumbar, or lumbar spine between 1985 and 1992. Diagnoses included idiopathic scoliosis in 100 adolescent or young adults, scoliosis in 63 mature adult patients, kyphosis in 61, neuromuscular scoliosis in 60, fracture in 47, a revision procedure in 39, tumor in 19, and vertebral osteomyelitis or diskitis in 8 patients. The anterior procedures were classified as combined, staged, or isolated. Complications were evaluated according to severity (major or minor) and type. Patients were divided into 4 age groups: 213 were 20 years of age or younger, 111 were 21 to 40 years of age, 98 were 41 to 60 years of age, and 25 were 61 to 85 years of age.

Results.—There were 60 major and 124 minor complications in 31% of the patients. The 2 postoperative deaths (0.4%) were the result of major pulmonary complications. Most of the major complications (37%) were categorized as pulmonary; genito-urinary problems accounted for 42% of minor complications. Patients with neuromuscular scoliosis had the highest rate of complications overall (52%) and of both major (18%) and minor (38%) complications. The lowest rate of complications was in young adults and adolescents with idiopathic scoliosis (16% overall, 3% major, and 14% minor). Type of operative procedure had a significant effect on blood loss and duration of operation, but not on the rate of complications. Combined procedures were associated with significantly more complications than staged or isolated procedures. In multivariate analysis, both combined procedures and an estimated blood loss >520 mL increased the risk of major complications. An age of 61 to 85 was associated with increased risk, whereas idiopathic scoliosis in patients 29 years of age or younger was associated with reduced risk of complications.

Discussion.—The rate of complications after anterior procedures on the spine compares favorably with that for other major orthopedic and non-orthopedic operations. Risk is increased in patients with a diagnosis of neuromuscular scoliosis, in those 61 years of age or older, when blood loss exceeds 520 mL, and when combined anterior and posterior procedures are performed.

▶ A large number of patients (447) with anterior procedures on their spine were reviewed. The complication rate was over 30% and this article nicely demonstrated that anterior procedures on the spine should be undertaken with caution. Its conclusion that these procedures are relatively safe should be put in context. I think that an anterior procedure for a tumor or an infection is certainly indicated. Anyone who starts to think about these procedures for degenerative disease should at least pause after they read this article and realize that the complication rate in some instances may out weigh the potential benefits for degenerative disk disease and its relief of symptoms.

S.W. Wiesel, M.D.

Tophaceous Gout of the Lumbar Spine Mimicking an Epidural Abscess: MR Features

Bonaldi VM, Duong H, Starr MR, et al (McGill Univ, Montreal; Anna Laberge Hosp, Quebec)
AJNR Am J Neuroradiol 17:1949–1952, 1996   4–10

Introduction.—Spinal involvement in tophaceous gout is not common, and the diagnosis often is missed before surgery. A case of tophaceous gout of the lumbar spine had cauda equina compression that mimicked an epidural abscess.

Case Report.—Man, 76, with long-standing peripheral gouty arthritis, was seen with a 1-week history of fever and lower back pain. Physical examination revealed tenderness to palpation on the right side. Multiple tophi were noted on the periphery, with a purulent discharge from the right big toe. Blood cultures were positive and antibiotics were given. Computed tomography scans showed spinal stenosis at the L3–L4 and L4–L5 levels. Laboratory findings included leukocytosis and elevated levels of serum uric acid. After 17 days, the patient's blood cultures were negative but back pain continued. Lumbar spine MR revealed an abnormal anterior epidural collection extending from the L3 to L4 levels, causing cauda equina compression (Fig 1). On T1-weighted images, the intensity was like soft tissue, but on T2-weighted images, it was relatively hyperintense. After contrast material was administered, the collection appeared multiloculated. These findings suggested infectious spondylodiskitis with an epidural abscess. Laminectomy did not reveal the expected abscess but uncovered a chalky granular substance. Multiple open biopsy specimens were collected, and histologic examination was consistent with tophaceous gout. The patient was treated with colchicine followed by allopurinol. Fever was alleviated, and the patient was discharged in stable condition.

Conclusion.—Findings such as those presented in this case report in patients with gouty arthritis and no neurologic symptoms should lead to suspicion of gouty involvement of the spine and permit more rapid diagnosis and treatment.

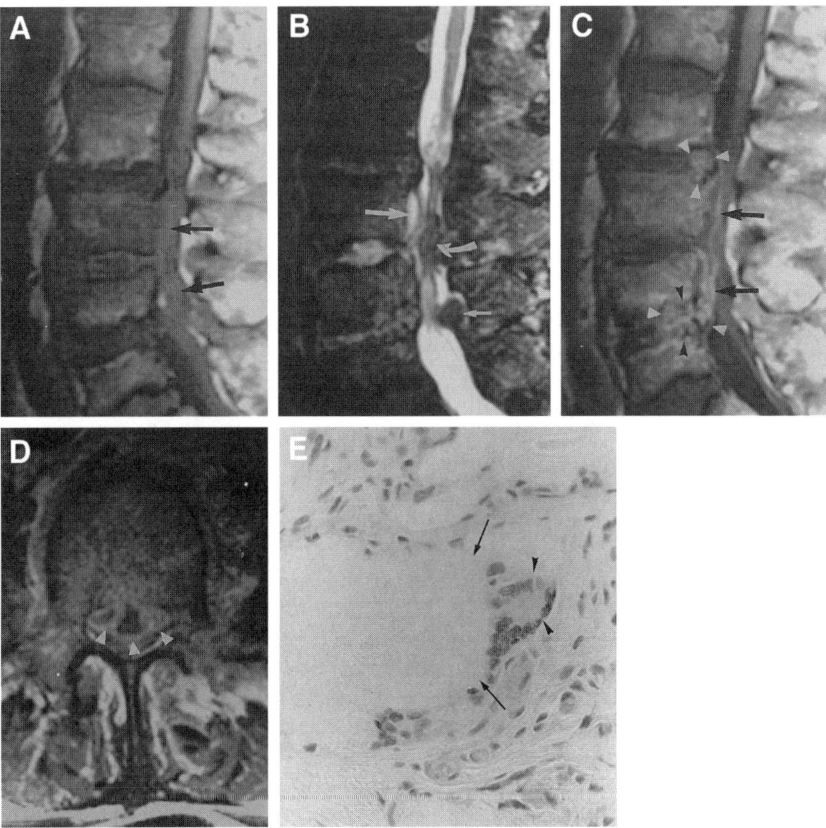

FIGURE 1.—Man, 76 years, with long-standing peripheral gouty arthritis and 1-week history of persistent fever and severe lower back pain. **A,** sagittal spin-echo T1-weighted (500/200 [repetition time/echo time]) MR image of the lumbar spine shows cauda equina compression by an epidural soft-tissue-intensity lesion at L3 and L4 (*arrows*). Note also herniation of the L2–L3 and L4–L5 disk and erosive changes at the L4 and L5 vertebral endplates. **B,** sagittal fast spin-echo T2-weighted (4000/102) MR image (echo train length, 8) of the lumbar spine shows abnormal hyperintense signal of the epidural collection at L3 (*long arrow*) and of the L3–L4 and L4–L5 intervertebral disks. Note the hypointense appearance of the compressed roots of the cauda equina (*curved arrow*). The hypointense structure at the posterior aspect of the spinal canal at L4–L5 represents partial volume averaging of the posterior elements (*short arrow*). **C,** contrast-enhanced sagittal spin-echo T1-weighted (500/20) MR image of the lumbar spine shows marginal enhancement of the epidural collection (*arrows*) and focal enhancement of the L2–L3 and L4–L5 disks and the L4 and L5 vertebral endplates (*arrowheads*). The L5 vertebral body is mildly compressed. **D,** contrast-enhanced axial spin-echo T1-weighted (500/20) MR image of the lumbar spine at L3 shows severe dural sac compression by the multiloculated epidural collection representing gouty tophaceous deposits (*arrowheads*). **E,** photomicrograph of biopsy specimen from the L2–L3 disk shows a large giant cell (*arrowheads*) adjacent to a tophaceous deposit (*arrows*). Several other multinucleated giant cells also are present; original magnification, ×200. (Courtesy of Bonaldi VM, Duong H, Starr MR, et al: Tophaceous gout of the lumbar spine mimicking epidural abscess: MR features *AJNR* 17(10):1949–1952, 1996, Copyright by American Society of Neuroradiology.)

▶ The key to appropriate treatment of any spinal condition is the correct diagnosis. One must always be on the alert for the unusual presentation of a disease as a routine low back condition. This particular article shows how gout can affect the spinal canal and be seen as a low back problem.

S.W. Wiesel, M.D.

Bone Graft

The Use of Bone Allografts in the Spine

Buttermann GR, Glazer PA, Bradford DS (Univ of California, San Francisco)
Clin Orthop 324:75–85, 1996   4–11

Background.—Bone allografts are used in spinal surgery primarily when insufficient autograft bone is available or when a structural element, such as an interbody graft that spans 1 disk space or a strut graft that spans more than 2 levels, is needed. Use of allografts avoids the donor-site discomfort and morbidity associated with autograft harvesting. Type of allograft bone used, patient age, and anatomical site influence the success of the fusion.

Applications.—Allograft bone is generally used for fusion in the posterior spine and for structural purposes in the anterior spine. Interbody allografts in the anterior cervical spine appear most effective for single-level fusions. Interbody autografts yield better results than do interbody allografts for multilevel fusions of cervical spine. For posterior cervical fusions, freeze-dried allograft bone should not be used.

Structural allografts in both interbody and strut-grafting procedures have been useful for deformity in the thoracolumbar region. For posterior thoracolumbar spinal fusions, the literature supports use of allograft bone in conjunction with segmental instrumentation. For pediatric deformity fusion procedures, use of cancellous allograft bone, especially if fresh-frozen, appears clinically comparable to that of iliac autograft bone. (Fusion rates are higher with fresh-frozen than with freeze-dried allografts; poor results are obtained with ethylene-oxide sterilized allografts.) In adults, marginal results occur with posterior fusion of allograft; in thoracolumbar deformity reconstructive procedures, anterior fusion with structural allografts may be done successfully, although supplementation with posterior instrumented fusions is recommended.

For posterolateral lumbar fusion in the adult patient, iliac autograft is the bone graft of choice. For anterior lumbar interbody fusions, maintenance of intervertebral distraction (despite delayed incorporation) has been achieved with structural allografts, such as femoral ring allografts.

Conclusions.—Allograft bone plays an important role in spinal surgery. Indications for use of allograft bone may evolve with the clinical availability of osteoinductive proteins, which may supplement or replace nonstructural allograft bone. The role of structural allografts may also change with use of supplemental osteoinductive protein and further evaluation of anterior interbody implants.

▶ There is continuous division of opinion regarding whether one should use allografts or autografts in spinal fusions. This study nicely demonstrates that allografts do have a place if the particular situation is selectively chosen. I personally believe that the use of an allograft can be undertaken but, as these authors indicate, only in specific situations.

S.W. Wiesel, M.D.

The Use of an Osteoinductive Growth Factor for Lumbar Spinal Fusion: Part I: Biology of Spinal Fusion
Boden SD, Schimandle JH, Hutton WC, et al (Emory Univ, Decatur, Ga; Veterans Affairs Med Ctr, Atlanta, Ga)
Spine 20:2626–2632, 1995   4–12

Introduction.—Posterolateral intertransverse process fusion is the most commonly performed type of lumbar spine fusion. Although the operation is usually successful, reported nonunion rates range as high as 35%. Biological methods of enhancing spinal fusion are being investigated as a means of overcoming the problem of nonunion. This 2-part study analyzed the histologic process of spinal fusion and then examined the use of an osteoinductive growth factor to enhance fusion.

Histologic Study.—The initial histologic study involved single-level posterolateral lumbar intertransverse process arthrodeses with iliac bone grafts in New Zealand white rabbits—a well-validated animal model. Histologic and quantitative analyses revealed 3 distinct and sequential phases of healing: inflammatory, reparative, and remodeling. All 3 processes were delayed in the central zone of the fusion mass compared with the outer transverse process zone. Healing occurred mainly through membranous bone formation, which first appeared at the ends of the fusion, emanating from the decorticated transverse processes., During weeks 3 and 4, the central zone underwent a period of endochondral bone formation in which cartilage formed and was converted to bone. By 10 weeks, the central and transverse process zones showed a similar extent of remodeling.

Growth Factor Study.—The second part of the study evaluated the effects of a bovine-derived osteoinductive bone protein extract delivered in various carrier materials and at varying doses. The experiments involved single-level posterolateral intertransverse process lumbar spinal arthrodeses performed in rabbits and rhesus macaques. In the rabbits, successful spinal fusions were demonstrated by manual palpation, radiography, biomechanical testing, and light microscopic examination. Both the bone protein and carriers were required to achieve solid fusion; stronger fusions were obtained when bone protein was delivered with carol or demineralized bone matrix than with autograft bone. This model showed a dose-dependent response to the osteoinductive growth factor. The technique was successfully extended to the macaques, which is important because of the relatively lower bone regeneration potential of primates. Monkeys treated with osteoinductive growth factor in a demineralized bone matrix carrier had spinal fusion within 12 wccks. Again, the effect of inducing new trabecular bone was dose dependent. The bone concentration needed to induce adequate bone formation in the monkey spine was 8 times higher than that required in rabbits, however.

Conclusion.—The histologic study shows that various factors related to the decorticated host bone and exposed marrow can affect lumbar intertransverse process spinal fusion and that some cases of nonunion may be related to a persistent central cartilage zone. The osteoinductive growth factor study shows that biological enhancement of spinal fusion is possible with implantation of both bone protein and a suitable carrier. The success of this technique in a primate model suggests that biological enhancement of spinal fusion may be achievable in humans.

The Use of an Osteoinductive Growth Factor for Lumbar Spinal Fusion: Part II: Study of Dose, Carrier, and Species
Boden SD, Schimandle JH, Hutton WC (Emory Univ, Decatur, Ga; Yerkes Regional Primate Ctr, Atlanta, Ga; Veterans Affairs Med Ctr, Atlanta, Ga)
Spine 20:2633–2644, 1995   4–13

Introduction.—Biological enhancement of spinal fusion could decrease the rate of nonunion in patients undergoing posterolateral lumbar spinal fusion. A bovine-derived osteoinductive growth factor to enhance lumbar fusion was studied in a rabbit model and in a nonhuman primate model. Investigators sought to determine the minimum effective dose of growth factor and the influence of different carrier materials on outcome.

Methods.—Experiments were carried out in 115 adult New Zealand white rabbits and 10 adult rhesus macaques. The animals underwent single-level posterolateral intertransverse process lumbar spinal arthrodesis to evaluate the different doses and carrier materials. Thirty-two rabbits received either 100 or 300 µg of an osteoinductive bone protein extract delivered in 1.2 g of rabbit demineralized bone matrix (DBM) carrier. The remaining 83 rabbits were randomized to receive 1 of 3 carrier materials: autogenous iliac bone, DBM, or Biocoral (a natural coral). Half received the carrier alone and half received 300 µg of the same growth factor. The monkeys were implanted with DBM carrier alone or DBM plus bone protein (3000, 6000, or 10,000 µg). Rabbit fusion masses were evaluated 5 weeks and monkey fusion masses 12 weeks after arthrodesis.

Results.—Manual palpation, radiography, biomechanical testing, and light microscopy confirmed successful posterolateral intertransverse process spinal fusions in the rabbit model. Response to the osteoinductive growth factor was dose dependent. The methodology transferred successfully to the rhesus monkey, an important consideration because the potential of bone regeneration is diminished in primates as compared with phylogenetically lower animals. In monkeys, spinal fusion was achieved in 12 weeks with use of the osteoinductive growth factor plus a demineralized bone matrix carrier.

Discussion.—The rabbit model demonstrated that solid fusion depended on implantation of both the bone protein and carriers. Bone protein delivered with either coral or DBM achieved fusion with a higher load to failure than did fusion achieved with an autograft. When compared with the rabbit, an 8-fold increase in bone protein concentration was needed to induce adequate bone formation in the rhesus monkey spine. The success of fusion in the rhesus monkey should contribute to the development of biological enhancement of spinal fusion in humans.

▶ The development of a bone-inductive substance is getting closer. This article reports on a bone morphogenic protein factor that can induce bone growth in a rabbit model as well as a monkey model. I believe that spinal fusions for degenerative disease will evolve in the next decade to the use of some form of bone morphogenic protein as the initiator of spinal fusion. This study is important in the sense that it demonstrates the evolution of this technique.

S.W. Wiesel, M.D.

Infection

Spinal Tuberculosis in Developed Countries: Difficulties in Diagnosis
Hayes AJ, Choksey M, Barnes N, et al (East London Tuberculosis Centre, London; London Chest Hosps, Whitechapel, London)
J R Coll Surg Edinb 41:192–196, 1996   4–14

Objective.—Surgery is advocated for patients with neurologic deficits, but some studies suggest that conservative treatment alone can be beneficial. Twenty-one cases of spinal tuberculosis (TB) were reviewed for the diagnostic methods employed, treatment options, surgical approaches, and outcome.

Methods.—The patients, 11 men and 10 women, were seen at the Royal London Hospital between 1985 and 1992. Data collected included patient age and racial origin, signs and symptoms of the disease, and findings of laboratory and radiographic studies. All but 1 patient were followed for 18 months. Outcome was considered favorable if the patient was pain-free, able to lead an independent life, had no significant neurologic deficit and no clinical evidence of sinuses, abscesses, or active TB; and had radiologically quiescent disease.

Results.—Spinal TB is much more common in developing countries than in the developed world. There was only 1 Caucasian in this series of patients; 16 were of Asian origin, 3 were African, and 1 was Vietnamese. The average age of the group was 38 years. Most patients experienced back pain and 15 also reported systemic symptoms. Neurologic deficits were present in 9 patients at admission and developed in 3 more during treatment. All patients had a raised erythrocyte sedimentation rate and a mild normocytic anemia. Pus or biopsy material was required for a microbiological diagnosis. Radiography often suggested metastatic cancer; only 8 patients had findings that allowed a confident diagnosis.

All patients received rifampicin, pyrazinamide, and isoniazid and 12 were also treated with intramuscular streptomycin. Treatment continued for 1 to 2 years, with the exception of pyrazinamide and streptomycin, which were discontinued by 3 months. Decompressive surgery was performed in 10 of the 12 patients with neurologic deficits. Eight initially had laminectomies and 2 had anterior fusion. Anterior fusion was subsequently performed in 4 patients who had undergone laminectomy. The second operation was required to limit kyphosis or because of a lack of neurologic improvement. Outcome was favorable in 19 patients.

Conclusion.—Spinal TB can be difficult to diagnose in the developed world because it is seen infrequently and can appear to be disseminated cancer. Diagnosis can be confirmed by tissue biopsy. Surgical treatment is indicated when neurologic deficits are present. The level of compression should be identified at preoperative imaging.

▶ It is important to be aware of spinal TB. This article nicely reviews the difficulty in diagnosis. The most important aspect is to think of the problem, and then it usually can be diagnosed without difficulty. Tuberculosis has become more and more common, and it needs to be very prevalent in our differential diagnosis.

S.W. Wiesel, M.D.

Pott's Paraplegia: 67 Cases
Moon M-S, Ha K-Y, Sun D-H, et al (Catholic Univ, Seoul, Korea)
Clin Orthop 323:122–128, 1996   4–15

Background.—Spinal deformity or paraplegia may occur as complications of tuberculosis of the spine. Two treatment approaches have been adopted for these cases of Pott's paraplegia: the conservative medical approach and the radical surgical approach. Results of both treatment approaches have varied widely. The effectiveness of these approaches was evaluated in patients who had early and late paraplegia.

Methods.—The records of 67 patients who had Pott's paraplegia that was treated since 1980 were reviewed. The patients included 9 children and 58 adults. Fifty-five adults and all 9 children had active tuberculosis seen within 2 weeks after the onset of paraplegia. The other 3 patients had healed tuberculosis, moderate to severe deformity, and gradual-onset complete paraplegia seen 3–6 months after onset of paraplegia. The indications for conservative treatment included children and adults with poor general conditions, minimal deformity, early and less severe paralysis with normal MRI scans of cord condition, and adult patients who refused surgery. Thirteen patients were treated with triple antituberculosis chemotherapy (isoniazid, ethambutol, and rifampicin) alone. Fifty-four patients underwent surgical treatment, including anterior radical surgery in 52 patients and posterior surgery in 2.

Results.—Overall, 93.8% of patients who had active tuberculosis had neurologic recovery. Only 1 patient who had healed tuberculosis and underwent a combined 2-stage procedure had minimal recovery; the other

2 patients had no recovery. All 13 conservatively treated patients, including 4 adults and the 9 children, had complete neurologic recovery, as did 45 of the 54 surgically treated patients. Neurologic recovery occurred in 2–6 months in adults and in 1–4 months in children treated conservatively. Among the surgically treated patients, neurologic recovery occurred within 2 months, with the quickest recovery in those who underwent the combined 2-stage procedure.

Conclusions.—In patients who have active disease, paraplegia can be treated successfully with either conservative treatment or surgical treatment, with careful patient selection of those receiving conservative treatment. The combined 2-stage surgical procedure is most useful for patients who have slight to moderate deformity. Because successful treatment is unlikely in patients who have paraplegia caused by healing in severely deformed spine, even with radical surgery, it is important to establish a diagnosis early.

▶ Tuberculosis is again being encountered in the spine. This is especially true in big city hospitals. In this study, patients who had chemotherapy were compared with those who had chemotherapy plus surgical intervention. Both regimens have their indications, and I think that the authors did a nice job in listing the indications for surgery as opposed to those for chemotherapy alone.

S.W. Wiesel, M.D.

Pathophysiology

Myeloscopic Observation of Adhesive Arachnoiditis in Patients With Lumbar Spinal Canal Stenosis
Kawauchi Y, Yone K, Sakou T (Kagoshima Univ, Japan)
Spinal Cord 34:403–410, 1996   4–16

Introduction.—A major factor that contributes to recovery after lumbar spinal canal stenosis (LSS) surgery is the severity of a patient's associated adhesive arachnoiditis. Success of the operation can often be predicted if the extent of adhesive arachnoiditis is accurately diagnosed. A myeloscope was used to examine 36 patients with LSS who were scheduled for surgery.

Patients and Methods.—The patients, 24 men and 12 women, ranged from 39 to 78 years of age. Ten had a degenerative type of LSS, 15 had the combined type, and 4 had the posttraumatic type. Symptoms in all cases had persisted despite conservative treatment. Twenty-nine patients had a partial laminectomy and 7 underwent total laminectomy. Myeloscopic examination, performed 1 or 2 weeks before surgery, was used to classify the degree of adhesive arachnoiditis as slight, moderate, or marked. Patients were evaluated for a mean period of 2 years and 9 months after surgery. Outcome was judged as good, fair, or poor according to Stauffer's criteria.

Results.—Adhesive arachnoiditis was slight in 7 patients, moderate in 16, and marked in 13. The degree of adhesive arachnoiditis was not significantly influenced by age, duration of symptoms, severity of clinical symptoms before surgery, or type of LSS. Both nocturnal pains and burning pains, however, affected only patients with moderate or marked adhesions. Patients whose myelograms revealed severe stenosis often had moderate or marked adhesions. Postoperative results were distinctly worse in patients with marked adhesions than in those with slight or moderate adhesions.

Discussion.—Adhesive arachnoiditis appears to be a major influence on postoperative results in LSS surgery. In this series of patients, good postoperative recovery was rare in those with marked adhesions. The marked adhesions discovered at myeloscopy may indicate a blocked cauda equina. Myeloscopy is useful to diagnose the extent of adhesions and predict the results of LSS surgery.

▶ This is a very interesting article. It examines severe LSS patients and demonstrates that they actually have scar tissue in the dura before any surgery is performed and that the worse the scar tissue, the worse the results. Additionally, it makes use of a new technical tool, the myeloscope, which I think will be involved in more and more of our procedures. It may certainly be used more often as a diagnostic procedure.

S.W. Wiesel, M.D.

Determinants of Lumbar Disc Degeneration: A Study Relating Lifetime Exposures and Magnetic Resonance Imaging Findings in Identical Twins
Battié MC, Videman T, Gibbons LE, et al (Univ of Alberta, Edmonton, Canada; Univ of Helsinki; Univ of Jyväskylä, Finland; et al)
Spine 20:2601–2612, 1995   4–17

Introduction.—The causes of most back symptoms are unknown. However, structural and biochemical changes associated with disk degeneration are strongly suspected to be the cause of back pain, particularly when associated with radicular pain. Several factors have been suggested as accelerators of degenerative disk changes. The effects of lifetime exposures to these commonly suspected risk factors on disk degeneration were studied in twins examined with MRI.

Methods.—Identical twin pairs were selected from the Finnish Twin Cohort. Data collected previously indicated discordance in the selected twin pairs in 1 of the following 5 risk factors: occupational materials handling, sedentary work, exercise participation, vehicular vibration, and cigarette smoking. A detailed, structured interview was conducted with each participant to review the lifetime work history and to collect data on sport and leisure time activities. Each job was then categorized by the type and degree of physical loading, and leisure time physical loading was evaluated. The participants were asked about their histories of back pain. All were examined with MRI to evaluate disk degeneration. The influence of the risk factors and the effects of twinship on the MRI findings were analyzed.

Results.—The identified risk factors were stronger determinants of upper than of lower lumbar disk degeneration. The only statistically significant associations were between disk height narrowing and occupational physical loading and between decreased signal intensity and greater leisure time physical loading. In multivariate analyses, occupational physical loading was the only significant predictor of twin differences in upper lumbar disk degeneration, and there were no significant predictors of twin differences in the lower lumbar region. Twinship, which reflects the influences of genetics and early shared environment, accounted for most variability in disk degeneration in both the upper and lower lumbar regions.

Conclusions.—The widely suspected environmental and behavioral factors have little effect on the process of disk degeneration. Disk degeneration is likely to be most dependent on genetic and early environmental influences, as well as on unidentified factors.

▶ This is an absolutely outstanding article. The authors gathered a unique set of individuals to study whether genetics or environmental influence is the most important in determining disk degeneration. The conclusion that genetics is the most important factor is, I think, extremely important as we advise our patients. This study was eloquently done.

S.W. Wiesel, M.D.

Orientation of the Lumbar Facet Joints: Association With Degenerative Disc Disease

Boden SD, Riew KD, Yamaguchi K, et al (Emory Univ, Atlanta, Ga)
J Bone Joint Surg (Am) 78A:403–411, 1996   4–18

Background.—The relationship betweeen facet tropism and intervertebral disk disease and between the orientation of the facet and degenerative spondylolisthesis is controversial, largely because of the lack of true normal controls in the studies. Magnetic resonance imaging has made it possible to identify true normal controls from an asymptomatic population. A technique for measuring the orientation of the lumbar facet joints on MR images was developed and validated, and the relationships between facet tropism and orientation and herniated disks and degenerative spondylolisthesis were analyzed.

Methods.—Magnetic resonance imaging scans were obtained of the lumbar spines of 46 asymptomatic volunteers who did not have a herniated disk, 21 asymptomatic volunteers who had a herniated disc, 46 patients who had operatively confirmed disk herniation, and 27 patients who had degenerative spondylolisthesis at the level of the fourth and fifth lumbar vertebrae. On axial MR images, the facet joint angle relative to the coronal plane was measured, and the difference between the right and left facet angles were calculated to determine tropism. The technique was validated by comparison with CT scans of 30 facet joints and by calculation of intra- and interobserver correlation. The median facet tropism was determined for each group, and the relationship between facet tropism at each level and disk herniation and between facet orientation at each level and degenerative spondylolisthesis was analyzed.

Results.—There was high intra- and interobserver correlation and high correlation between MRI and CT measurements of facet angles. The median facet tropism was significantly higher in patients who had confirmed disk herniation than in asymptomatic individuals who did not have disk herniation. The relationship between disk herniation and the severity of facet tropism was significant only in symptomatic patients who had herniated disks at the level of the fourth or fifth lumbar vertebrae. A sagittal orientation of more than 45 degrees in both the left and right facet joints at the level of the fourth and fifth lumbar vertebrae was significantly associated with symptomatic disk herniation at that level, which increased the odds ratio to 2.9. Patients who had degenerative spondylolisthesis also had a significantly greater mean facet angle than did the asymptomatic individuals, particularly at the level of the slip. A sagittal orientation of more than 45 degrees of both the left and right facets was strongly related to degenerative spondylolisthesis; this orientation occurred in 22 of 27 patients, compared with 10 of 66 asymptomatic individuals.

Conclusions.—Patients who have herniated disks have a doubled magnitude of facet tropism at the level of the fourth and fifth lumbar vertebrae compared with asymptomatic individuals. Significant sagittal orientation of the facet joints at the level of the fourth and fifth lumbar vertebrae is highly associated with both disk herniation and degenerative spondylolisthesis. Because facet sagittal orientation occurred both at involved vertebrae and at levels with no evidence of degenerative spondylolisthesis, this orientation is probably part of the pre-existing morphology rather than secondary to the spondylolisthesis.

▶ As our population lives longer, we are seeing more and more patients who have degenerative spondylolisthesis at the L4-5 level. In addition, some of these patients undergo simple laminectomy for herniated disk earlier in life. This study nicely demonstrates that if the facet joint angles are more than 45 degrees relative to the coronal plane, degenerative spondylolisthesis is 25 times more likely to develop over time. This raises the question of whether a patient should have a bilateral lateral fusion with this finding if he or she has to have a simple laminectomy early in life. Long-term follow-up is necessary.

S.W. Wiesel, M.D.

Is Pathology Examination of Disc Specimens Necessary After Routine Anterior Cervical Discectomy and Fusion?
Daftari TK, Levine J, Fischgrund JS, et al (Georgia Orthopaedics Sports Medicine, Austell; Nova Southeastern Univ, Miami, Fla; William Beaumont Hosp, Royal Oak, Mich)
Spine 21:2156–2159, 1996   4–19

Background.—Most hospital and nursing policies require routine submission of disk specimens obtained during anterior cervical diskectomy and fusion for histologic examination. However, there have been no published studies examining the need for routine pathologic examination of disk specimens in this setting. To investigate this need, the outcomes of these pathologic examinations were studied retrospectively.

Methods.—A total of 394 patients undergoing cervical fusion and cervical diskectomy between 1990 and 1994 were identified, and their records were reviewed. Data were collected on symptoms, clinical and final diagnoses, and operative procedures.

Results.—All of the patients had symptoms and physical examination findings that were consistent with cervical radiculopathy. The clinical diagnoses included herniated cervical disk in 334, cervical spondylosis in 47, stenosis in 3, and other diagnoses (including neuritis, myelopathy, and spondylopathy) in 10. Operative findings in all patients were also consistent with a herniated soft disk or degenerative spondylosis. No operative reports contained unexpected findings suggesting an infectious or pathologic process. The pathology reports contained diagnoses including intervertebral disks, degenerative changes, and degenerative fibrocartilage, with occasional notations of calcification, cartilage, or vessels. There was complete concordance between the histologic and clinical diagnoses. By using a 95% confidence interval, the chance of a positive finding in 394 patients is 7.5 in 1,000.

Conclusions.—The concordance seen between histologic and clinical diagnoses suggests that disk specimens need not be routinely submitted for pathologic examination after anterior cervical diskectomy. Changing this policy would result in substantial savings in time and expense.

▶ In this era of managed care, we are all trying to look objectively at what tests are necessary. Our surgical training has embedded in us that it is always necessary to send our specimens to pathology. In many instances—particularly in the situation described in this paper—there is no information gathered that aids in the care of the patient. I thought the study was well done, and I firmly believe in the outcome. This probably can be translated to diskectomies in the lumbar spine as well but that study still needs to be performed.

S.W. Wiesel, M.D.

Osteoarthrosis of the Atlanto-Axial Joints: Long-Term Follow-up After Treatment With Arthrodesis

Ghanayem AJ, Leventhal M, Bohlman HH (Case Western Reserve Univ, Cleveland, Ohio; VA Med Ctr, Cleveland, Ohio)
J Bone Joint Surg Am 78A:1300–1306, 1996   4–20

Background.—Osteoarthrosis of the atlantoaxial joints without trauma is an uncommon cause of occipitocervical pain and atlantoaxial instability. A series of patients with occipitocervical pain caused by osteoarthrosis were treated with arthrodesis. The long-term results are reported.

Methods.—Fifteen patients with occipitocervical pain not diminished after nonoperative treatment and with osteoarthrosis of the atlantoaxial joints underwent an arthrodesis between 1973 and 1990. Four of the patients also had atlantoaxial instability. Their average age was 72 years (range, 54–86 years). The indications for surgery were refractory pain in 14 patients and acute quadriparesis in 1 patient. The procedures performed were posterior arthrodesis in 14 and anterior transoral arthrodesis in 1 patient. Two patients died: 1 of cardiopulmonary arrest 4 days after surgery and 1 of complications of bladder cancer 1 year and 8 months after surgery. The other 13 patients were monitored for an average of 7 years and 2 months. The radiographs were reviewed, as well as pain and functional outcome at the final follow-up.

Results.—Twelve of the 13 patients with long-term follow-up had solid fusion. The remaining patient had a pseudarthrosis without atlantoaxial instability. One patient had preoperative cerebellar degeneration that progressed postoperatively. The patient with quadriparesis recovered normal neurologic function. The remaining 11 patients maintained normal neurologic function. No patient had a poor result.

Conclusions.—A trial of nonoperative treatment with immobilization in a collar and analgesic medication is recommended as the initial management of patients with occipitocervical pain only. Arthrodesis can be safely performed with excellent long-term results in patients with refractory pain, instability, or neurologic deficit related to osteoarthrosis of the atlantoaxial joints.

▶ The incidence of primary arthritis between C1 and C2 is relatively low. However, the symptoms can be excruciating. This is a very nice series of patients who were treated with fusions. The study was well done and the outcomes well documented.

S.W. Wiesel, M.D.

Lumbar Motion Segment Pathology Adjacent to Thoracolumbar, Lumbar, and Lumbosacral Fusions

Schlegel JD, Smith JA, Schleusener RL (Univ of Utah, Salt Lake City)
Spine 21:970–981, 1996

4–21

Background.—There has been an increase in the number of surgical fusions of the lumbar spine, despite reports of poor results. In appropriately selected patients with certain categories of lumbar instability, however, spinal fusion can be successful. The records of 58 patients with symptoms that appeared more than 2 years after a previously fused thoracic or lumbosacral segment were reviewed to evaluate risk factors for adjacent segment abnormalities after an initially successful procedure.

Methods.—Principal diagnoses at the time of the index procedure were spinal stenosis in 25 patients, herniated nucleus pulposus in 18, kyphoscoliosis in 10, spondylolisthesis in 8, and spinal fracture in 5. The symptom-free period after spinal fusion averaged 13.1 years. Conservative treatment had failed to resolve severe back and leg pain, and all patients had functional limitations. Data analyzed included radiographs and other imaging studies, results of follow-up evaluations, and patient demographics.

Results.—The most common finding at follow-up was spinal stenosis (50 patients). In this group of patients, the segment adjacent to the adjacent segment was almost as likely to break down as the adjacent segment itself. Listhesis was present in 13 patients and herniated nucleus pulposus in 7; some were in a combined category. Thirty-seven patients were followed for 2 years after they sought treatment for late segmental abnormalities. Fourteen underwent a decompression and fusion procedure and 23 had a decompression procedure only; 7 required an additional surgical procedure during follow-up. Twenty-six of these patients described their current functional status as good or excellent.

Discussion.—The number of spinal fusions performed in the United States has grown at an increasingly rapid rate in recent years. In this series of patients, a long symptom-free period was followed by severe back and leg pain and functional limitations. When diagnostic category and surgical procedure were analyzed (decompression, decompression with fusion, decompression with fusion ± instrumentation), there appeared to be no significant trend in outcome. Time to breakdown was shorter in patients who had initially undergone floating fusion.

▶ Every time a free fusion is performed in the lumbar spine, one wonders if the level above or level below will eventually become unstable. This article definitively demonstrates that this is a real possibility, and not only should this be discussed in advance with the patient as a possibility, but as the patient is followed over time, appropriate x-ray examinations should be obtained. Once patients are fused, they should understand that they need to be followed long-term. In this particular study, the average instability occurred 13 years after the primary fusion.

S.W. Wiesel, M.D.

Treatment

Manipulation and Mobilization of the Cervical Spine: A Systematic Review of the Literature
Hurwitz EL, Aker PD, Adams AH, et al (RAND, Santa Monica, Calif; Univ of California, Los Angeles; Canadian Mem Chiropractic College, Toronto; et al)
Spine 21:1746–1760, 1996   4–22

Background.—Spinal manipulation and mobilization are common treatment modalities for patients with neck pain and headache. The efficacy of these approaches has been well documented in patients with low back pain but has not been widely studied in patients with neck pain and headache. The efficacy and complications of cervical spinal manipulation and mobilization in these patients were surveyed in a literature review.

Methods.—Computerized searches were done to identify 67 studies or reports addressing either the efficacy or complications of cervical spinal manipulation, mobilization, or both in patients with neck pain or headache. The reviewed studies included 14 randomized controlled trials, 2 cohort studies, 14 case series, and 37 case reports. The studies were assessed for quality. Efficacy was analyzed with the random effects method. Complication rates and types were analyzed.

Results.—Study quality varied, and many studies had significant methodological problems. There were no randomized trials assessing the efficacy of cervical spinal manipulation for the treatment of acute neck pain. However, limited data indicate a potential benefit associated with mobilization in patients with acute neck pain. Manipulation, mobilization, or physiotherapy all were shown to be more effective than muscle relaxants or usual medical care in the management of subacute or chronic neck pain, with manipulation probably the most effective approach. There also is some evidence that manipulation or mobilization can be beneficial in the management of headache, but the data are sparse and of poor quality.

Serious complications of cervical spinal manipulation occurred at a rate of 6 per 10 million manipulations, and death occurred at a rate of 3 per 10 million manipulations. Most of the complications of cervical spinal manipulation involved vertebrobasilar accidents that resulted in brain stem and/or cerebellar infarction, Wallenberg's syndrome, and locked-in syndrome. Other complications were spinal cord compression, vertebral fracture, tracheal rupture, diaphragm paralysis, internal carotid hematoma, and cardiac arrest.

Conclusions.—It is likely that mobilization has at least short-term benefits in the management of acute neck pain. Manipulation appears to be somewhat more effective than mobilization or physical therapy in the treatment of subacute or chronic neck pain. Either manipulation or mobilization may be effective in the management of muscle tension headache.

Complications are rare but must be considered because of their potential seriousness.

▶ This is an up-to-date overview of the indications of manipulation of the cervical spine. The references by themselves make it worth reviewing the article. Additionally, I thought the presentation of the complications of cervical manipulation was excellent. The bottom line is that there can be significant complications, although the percentage is low, and one should not undertake this therapeutic modality lightly.

S.W. Wiesel, M.D.

Cervical and Lumbar MRI in Asymptomatic Older Male Lifelong Athletes: Frequency of Degenerative Findings

Healy JF, Healy BB, Wong WHM, et al (Univ of California, San Diego)
J Comput Assist Tomogr 20:107–112, 1996   4–23

Background.—The cervical and lumbar spine are among the first areas to show evidence of degenerative joint disease on imaging studies. On MRI scans of the older spine, various abnormalities can be seen that produce no symptoms. These abnormalities may confuse the evaluation of spinal symptoms. The prevalence of asymptomatic abnormalities seen in cervical and lumbar spine imaging was determined.

Methods.—An MRI of the spine was performed in 19 male athletes between 41 and 69 years of age who were highly active. Participants were asymptomatic and were performing at their normal athletic activity. Spine, athletic, and sports injury histories were taken.

Results.—The prevalence of asymptomatic degenerative findings on MRI scans was similar to that seen in other populations. Degenerative

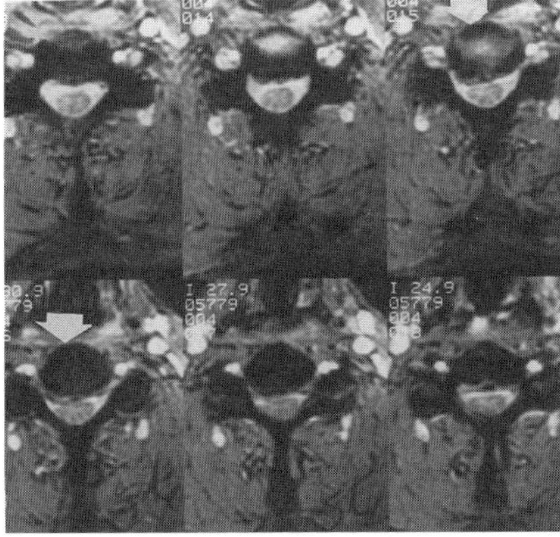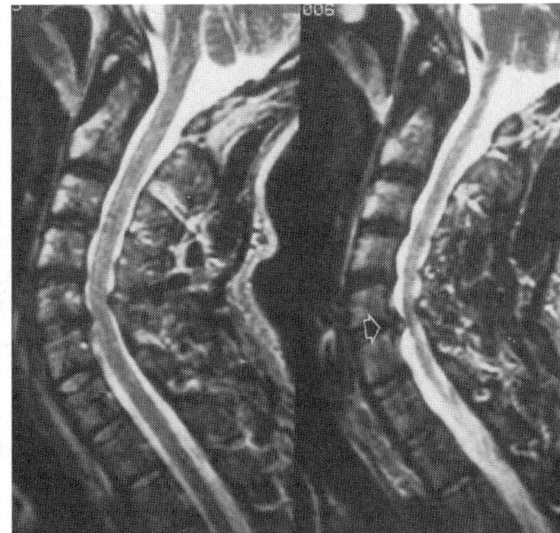

FIGURE 3.—A 45-year-old triathlete and former Olympic cyclist. Magnetic resonance imaging (T2 axial and sagittal) revealed right posterolateral disk herniation at C5 and C6 (*arrows*). (Courtesy of Healy JF, Healy BB, Wong WHM, et al: Cervical and lumbar MRI in asymptomatic older male lifelong athletes: Frequency of degenerative findings. *J Comput Assist Tomogr* 20:107–112, 1996.)

changes included disk protrusion and herniation, spondylosis, and spinal stenosis. The prevalence of these changes increased with older age. The cervical disk protrusion with the most dramatic appearance was seen in a 45-year-old triathlete (Fig 3). This participant had excellent strength and flexibility, but reported a mildly stiff neck after he rode a bicycle more than 80 miles or hang-glided more than 3 hours. He had raced more than 700,000 miles with his head in extreme extension. In these subjects, all imaging findings were asymptomatic and did not interfere with athletic activity.

Discussion.—The findings in this study group were similar to those in other populations. However, these subjects are asymptomatic and very active. Therefore, MRI findings must be evaluated with a clinical history and results of a physical examination. An MRI of the spine can show many abnormalities that do not produce signs or symptoms. These findings may be given undeserved importance by personal injury litigators, worker's compensation authorities, and others.

▶ This article reinforces that findings on diagnostic studies cannot be interpreted in isolation. The normal aging process produces definite changes on the MRI that, if taken in and of themselves, can result in inappropriate intervention. This particular group of patients happened to be athletes. They demonstrated the same changes as other groups of patients that have been similarly studied.

S.W. Wiesel, M.D.

Burst Fractures of the Second Through Fifth Lumbar Vertebrae: Clinical and Radiographic Results
Andreychik DA, Alander DH, Senica KM, et al (Southern Illinois Univ, Springfield)
J Bone Joint Surg Am 78A:1156–1166, 1996   4–24

Background.—The optimal treatment for lumbar burst fractures is controversial. Decision making may be further complicated in those cases with a neurologic deficit. The long-term radiographic and functional outcomes of operative and nonoperative treatments of lumbar burst fractures were evaluated in a retrospective study.

Methods.—The records of 55 patients with a burst fracture at the second, third, fourth, or fifth lumbar level treated between 1976 and 1992 and followed for more than 2 years were reviewed. Of the 55 patients, 30 were managed nonoperatively and 25 were managed operatively. The nonoperative approaches included a body cast (20 patients), a custom-molded thoracolumbosacral orthosis (7 patients), or bed rest for more than 4 weeks (3 patients with associated pelvic fracture). Operative management included posterior arthrodesis with long-segment hook-and-rod fixation (8 patients), posterior arthrodesis with short-segment transpedicular fixation (8 patients), posterior arthrodesis and instrumentation followed by anterior decompression and arthrodesis (6 patients), and anterior decompression and arthrodesis alone (3 patients). The initial and follow-up radiographs were reviewed to measure kyphosis, compression, scoliosis, and the vertebral wedge index. Neurologic, pain, and functional outcomes at the most recent follow-up evaluation were reviewed.

Results.—There were 36 patients who were initially neurologically intact; all remained neurologically intact. These included 23 patients managed nonoperatively and 13 managed with posterior arthrodesis. Of the 19 patients with an initial neurologic deficit, 10 had an isolated single nerve root deficit (8 with partial paralysis and 2 with complete paralysis) and 9 had diffuse multiple nerve root dysfunction. The single nerve root deficits with partial paralysis resolved in all 8 patients, including 6 who had been treated nonoperatively, 1 treated with posterior arthrodesis, and 1 treated with anterior decompression and arthrodesis. All 9 patients with multiple nerve root deficits were managed surgically: 2 with posterior arthrodesis and 7 with anterior and posterior arthrodesis or anterior decompression and arthrodesis alone. Neurologic recovery was best in the patients who underwent anterior decompression and arthrodesis. Radiographic evaluation revealed significantly better anatomical results among those managed operatively than among those managed nonoperatively. However, there were no significant differences in pain or functional outcome among the treatment groups.

Conclusion.—Nonoperative management with early protected mobilization is recommended for lumbar burst fracture in patients with no neurologic deficit or with a partial single nerve root paralysis. However, patients with a complete single nerve root paralysis or a multiple nerve root paralysis may benefit from anterior decompressive procedures.

▶ There is constant discussion regarding when to openly treat lumbar burst fractures. As we have become more sophisticated in our instrumentation technique, many physicians have become much more aggressive. This article is very thoughtful and gives an excellent presentation regarding the fact that nonoperative treatment has its appropriate place. I think the outcomes are well documented and that it is a very good lesson for all of us.

S.W. Wiesel, M.D.

Nonoperative Management of Types II and III Odontoid Fractures: The Philadelphia Collar Versus the Halo Vest
Polin RS, Szabo T, Bogaev CA, et al (Univ of Virginia, Charlottesville)
Neurosurgery 38:450–457, 1996   4–25

Introduction.—There have been many attempts to find options to the halo apparatus for the nonsurgical management of odontoid fractures. The nonsurgical management of these fractures was compared in 54 patients treated with cervical orthoses and halo vests.

Methods.—Thirty-six patients had type II fractures, and 18 had type III fractures. Average patient age was 50.7 years. Patients were nonrandomly assigned by their attending physician into halo vest and rigid orthosis groups.

Results.—Twenty patients in the type II fracture group were treated with the halo vest, and 16 were treated with a neck orthosis. Five patients in the type II group showed a persistent, unhealed fracture line but were stable to flexion and extension, 7 remained unstable to flexion and extension, and 4 eventually required late surgical intervention for persistent instability. One patient died of aspiration pneumonia after receiving a closed head injury in the hospital when attempting to walk while in the halo vest. Significantly more patients younger than 40 years of age in the type II group achieved fracture union (9 of 11 [82%]), compared with patients aged 60 years or older (7 of 14 [50%]).

Five of 18 patients in the type III fracture group were treated with the halo vest. The remaining 5 wore a rigid orthosis. All patients who had type III odontoid fractures showed fracture healing and stability to flexion and extension on postimmobilization radiographs.

A comparison of 16 patients treated with the rigid cervical orthosis and 20 patients placed in the halo vest for type II fractures showed similar rates of late surgical intervention. The overall rate of instability was 27% (4 of 15) in the cervical orthosis group and 16% (3 of 19) in the halo vest group. Treatment failures were observed in 7 of 15 patients treated with a rigid collar and in 5 of 19 patients with halo vests. This difference in healing between groups was not significant. The mean ages of type II patients treated with a rigid collar and halo vest were 69 and 48.5, respectively; this age difference was significant.

Conclusion.—There was an overall 23% incidence of late instability to flexion and extension in patients with type II odontoid fractures. In patients who had type III fractures, there was a 34% rate of fracture line persistence with no late instability. Four patients who had type II fracture required late fusion. No patients who had type III fracture required surgery. There was no significant between-group difference in the rate of instability and the need for late fusion in patients treated with a rigid collar or halo vest. Because the halo vest is associated with morbidity and discomfort, all patients who have type III fractures should be treated with a rigid collar. In the nonoperative management of type II fractures, the rigid collar orthosis should be used instead of the halo vest because there was no difference in patient outcome in this series.

▶ The traditional management of type II, and some type III, odontoid fractures has been surgical. This article demonstrates nicely that one can treat a type II fracture nonoperatively. I think that this should be taken into consideration when one offers the various alternatives to a particular patient.

S.W. Wiesel, M.D.

Nonoperative Management of Herniated Cervical Intervertebral Disc With Radiculopathy

Saal JS, Saal JA, Yurth EF (SOAR, Menlo Park, Calif; Mapleton Hill Orthopaedics PC, Boulder, Colo)
Spine 21:1877–1883, 1996   4–26

Objective.—There have been few studies of nonoperative treatment of cervical herniated nucleus pulposus (CHNP) and radiculopathy. Results of a longitudinal cohort study of symptom resolution, function, and patient satisfaction in CHNP with extremity pain treated nonoperatively and the effectiveness of nonsurgical treatment of patients with extruded cervical disks were evaluated.

Methods.—A total of 26 patients with CHNP, aged 22–58 years, with arm pain were treated with ice, relative rest, a hard cervical collar worn for up to 2 weeks in a position that maximized arm pain reduction, nonsteroidal anti-inflammatory drugs for 6–12 weeks, manual and mechanical traction in physical therapy, home cervical traction, and exercises to strengthen the shoulder girdle and chest and improve posture control and body mechanics. Twenty patients had an extruded disk, and 6 had a herniated disk. Twenty patients had neurologic loss. One week of prednisone treatment (maximum of 60 mg/day for 3 days followed by rapid tapering) was provided to 22 patients when pain control was not adequate. An additional epidural or selective nerve corticosteroid injection was administered to 9 patients to control symptoms. Patients evaluated symptoms, function, satisfaction, use of medication, and other medical and surgical treatment in a questionnaire. Outcome was rated as excellent, good, fair, or poor. Patients were studied for an average of 2.3 years.

Results.—Twenty-four patients were successfully treated for CHNP without surgery with 22 returning to work, 21 returning to the same job, 1 retiring, and 1 working part-time. A good or excellent outcome was achieved by 20 nonoperatively treated patients, 19 patients with an extruded disk, and 5 patients with a herniated disk. Four patients with a fair outcome had multilevel degenerative problems. Two patients had spinal surgery. Neurologic deficits resolved in all patients with neurologic loss.

Conclusion.—Twenty-four patients with CHNP were successfully treated nonoperatively. Twenty had a good or excellent outcome, 19 of whom had disk extrusions. Four patients had a fair outcome, and 2 had spinal surgery.

▶ It has long been known that nonoperative treatment of lumbar disks proves quite successful. This is a well-conceived article that demonstrates the same process occurs in the cervical spine. Radiculopathies in the cervical spine with or without neurologic deficits have an excellent chance to be successfully treated with noninvasive measures. The goal is the relief of pain. A neurologic deficit may or may not return.

S.W. Wiesel, M.D.

Reduction of High-Grade Spondylolisthesis Using Edwards Instrumentation

Hu SS, Bradford DS, Transfeldt EE, et al (Univ of California, San Francisco; Univ of Minnesota, Minneapolis)
Spine 21:367–371, 1996   4–27

Background.—Various surgical options are available for patients with high-grade spondylolisthesis. In those with a loss of sagittal balance, intractable pain, and/or neurologic deficit, surgical reduction may be considered. Techniques for reduction include cast reduction, Harrington rod distraction, and posterior translation through instrumented segments. Posterior decompression and reduction with the Edwards Modular Spine System was reported.

Methods.—Sixteen patients had Grade III or higher spondylolisthesis and all but 1 experienced leg and back pain. Six were unable to stand upright with the knees straight and 9 had progression of slippage. Average age of the patients was 20 years. Seven had previously undergone a total of 12 surgical procedures for spondylolisthesis. Clinical data were obtained from charts, telephone interviews, and/or office visits. Pre- and postoperative radiographic films were examined and the percent slip and slip angle measured before and after reduction.

Results.—The average slip was reduced from 89% preoperatively to 29% postoperatively. The average slip angle, 50 degrees preoperatively, improved to 24 degrees after posterior decompression and reduction. Surgery time and blood loss averaged 8.2 hours and 2,760 cc, respectively. Complications included 4 failures of fixation with screw pullout. Four patients had neurologic defects; 2 of 3 cases of unilateral weakness resolved entirely and 1 resolved only partially. Eight patients had no postoperative complications. Results were judged excellent in 10 patients (all were pain free, took no medication, and had no activity restrictions). Five patients with good results had mild pain and took medicine occasionally or had minor activity limitations. One patient had only a fair result; although limitations were minor in this case, revision surgery was required and there was a residual neurologic deficit.

Discussion.—Reduction of high-grade spondylolisthesis may be considered for patients with severe pain and/or deformity. The Edwards Modular Spinal System for reduction is technically demanding and carries risks similar to other methods of reduction. With proper patient selection, however, good to excellent results can be expected. The rate of hardware-related complications may be reduced with improved sacral fixation. Reduction of the slip angle to less than 45 degrees is essential.

▶ This study demonstrated that partial reduction of a high-grade slip is technically possible. Is it necessary, however, to reduce these high-grade slips? Traditionally, these patients have been fused in situ and they clinically do well. Unfortunately, they are still left with a deformity that is partially relieved with instrumented reduction. As the authors point out, it is a technically demanding procedure with high risks. It is, however, important to be aware that this type of procedure is available and that in the proper hands the results are reasonable.

S.W. Wiesel, M.D.

Miscellaneous Conditions

Primary Bone Tumors of the Pelvis Presenting as Spinal Disease
Thompson RC Jr, Berg TL (Univ of Minnesota, Minneapolis)
Orthopedics 19:1011–1016, 1996   4–28

Background.—Tumors of the pelvis may cause symptoms such as low back pain or radicular pain, which suggest localized structural pathology. In a review of 14 patients with pelvic tumors who were seen with spinal symptoms, common features were identifed and appropriate diagnostic studies were suggested.

Study Design.—The medical records and radiographs of 14 cases of pelvic bone malignancies with spinal symptoms between 1978 and 1992 were reviewed.

Findings.—The patient series consisted of 8 men and 6 women, with an average age of 56 years at symptom onset. Thirteen of these 14 patients were older than 45 years. Five patients had previous histories of back pain. The average time from onset of symptoms to diagnosis was 1 year. In all cases, pain, without antecedent trauma, was the initial symptom and became constant, progressive, and intractable over time. Radicular pain occurred in 12 cases. Anorexia, malaise, and night pain occurred in 7 patients. Tenderness in the pelvic region was an early symptom, whereas neurologic findings, palpable masses, pain on weight-bearing, and decreases in hip motion occurred later. Spinal radiographs were insufficient to diagnose tumor. Tumor was visible on all CT scans of the pelvis and was diagnosed. All treatment with conservative therapy failed.

Conclusions.—In 14 cases of pelvic malignancies that were seen with low back pain or radicular symptoms, the symptoms resulted in a significant diagnostic delay. Physicians treating patients older than 45 years who have progressive back pain that does not respond to conservative treatment should consider this alternative diagnosis. The timing, character, and progression of pain is important for differential diagnosis. Abnormal laboratory findings, such as elevated erythrocyte sedimentation rate or serum alkaline phosphastase levels, may also indicate neoplasm. All radiographic studies should include the pelvis. If no lesions are detected by radiography, a bone scan or CT or MRI scan may be necessary to identify the lesion.

▶ This is an excellent article showing that other diseases can be seen initially as back pain with or without sciatica. One must constantly be on the alert for these cases. My feeling is that all of us who see patients with low back pain should have in our mind an algorithm to make sure that we do not misdiagnose these types of cases. The algorithm should include spondyloarthropathy, metabolic disease, tumors, and peripheral neuropathies, at a minimum.

S.W. Wiesel, M.D.

Survival Rates of Patients With Metastatic Spinal Cancer After Scintigraphic Detection of Abnormal Radioactive Accumulation
Tatsui H, Onomura T, Morishita S, et al (Osaka Med College, Japan)
Spine 21:2143–2148, 1996   4–29

Objective.—Predicting survival for patients with metastatic spinal cancer is important to the design of any treatment plan. Bone scintigraphy is a useful tool for detecting metastatic bone cancer. Results of a retrospective analysis of timing of spinal metastases and survival of patients from bone scintigraphy data were presented.

Methods.—Within 3 months of diagnosis of primary disease, whole body and spot scintigraphy were performed on 2,372 patients, aged 17 to 88 years, with breast (N = 114), lung (N = 149), cervical (N = 46), stomach (N = 28), prostate (N = 59), or kidney cancer (N = 29) 2½ to 3 hours after intravenous administration of 20 mCi of technetium-99m methylene diphosphate. Abnormal spinal or sacroiliac joint uptake was detected in 766 patients and confirmed to indicate metastatic tumors in 425. The incidence of spinal accumulation varied from 30% to 54%. Scintigraphy was repeated at 6- to 12-month intervals. Survival was calculated using the Kaplan-Meier method. Operative technique, postoperative survival and symptomatic progression were analyzed in patients who had surgery.

Results.—The interval from diagnosis to spinal accumulation was significantly shorter for patients with lung cancer (3.6 months) that for those with breast cancer (29.4 months), cervical cancer (21.4 months), or renal cancer (13.9 months). The interval for breast cancer was significantly longer than for lung cancer, gastric cancer (6.9 months), and prostate cancer (12.8 months). The 1-year survival rates were highest for breast (77.7%) and prostate cancers (83.3%), intermediate for cervical (44.6%) and renal (51.2%) cancers, and lowest for pulmonary (21.7%) and gastric (0%) cancers. The 6-month survival rate for gastric cancer was 15.3%.

Conclusion.—When metastatic spinal tumors are discovered, the aggressiveness of treatment depends on expected survival rates that, in turn, depend on the type of primary cancer.

▶ The question constantly arises once metastases in the spine are identified as to how aggressive treatment should be. This article attempts to answer that question. It covers a 10-year period involving more than 400 patients with metastases. Although retrospective, I thinks it gives us some good basic guidelines as to when to be aggressive and when to just treat symptomatically.

S.W. Wiesel, M.D.

Spinal Stenosis and Neurogenic Claudication

Porter RW (Royal College of Surgeons, Edinburgh, Scotland)
Spine 21:2046–2052, 1996   4–30

Introduction.—Claudication symptoms can result from a structural narrowing of the vertebral canal, which compresses the cauda equina. The clinical presentation, pathophysiology, and management of this neurogenic claudication were reviewed.

Clinical Presentation.—Neurogenic claudication is most common among men older than 50 years. Usually, bilateral or unilateral symptoms of weakness, tiredness, or heaviness of the legs are not present at rest, are manifested after walking a short distance, and are relieved again by rest. Patients typically are unable to stand erect, with gradually increasing stooping while walking. Evaluation should include treadmill testing to establish objective evidence of symptom development and changing posture. Plain radiography may reveal a shallow vertebral canal, degenerative spondylolisthesis, or structural lumbar scoliosis; these are present in a substantial portion of patients. Doppler studies of the peripheral circulation and arteriography are also useful, as is a CT or MRI scan. The differential diagnosis includes intermittent claudication from peripheral vascular disease, sciatic claudication, referred pain from the lower lumbar region, root pain, and multiple root pathology.

Pathophysiology. —Spinal stenosis is only 1 factor contributing to neurogenic claudication. Other factors include degenerative soft tissue, bony pathology, and vertebral displacement with an intact neural arch. There are usually at least 2 levels of low pressue stenosis, between which venous pooling occurs in the cauda equina, resulting in a failure of arterial vasodilatation of the affected congested roots during exercise.

Management—Typically, symptoms do not progress. Therefore, clinical observation may be reasonably recommended in the absence of severe disability. Some patients have responded to calcitonin administration, but this treatment has not yet been adequately studied. However, if the symptoms require a substantial reduction of activities or lifestyle alteration, surgery may be recommended. Surgical decompression must be extensive enough to completely free the dura but should not produce instability or an excessively shallow spinal gutter. In patients with a degenerative spondylolisthesis, posterolateral spinal fusion may be combined with decompression.

▶ I do not ordinarily choose review articles for the YEAR BOOK. However, this one was succinct, informative, and up to date on spinal stenosis. Richard Porter is a world-renowned spinal surgeon. I have heard him lecture with distinction. The information presented in this article is, in my view, accurate with excellent insights. I think it is well worth reviewing.

S.W. Wiesel, M.D.

The Significance of an Absent Ankle Reflex

Bowditch MG, Sanderson P, Livesey JP (Northern Gen Hosp, Sheffield, England)
J Bone Joint Surg (Br) 78B:276–279, 1996   4–31

Background.—An absent ankle reflex has been reported to be a definite neurologic sign that indicates a possible nerve-root compression. The significance of a clinical test depends on its sensitivity, specificity, and positive and negative predictive values. Because predictive values are strongly dependent on prevalence, the prevalence of absent ankle reflexes was investigated in a normal orthopedic population through the full range of adult ages.

Methods.—During a 6-month period, the presence or absence of ankle reflexes in 1,074 adult patients who did not have systemic diseases associated with absent reflexes was determined prospectively in the orthopedic outpatient department in 2 hospitals. Reflex findings were assessed in age subgroups. Associations between the prevalence of absent unilateral and bilateral ankle reflexes and increasing age were analyzed.

Results.—The prevalence of absent ankle reflexes increased significantly with increasing age. This pattern was particularly dramatic for bilateral absence, which increased steadily with age; a significant increase was noted between the fifth and sixth decades of life and again between the seventh and eighth decades. The prevalence of unilateral absence also increased steadily but to a lesser degree and without any significant increases in particular decades. There were no significant gender-related differences at any age.

Conclusions.—The differences in prevalence of bilateral and unilateral absence of ankle reflex suggest that they have different etiologies. Unilateral loss of ankle reflex was present in 1% to 10% of patients older than 40 years of age. This finding indicates that the unilateral, but not bilateral, absence is a useful neurologic sign. Previous reports of the predictive value of the absent ankle reflex in the diagnosis of herniated lumbar disk of 90% between ages 20 and 45 years and 60% beyond age 50 years are supported.

▶ An isolated neurologic deficit, such as an absent ankle jerk or weak extensor halluces longus, is not in itself a justification for surgery. This article nicely demonstrates that some individuals have this finding in isolation. As is stated, the finding should be taken in the light of the total clinical picture. It is generally believed that pain, not a single neurologic deficit, is the primary reason for surgical intervention.

S.W. Wiesel, M.D.

5 General Adult Reconstruction

Introduction

As it has in the past, this section primarily includes articles relating to total knee arthroplasty and its complications. In addition, there are sections on injuries to the anterior cruciate ligament and problems of the patellofemoral joint.

It is hard to generalize about these somewhat disparate articles, but they do demonstrate continued improvement in the quality of clinical studies being reported in orthopedic surgery. More and more papers include the inclusion criteria for the study, are prospective in nature, and have appropriate control groups. In addition, patient satisfaction and patient assessment of outcome are being included more frequently in the orthopedic literature.

Total knee arthroplasty appears to have matured considerably in the past several years, and we now have the advantage of several long-term follow-up studies, including some as long as 15 years. These studies have served to indicate directions for change to improve survivorship and function; current designs appear to have excellent durability. In fact, the durability of total knee arthroplasty as performed in 1997 is probably at least equivalent to that of total hip arthroplasty.

Clement B. Sledge, M.D.

General Considerations in Total Joint Replacement

Randomized Trial of Epidural Versus General Anesthesia: Outcomes After Primary Total Knee Replacement
Williams-Russo P, Sharrock NE, Haas SB, et al (Cornell Univ, New York)
Clin Orthop 331:199–208, 1996   5–1

Background.—Epidural anesthesia may have several advantages over general anesthesia in total knee replacement surgery. The effects of epidural and general anesthesia on early postoperative outcomes after unilateral primary total knee replacement were compared.

Methods and Findings.—Two hundred sixty-two patients were randomly assigned to epidural or general anesthesia. After surgery, patients receiving epidural anesthesia achieved all rehabilitative milestones earlier than did patients receiving general anesthesia. The difference was significant for stair climbing. The incidence of deep vein thrombosis was 40% in the epidural anesthesia group and 48% in the general anesthesia group. No clots occurred proximal to the popliteal veins. The incidences of pulmonary embolism on lung scan were 12% and 9%, respectively, in the epidural and general anesthesia groups.

Conclusion.—The use of epidural anesthesia is associated with a faster attainment of rehabilitation goals after total knee replacement and a minor, nonsignificant decrease in the rate of deep vein thrombosis. The 2 types of anesthesia were comparable in the occurrence of early postoperative pulmonary embolism.

▶ It is generally held that the use of regional and epidural anesthesia decreases the incidence of postoperative deep venous thrombosis and pulmonary embolism. In this study, no difference was found in these complications whem comparing patients undergoing knee replacement under epidural anesthesia with those undergoing the same operation under general anesthesia. It should be noted, however, that both groups of patients had standard postoperative prophylaxis consisting primarily of warfarin. The authors point out that in other studies of the incidence of thromboembolic complications after hip surgery, the incidence is diminished by the use of epidural anesthesia. They postulate that the use of a tourniquet contributes an additional risk factor in knee surgery, that is not addressed by epidural anesthesia. The patients who underwent epidural anesthesia in this study did have a quicker postoperative rehabilitation, shorter length of stay, and earlier achievement of functional goals.

C.B. Sledge, M.D.

The Effect of Preoperative Exercise on Total Knee Replacement Outcomes
D'Lima DD, Colwell CW Jr, Morris BA, et al (Scripps Clinic and Research Found, La Jolla, Calif)
Clin Orthop 326:174–182, 1996   5–2

Background.—The progressive decline in physical fitness in the elderly can be caused by simple deconditioning because of diminished exercise. The effect of preoperative physical therapy or general cardiovascular conditioning on the outcome of total knee replacement was evaluated.

Methods.—Thirty patients older than 55 years scheduled for elective primary unilateral total knee replacement were randomly assigned to 1 of 3 preoperative treatment groups. The control group was given no recommendations for preoperative exercise or physical therapy. The patients in group 2 were given physical therapy to strengthen the upper and lower extremities and improve the range of motion in the knee 3 times weekly for eighteen 45-minute sessions. The patients in group 3 participated in three 45-minute cardiovascular conditioning sessions per week for 18 weeks, which emphasized arm and cycle ergometry. The patients were evaluated at 6 weeks before surgery and 1, 3, 12, 24, and 48 weeks postoperatively, using the Hospital for Special Surgery Knee Rating, the Arthritis Impact Measurement Scale, and the Quality of Well Being.

Results.—There were no significant differences among the 3 groups in age, length of hospital stay, or complication rate. Pain increased preoperatively in the control and cardiovascular condition groups and decreased slighty preoperatively in the physical therapy group. Postoperatively, pain relief was greatest in the control group at week 3, comparable in the 3 groups at weeks 12 and 24, and greater in the cardiovascular conditioning and physical therapy groups at week 48. Function declined most precipitously in the 2 exercise groups immediately postoperatively but was similar in the 3 groups at 48 weeks. The patients tolerated both exercise programs well without experiencing adverse events.

Conclusions.—Neither the physical therapy program nor the cardiovascular conditioning program administered preoperatively resulted in an outcome benefit in elderly patients undergoing total knee replacement.

Clinical Significance.—Although improved surgical outcome associated with preoperative strengthening programs makes intuitive sense, the data do not support this association in elderly patients requiring knee surgery. Preoperative physical therapy does not effectively improve the outcome or reduce the hospital stay in patients undergoing total knee replacement.

▶ The authors of this paper are unable to show any benefit of preoperative exercise in a group of patients undergoing total knee arthroplasty. Possible explanations are (1) there is no benefit to such exercise; (2) these patients were so chronically disabled that a short period of exercise before surgery had no measurable effect; or (3) the size of the experimental groups, 10 patients in each of 3 groups, was insufficient to show statistical differences. Nevertheless, this study does bring into question the expenditure of time, effort, and professional expertise in having patients participate in preoperative exercise programs before undergoing total knee arthroplasty.

C.B. Sledge, M.D.

Bladder Management After Total Joint Arthroplasty
Knight RM, Pellegrini VD Jr (Pennsylvania State Univ, Hershey; Milton S Hershey Med Ctr, Pa; Univ of Rochester)
J Arthroplasty 11:882–888, 1996   5–3

Introduction.—A common organism is often present in patients with joint arthroplasty who have urinary tract infections (UTIs). Indwelling bladder catheterization and intermittent catheterization were prospectively compared to determine the impact of each on bladder dysfunction and the incidence of UTIs after total joint arthroplasty.

Methods.—A total of 174 patients undergoing either total hip arthroplasty or total knee arthroplasty were randomized to 48 hours of either an indwelling Foley catheter (group 1) or intermittent straight catheterization every 6 hours if unable to void or void adequate amounts (group 2). Postoperative urine specimens were collect for culture on days 2 and 5. A cost-effectiveness analysis was performed.

Results.—Of 174 patients, complete data were available for 119. Group 1 patients had a UTI rate of 8% (5 of 62 patients), and group 2 patients had a rate of 12% (7 of 57 patients). No patients had prosthetic joint infections. Straight catheterization was needed for inability to void 48 hours after surgery by significantly less group 1 than group 2 patients (19% vs. 35%). Significantly less group 1 patients required catheterization after epidural analgesia was discontinued compared with group 2 patients (35% vs. 16%). Using indwelling Foley catheters instead of intermittent catheterization saved 150 minutes per patient and $3,000 per patient.

Conclusion.—Use of an indwelling Foley catheter in the first 48 hours after total hip arthrolasty and total knee arthroplasty was associated with a significantly quicker return of normal bladder function and was less labor intensive and less expensive than use of intermittent straight catheterization.

▶ One of the most common complications of joint replacement in the usual population undergoing such procedures is urinary retention, especially in males. There has been no consensus regarding whether to use intermittent catheterization or an indwelling catheter. In this study, the routine use of an indwelling catheter reduced the frequency of UTIs, was less labor intensive and, therefore, less expensive that intermittent catheterization, and carried no increased risk of UTIs. Although comfort was not addressed in this study, I'm sure the patients who had an indwelling catheter were more comfortable than those who faced repeated intermittent catheterization.

C.B. Sledge, M.D.

Blood Management in Orthopedic Surgery
Sculco TP (Hosp for Special Surgery, New York)
Am J Surg 170:60S–63S, 1995   5–4

Introduction.—Blood management in orthopedic procedure is focused on reducing blood loss and preventing allogeneic transfusions. Blood management strategies for orthopedic surgery are discussed.

Preoperative Autologous Donation (PAD).—Advantages of PAD include no transmission of infectious disease, no transfusion reaction, no immunomodulation, and decreased red blood cell (RBC) mass. Only 5% of all transfusions are autologous, reflecting the emergent need of most blood transfused. The cost of PAD is well-justified when the cost of managing transfusion-transmitted infectious disease is considered.

Hemodilution.—Hemodilution gives the advantage of reduced RBC mass, which means reduced RBC loss during surgery. The method is used infrequently in orthopedic surgeries. Optimal hemodilution needs a dedicated anesthesia team, meticulous monitoring, and an efficient protocol to avert delays and minimize surgical morbidity.

Intraoperative Blood Salvage.—Intraoperative blood salvage is expensive, but it is useful in orthopedic procedures in which the anticipated blood loss exceeds 1,000 mL. It should not be used in patients with active infections or neoplasms.

Postoperative Reinfusion.—Blood transfusion requirements are the same regardless of whether postoperative drainage is reinfused or not used. Patients must be monitored carefully when undergoing postoperative reinfusion of wound drainage. The drainage should be washed before reinfusion to improve the quality of the reinfused blood.

Recombinant Human Erythropoietin (Epoetin alfa).—Epoetin alfa may be used preoperatively to enhance autologous blood collection and to increase perioperative RBC mass in patients with anticipated large blood losses. Epoetin alfa may be used in patients who are of the Jehovah's Witness faith.

Conclusion.—The orthopedic surgeon needs to be well versed in techniques that reduce the need for allogeneic RBC transfusion. An important advance in blood management is allowing hematocrit levels to be below 30% without transfusion of unnecessary units of allogeneic blood.

▶ This review addresses the usefulness of preoperative autologous donation of blood, hemodilution, and intraoperative and postoperative blood salvage, as well as the use of erythropoietin to increase RBC mass. The author provides guidelines for each of these techniques and reminds us that the surgeon is in the key position to determine which of these techniques is used and to diminish the use of homologous blood with its attendant risks.

C.B. Sledge, M.D.

Postoperative Blood Salvage in Total Knee Arthroplasty Using the Solcotrans Autotransfusion System
Marks RM, Vaccaro AR, Balderston RA, et al (Thomas Jefferson Univ, Philadelphia; Jefferson Med College, Philadelphia; Rothman Inst, Philadelphia; et al)
J Arthroplasty 10:433–437, 1995   5-5

Introduction.—The Solcotrans system is an autotransfusion system that reinfuses postoperative wound drainage. The safety, efficacy, and effect on postoperative blood requirements of the Solcotrans system was evaluated in patients undergoing primary total knee arthroplasty (TKA).

Methods.—One-hundred forty-four patients undergoing TKA were placed in either a Hemovac group (group 1) or a Solcotrans group (group 2). Group 2 patients with inadequate drainage to autotransfuse were added to group 1 patients.

Results.—Of 81 patients assigned to group 2, 56 (39%) were able to autotransfuse and 25 were added to group 1. There were 88 (61%) group 1 patients. Total drainage for the Hemovac group averaged 718 mL, and drainage for the Solcotrans group averaged 1,141 mL. Patients in group 2 autotransfused on average of 524 mL of Solcotrans drainage. Methyl methacrylate was found in the postoperative drainage of 3 patients from group 2. No adverse reactions were observed in the 3 patients with methyl methacrylate-laden drainage. There were no significant between-group differences in preoperative or postoperative hemoglobin or hematocrit levels. Thirteen (9%) patients received 24 units of homologous blood: 8 group 1 patients received 16 units and 5 group 2 patients received 8 units. Only 2 (1.6%) of 122 patients who autodonated 2 units of blood required homologous blood. Of the 22 patients who autodonated only 1 unit or did not autodonate, 11 (50%) required homologous blood.

Conclusion.—No adverse sequelae were associated with the use of Solcotrans drainage. The use of the Solcotrans system did not lower homologous blood requirements; thus, its use in the postoperative management of patients with TKA is not recommended.

▶ Because the authors were unable to show a decreased need for homologous blood transfusion when comparing a group of patients who underwent postoperative salvage and reinfusion with those in a control group, they do not recommend this technique, which is expensive and labor intensive.

C.B. Sledge, M.D.

Improvement in Cardiovascular Fitness After Total Knee Arthroplasty

Ries MD, Philbin EF, Groff GD, et al (Mary Imogene Bassett Hosp, Cooperstown, NY)

J Bone Joint Surg (Am) 78A:1696–1701, 1996   5–6

Introduction.—The impact of total knee arthroplasty (TKA) for severe osteoarthritis of the knee on health, fitness, and the risk of coronary heart disease is not known. The effect of TKA on cardiovascular fitness was evaluated in 19 patients undergoing TKA.

Methods.—Cardiopulmonary fitness was evaluated at baseline in 19 patients undergoing TKA and in 16 patients being treated medically for severe osteoarthritis of the knee. Patients in both groups were reevaluated 1 and 2 years later. A progressive maximum exercise test using a bicycle ergometer and a metabolic test was performed to determine physical fitness. Patients completed an Arthritis Impact-Measurement Scales questionnaire at each assessment. The questionnaire evaluates health status and activity for patients with osteoarthritis. Of 19 patients in the TKA group, 16 were reevaluated at 1 year, and 13 were reevaluated at 2 years after surgery. Of 16 patients in the control group, 16 were reevaluated at 1 year, and 9 were reevaluated at 2 years.

Results.—At a 1-year follow-up, the TKA group had near-significant improvement in maximum oxygen consumption, maximum oxygen consumption corrected for body weight, and the percentage of predicted maximum oxygen consumption. In 2 years, there were significant improvements in these variables. There were no significant changes in maximum oxygen consumption or maximum oxygen consumption corrected for body weight in the control group. The control group experienced significant decreases in duration of exercise and maximum workload at both 1 and 2 years. Physical activity increased significantly at 1 and 2 years in the TKA group but not in the control group.

Conclusion.—Patients undergoing TKA for severe osteoarthritis had improvement in cardiovascular fitness at 1 year and significant improvement at 2 years. A decline in physical fitness was seen in the control group of patients managed medically. The group evaluated was small, but it may be that TKA can be used as a therapeutic measure to improve cardiopulmonary fitness in patients with osteoarthritis that severely limits physical activity because of knee pain.

▶ A small number of patients undergoing TKA for osteoarthritis were compared with a matched group of controls who underwent medical management of their osteoarthritis. The patients undergoing surgery, as a result of their increased functional level and absence of pain, showed improved cardiovascular fitness by 1 year after surgery, and this continued for 2 years. Perhaps cardiovascular limitation will become an *indication* for joint arthroplasty in patients severely disabled by osteoarthritis of the hip or knee.

C.B. Sledge, M.D.

The Influence of Total Knee Arthroplasty on Lower Limb Blood Flow

Scriven MW, Fligelstone LJ, Oshodi TO, et al (Univ Hosp of Wales, Cardiff)
J R Coll Surg Edinb 41:323–324, 1996   5–7

Introduction.—Little is known about the effects of total knee arthroplasty (TKA) on distal perfusion in patients who do not have peripheral vascular disease (PVD). Forty-four patients with no evidence of PVD were evaluated to determine the effect of TKA, under tourniquet control, on blood flow.

Methods.—Ankle and brachial systolic pressures were measured, and the ankle–brachial index was calculated using a hand-held Doppler probe. Full arterial duplex scanning was performed with an emphasis on femoral and distal waveform analysis. Patients with symptoms and signs of lower limb arterial impairment were excluded. Patients underwent standard

TKA with a tourniquet applied to mid-thigh and inflated to a pressure above that of systolic blood.

Results.—Three of 44 patients evaluated were eliminated because symptomatic deep vein thromboses prevented ankle pressure measurement. The remaining 41 patients underwent 45 TKA procedures (3 simultaneously and 1 on separate occasions). No abnormalities in waveform analysis were detected in the femoral or distal segments preoperatively or postoperatively. There were no significant preoperative or postoperative differences in ankle brachial indices. There were no significant differences in outcome among patients with or without the atherosclerotic risk factors of smoking, hypertension, ischemic heart disease, or diabetes mellitus.

Conclusion.—Patients with no evidence of PVD had no adverse effects from the use of a mid-thigh tourniquet during TKA. It is recommended that any patient with actual or suspected PVD be thoroughly evaluated (including Duplex scanning and ankle brachial index measurements) by a vascular surgeon before planning TKA.

▶ In the age range of patients undergoing knee arthroplasty, PVD is quite common. A concern in such patients is the effect of a tourniquet on blood supply to the lower extremity. In this group of 41 patients, none of whom had obvious PVD before surgery, no deleterious effect on lower limb blood flow was shown. Unknown is the effect on patients *with* PVD. Most vascular surgeons recommend minimal use of the tourniquet in terms of both inflation pressure and duration of use in such patients. Until a study similar to the one presented here is carried out on patients with pre-existing PVD, caution will still be necessary when using tourniquets on patients with compromised vascularity.

C.B. Sledge, M.D.

Thickness of Tibial Inserts in Total Knee Arthroplasty

Weber AB, Morris HG (St Vincent's Hosp, Victoria, Australia)
J Arthroplasty 11:856–858, 1996   5–8

Introduction.—There is a lack of standardization between manufacturers regarding the actual thickness of ultrahigh molecular weight polyethylene used in tibial inserts of knee prostheses. The thickness of tibial inserts and metal trays from 8 manufacturers was measured to determine actual thickness.

Methods.—Samples of medium-sized metal tibial trays and 3 standard polyethylene inserts were requested from manufacturers. Companies were asked for samples that were at least 6 mm thick and for a sample of the thinnest tibial insert on the market if it differed from what was requested. Metal trays and inserts were measured using a micrometer that measured to 0.01 mm. Metal trays were measured 6 times, and the mean was recorded. Measurements of the porous surface were taken independently, if possible. The smallest measurement was recorded, as was the named

TABLE 1.—Component Measurements

Prosthesis	Metal (mm)	"Size"	Width	Polyethylene (mm)
AMK (DePuy, Warsaw, IN)	4.1	10	1	5.9 (5.0)*
			3	6.2 (5.9)*
			5	6.2
Duracon (Howmedica, Rutherford, NJ)	3.3	9	Small	6.1
			Medium	5.9
			Large	5.9
Genesis (Smith & Nephew Orthopaedics, Memphis, TN)	4.2	8	Medium	5.4
		10	Small	7.4
			Medium	7.4
			Extra large	7.3
Ir.sall-Burstein II (Zimmer, Warsaw, IN)	2.5	10	54	7.4
			64	7.3
			74	7.3
Kinemax (Howmedica)	2.2	8	Extra small	6.1
			Medium	6.1
			Extra large	6.0
Miller-Galante II (Zimmer)	3.9/3.8†	9	EF green‡	5.3
		11	AB purple‡	7.2
			EF green‡	7.3
			GHJK blue‡	7.3
Natural-Knee (Intermedics, Austin, TX)	3.6	7	A	4.0
		11	O	7.5
			A	7.5
			B	7.5
Osteonics (Allendale, NJ)	3.8	8	5	6.5
		10	3	7.6
			7	7.5
			11	7.6

*The AMK has a "dovetail"-type articulation with the metal baseplate. The first figure represents the thinnest measurement in a vertical plane; the figure in parentheses represents an oblique measurement to the dovetail, which was the thinnest margin in the smaller sizes.

†Second figure represents measurement of metal tray without the porous surface.

‡Descriptive color coding used by Zimmer.

(Courtesy of Weber AB, Morris HG: Thickness of tibial inserts in total knee arthroplasty. *J Arthroplasty* 11:856–858, 1996.)

"thickness" of the insert. The accuracy of measurements was within 0.1 mm.

Results.—Considerable differences in the thickness of metal trays was observed (Table 1). It appears that the industry practice is to refer to the "size" of the insert as the combined thickness of metal and polyethylene.

Discussion.—In choosing appropriate prostheses for patients, surgeons need to understand that there are differences in metal and polyethylene dimensions among manufacturers. Inserts should be labeled to indicate the minimum thickness, not what they become in combination with a metal baseplate.

▶ A number of studies have shown that polyethylene tibial inserts of total knee implants should be at least 6 mm thick to avoid premature failure. With the advent of modular tibial components and metal trays, that recommendation has recently been increased to 8 mm. There has been confusion regarding the relationship between the *nominal* size of the tibial component and the actual thickness of polyethylene. In most, if not all, systems, the nominal thickness includes the metal tray and the thickness of polyethylene where it is greatest. Table 1 shows that anywhere from 2.2 to 4.2 mm of the nominal size may be occupied by the metal tray, which thereby reduces the thickness of the polyethylene insert to less than the recommended 8 mm even when the nominal size is 11 mm. Because there is variation from manufacturer to manufacturer, the surgeon should be aware of these measurements and should choose a tibial component with adequate (6–8 mm) *polyethylene* thickness in the *thinnest* areas of the insert.

C.B. Sledge, M.D.

The Effects of Particulate Polyethylene at a Weight-bearing Bone-Implant Interface: A Study in Rats

Allen M, Brett F, Millett P, et al (Addenbrooke's Hosp, Cambridge, England)
J Bone Joint Surg Br 78:32–37, 1996   5–9

Introduction.—Particulate wear debris is probably an important factor in the pathogenesis of aseptic loosening of arthroplasty components. Described is an animal model on which the effects of particulate debris can be tested in isolation or in combination.

Methods.—Ceramic "drawing-pin" implants were inserted in weight-bearing positions in the right proximal tibia of 10 male Sprague-Dawley rats. At 8, 10, and 12 weeks after surgery, animals underwent intra-articular injections of either high-density polyethylene (HDP) (4 rats), saline (2 rats), or no injection (4 rats). Two animals each were sacrificed at 6 weeks and 14 weeks after surgery. Postmortem examinations were performed. The femur and tibia were disarticulated, and high-definition cranocaudal radiographs of the right tibia were taken to determine placement of the implant. The bone–implant interface underwent histopathologic examination.

Results.—Animals were able to bear weight on the operated leg within 72 hours of surgery. Postmortem examination indicated healing of the surgical wounds with no evidence of adverse tissue reactions around the monofilament nylon sutures. Radiography revealed correct placement of the implant in all animals. At 6 weeks after surgery, there was appositional bone growth up to and around the prosthesis at all levels under the head of the pin, which was surrounded by articular cartilage of normal appearance. At 14 weeks, the amount of new bone growth had increased, and active bone remodeling was seen. The histologic responses were similar for the saline-injected and noninjected controls. A chronic inflammatory response with numerous foreign-body giant cells in periprosthetic tissues was observed in the HDP-injected group.

Conclusion.—The rat model used is appropriate for testing the relationship between a weight-bearing implant and particulate wear debris. More relevant information can be gathered by injecting test materials into a joint containing a weight-bearing implant than by injecting into a healthy joint.

▶ This study provides a very clever and useful model to examine the effects of polyethylene debris at the bone–implant interface with micro-motion as a factor. There have been recent suggestions that pharmacologic management of bone loss around a loose implant, using bisphosphonates, is effective. The model proposed in this study would be a useful way to determine the effectiveness of such management before widespread application to humans.

C.B. Sledge, M.D.

Results of Total Knee Arthroplasty

Survivorship Analysis of Cemented Total Condylar Knee Arthroplasty
Nafei A, Kristensen O, Knudsen HM, et al (Aarhus Univ, Denmark)
J Arthroplasty 11:7–10, 1996   5–10

Background.—Few authors have reported long-term survival analysis of cemented total condylar knee arthroplasty. The modified Insall-Burstein prosthesis, a semiconstrained, cruciate ligament–sacrificing, cemented prosthesis without metal backing, is used in the authors' center for total knee resurfacing arthroplasty. The survival rate of a large series of these prostheses was reported.

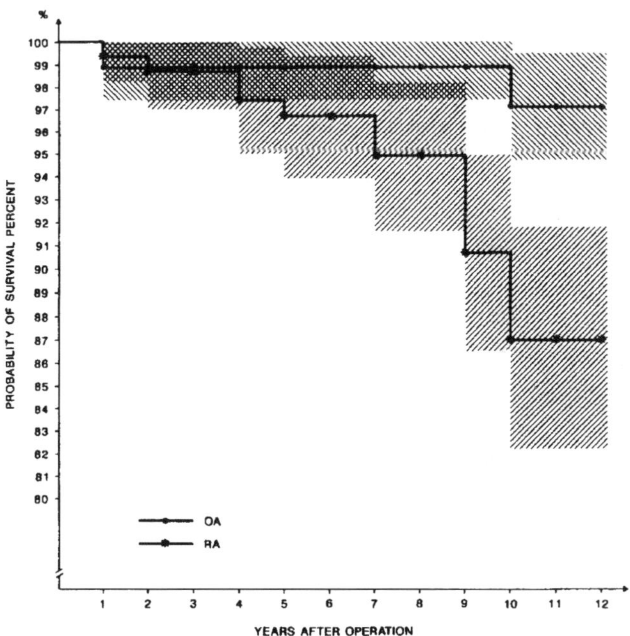

FIGURE 2.—Cumulative survival rates of the osteoarthrosis (*OA*) and the rheumatoid arthritis (*RA*) groups. Hatched areas represent 95% confidence limits. *P* = 0.005. (Courtesy of Nafei A, Kristensen O, Knudsen HM, et al: Survivorship analysis of cemented total condylar knee arthroplasty. *J Arthroplasty* 11:7–10, 1996.)

Methods.—Three hundred forty-eight consecutive primary total condylar knee arthroplasties performed on 235 patients during 27 months were analyzed. The maximum follow-up was 12 years. One hundred eighty-four knees were given a diagnosis of osteoarthrosis and 164 had rheumatoid arthritis. Ten patients, with 10 total knee arthroplasties, were lost to follow-up.

Findings.—The overall cumulative survival rate was 92%. The osteoarthrosis group had a significantly higher survival rate (97%) than did the rheumatoid arthritis group (87%). The survival rate was not significantly affected by age, sex, or body mass index (Fig 2).

Conclusion.—The most important finding in this study was the significant difference between survival rates in the 2 diagnostic groups. None of the other variables studied affected survival.

▶ A total of 348 consecutive total condylar knee arthroplasties were followed for a maximum of 12 years. The overall cumulative survival rate was 92.3%, with a large difference between patients with osteoarthritis and those with rheumatoid arthritis; the cumulative success rate in the later group was 87% at 12 years. This finding is in contrast to previous articles found in the literature, and the authors point out the need to stratify patients into similar groups (age, preoperative alignment, weight, etc.) before drawing conclusions about any single variable, such as diagnosis.

C.B. Sledge, M.D.

Kinematic Condylar Total Knee Arthroplasty: 14-year Survivorship Analysis of 208 Consecutive Cases

Weir DJ, Moran CG, Pinder IM (Freeman Hosp, Newcastle Upon Tyne, England)
J Bone Joint Surg Br 78B:907–911, 1996   5–11

Background.—The unconstrained condylar prosthesis is the preferred implant in many treatment centers for arthritis of the knee. There is little information on long-term survival of knee replacement. The long-term outcome of the Kinematic Condylar Total Knee Replacement was evaluated.

Methods.—The Kinematic Condylar Total Knee Replacement was used in 208 primary total knee arthroplasties in 177 consecutive patients. There were 47 men and 130 women; the mean patient age was 65 years.

Results.—The minimum follow-up was 10 years and the mean follow-up was 12 years. Data were not available for 7 patients. Revision was required in 22 knees; the time between replacement and revision was 8 years. The 10-year survival rate was 92%. There was no difference in survival of knees with osteoarthritis or rheumatoid arthritis when survival was stratified by diagnosis and thickness of polyethylene.

Discussion.—These results are poorer than results of other studies, although many did not report how many patients were lost to follow-up.

The results of the original Condylar Knee Replacement were good. New implant designs should be thoroughly evaluated clinically and in the laboratory before being introduced.

▶ A total of 208 knee replacements were followed for a minimum of 10 years and a mean of 12 years with only 7 patients lost to follow-up. Overall survival was 92% at 10 years. The authors were unable to show a difference in survival based on diagnosis or thickness of the polyethylene insert. They stress that patients lost to follow-up should be considered failures. Following their own advice makes the survival at 10 years drop to 89% in this series. The authors conclude that "Widespread introduction of new designs should be allowed only after adequate laboratory and clinical evaluation of the implant." Given the excellent results of this series and numerous reports of disastrous results of modifications to implants, their statement appears to be appropriate. Changes in prosthesis design should address specific identified problems in the predecessor design and be followed by evidence that the modification has solved the problem.

C.B. Sledge, M.D.

Long-term Results of Total Knee Arthroplasty in Class 3 and 4 Rheumatoid Arthritis
Rodriguez JA, Saddler S, Edelman S, et al (Lenox Hill Hosp, New York; Cincinnati Sportsmedicine and Orthopaedic Ctr, Ohio)
J Arthroplasty 11:141–145, 1996
5–12

Background.—Total knee arthroplasty can relieve pain and restore functional ability in patients with rheumatoid disease. The polyarticular nature of rheumatoid arthritis distinguishes it from the more common osteoarthritis. Many patients with rheumatoid disease require multiple joint arthroplasties to improve functional ability. There is little information on the outcome of total knee arthroplasty beyond 10 years. Results of total condylar knee arthroplasty at 13 years were reported.

Methods.—The results of 104 total condylar knee arthroplasties in 67 patients were reviewed clinically and radiographically. Patients had class 3 or 4 rheumatoid arthritis; 91 procedures were done in women. The average patient age was 52 years. The average follow-up was 12.7 years.

Results.—The Hospital for Special Surgery knee scores were good-to-excellent in 84 knees, fair in 17 knees, and poor in 3 knees. The average range of motion was 95 degrees. No flexion contracture was greater than 5 degrees. Of 8 failures, 6 were from delayed sepsis and 2 were from aseptic loosening. At 15 years, there was a 91% probability of the arthroplasty remaining functional in situ. In a questionnaire, 70% of patients reported that they were pain free, and 30% reported that they had occasional knee pain.

Discussion.—All patients in this series reported total or partial relief of pain after total condylar knee arthroplasty. Pain relief was sustained at nearly 13 years, and functional status also improved. Late failure of total knee arthroplasty usually results from delayed infection.

▶ This study addresses total knee arthroplasty in patients with rheumatoid arthritis with clinical and radiographic follow-up averaging 12.7 years. The results were excellent, with a 91% probability of survival at 15 years. The authors do not comment on patients lost to follow-up or state whether they were included in the survival analysis. The most common cause of failure was late infection, occurring in 4.1% of knees at an average of 7 years after the index operation.

It must be pointed out that these patients were severely disabled by their rheumatoid arthritis and placed low functional demand on the implant. This would be one reason why aseptic loosening was a rare cause of failure in this series.

C.B. Sledge, M.D.

Functional Outcome and Patient Satisfaction in Total Knee Patients Over the Age of 75
Anderson JG, Wixson RL, Tsai D, et al (Northwestern Univ, Chicago)
J Arthroplasty 11:831–840, 1996   5–13

Background.—Total knee arthroplasty can reduce deformity, improve function, and relieve pain in patients with degenerative or rheumatoid arthritis. Most studies have assessed the outcome of total knee arthroplasty by means of traditional orthopedic criteria and standardized knee-scoring systems. There is little information on patient-reported functional status or patient satisfaction. Several instruments have been developed to describe functional status and patient satisfaction from the patient's perspective.

Methods.—The outcome of 98 total knee arthroplasties in 74 patients with degenerative or rheumatoid arthritis of the knee was reviewed. All patients were aged 75 years or older. A validated questionnaire evaluated pain, function, satisfaction, and mental health. The average follow-up was 34 months.

Results.—At follow-up, 90.8% of patients reported improvement after total knee arthroplasty, 88.8% were satisfied with results, and 91.8% believed they made the right decision in having the procedure. There was a correlation between dissatisfaction with results and lower mental health scores, decreased physical function, and increased pain. There was a correlation between satisfaction with results and better pain scores on the Western Ontario and McMaster Universities Osteoarthritis Index and the SF-36 Health Status questionnaire, but not for the Hospital for Special Surgery scoring system. Revision was associated with preoperative deformity greater than 20 degrees.

Discussion.—These findings indicate that total knee arthroplasty in the elderly is safe, can relieve knee pain, and can restore function. Patient satisfaction is high after this procedure, especially in those with good emotional, physical, and social well-being. Conventional knee-scoring systems may not accurately reflect patient satisfaction.

▶ This paper reports excellent pain relief and satisfaction scores in a group of patients 75 years of age or older undergoing total knee arthroplasty. It is important to note that the overall patient satisfaction correlated with both the Western Ontario and McMaster Universities Osteoarthritis Index and the SF-36 scores but not with the Hospital for Special Surgery (HSS) knee score. If these 2 outcome measures had not been added to the more typical HSS evaluation, an important correlation would have been missed.

C.B. Sledge, M.D.

Total Knee Replacement After Arthrodesis

Results of Total Knee Arthroplasty Following Takedown of Formal Knee Fusion
Cameron HU, Hu C (Orthopaedic and Arthritic Hosp, Toronto)
J Arthroplasty 11:732–737, 1996
5–14

Background.—The senior author reported results of knee fusion takedown in 4 cases of total knee insertion. An additional 14 procedures have been performed. Studies of formal knee fusion takedown were reviewed.

Methods.—A review was conducted of 17 cases of formal knee fusion takedown with follow-up from 1 to 10 years. There were 10 men and 7 women. The average patient age was 59 years. The length of time fused was 1 to 40 years. Patients with spontaneous bony ankylosis or with a jog of motion were excluded.

Results.—In 2 patients, refusion was done for patellar tendon loss and sepsis. One patient had a chronic infection but refused the refusion procedure. Two patients who were immobilized for the first 10 days after total knee arthroplasty had a range of flexion of 35 degrees. In the other patients, the mean range of flexion was 84 degrees. On the Hospital for Special Surgery scoring system, 29.4% cases were excellent, 29.4% were good, 17.6% were fair, and 17.6% were poor; this included the 2 patients who had refusion. Nine patients had complications; surgery resolved the complications in 6.

Discussion.—These patients preferred the mobile knee to the fused knee. The authors remain ambivalent about knee fusion takedown because of the high rate of complications. Extreme caution is recommended when offering this procedure to patients with a fused knee.

Total Knee Arthroplasty in a Previously Ankylosed or Arthrodesed Knee
Naranja RJ Jr, Lotke PA, Pagnano MW, et al (Univ of Pennsylvania, Philadelphia; Mayo Clinic, Rochester, Minn)
Clin Orthop 331:234–237, 1996   5–15

Background.—Because of the success of primary total knee arthroplasty, it is now being used in younger patients, patients needing revision arthroplasty for aseptic loosening, and patients with previous infection. There is little information regarding total knee arthroplasty in a previously ankylosed or arthrodesed knee. Long-term results and complications in patients with a previously ankylosed or arthrodesed knee converted to a total knee replacement were reported.

Methods.—A review was conducted of total knee arthroplasty in 37 knees in 35 patients who had no knee motion. The average patient age was 53 years; 28 patients were women. The average follow-up was 90 months.

Results.—At follow-up, the range of motion averaged 7 degrees lack of full extension and 62 degrees flexion. The rate of total complications was 57%. The short-term complication rate was 24% and the major complication rate was 35%. The infection rate was 14%. A satisfactory outcome consisting of no pain and unlimited walking distance was seen in 29% of patients. In patients with a satisfactory outcome, the average patient age was 45 years and the average postoperative knee flexion was 87 degrees. This was significantly different from results in patients who had an unsatisfactory outcome. There was no association between results and the angle at which the knee had been ankylosed.

Discussion.—Total knee arthroplasty in a previously ankylosed or arthrodesed knee is a difficult procedure which has a high complication rate and compromised results. In these patients, a consistent lack of adequate motion was seen. Surgeons should carefully consider the risks and benefits of this procedure.

▶ Both of these articles,—(Abstracts 5–14 and 5–15) the first reporting 17 cases of conversion of knee fusion to total knee arthroplasty and the second reporting total knee arthroplasty 37 knees—urge extreme caution. The paper by Cameron and Hu, covering patients with formal knee fusion, reported a 53% complication rate with 18% of the patients achieving a poor result. The authors remain "ambivalent" regarding the procedure.

The larger, multi-center report by Naranja et al. describes 37 knees without any motion in the knee; not all of the patients had undergone formal arthrodesis. The complication rate was 57%, and a satisfactory outcome was attained in only 29% of the patients. These authors, too, suggest great caution before undertaking this procedure.

C.B. Sledge, M.D.

Tubercle Osteotomy

Extended Tibial Tubercle Osteotomy in Total Knee Arthroplasty

Ries MD, Richman JA (Mary Imogene Bassett Hosp, Cooperstown, NY)
J Arthroplasty 11:964–967, 1996   5–16

Background.—Many primary and revision total knee arthroplasties can be exposed through a conventional medial prepatellar arthrotomy. Extension of the approach proximally with rectus tendon transection or distally with tibial tubercle osteotomy may be necessary if soft-tissue contracture or scarring impairs lateral patellar eversion and if patellar tendon rupture is a possibility. When patellar eversion is difficult, some surgeons transect the rectus tendon in a V–Y or transverse manner because of the possibility of tibial tubercle avulsion with catastrophic loss of extensor mechanism function complicating tibial tubercle osteotomy. Results of a long tapered tibial tubercle osteotomy and repair with screws in difficult total knee arthroplasty are reported.

Methods.—In 29 patients, 30 consecutive tibial tubercle osteotomies were performed during total knee arthroplasty. Revision total knee arthroplasty was performed in 18 patients, primary total knee arthroplasty was performed in 9 patients, and extensor mechanism realignment for patellar instability after total knee arthroplasty was performed in 2 patients. The average patient age was 65 years, and the average follow-up was 18 months.

Technique.—The conventional medial parapatellar approach was used routinely during total knee arthroplasty. In cases of difficult patellar eversion, the soft tissues were elevated subperi-

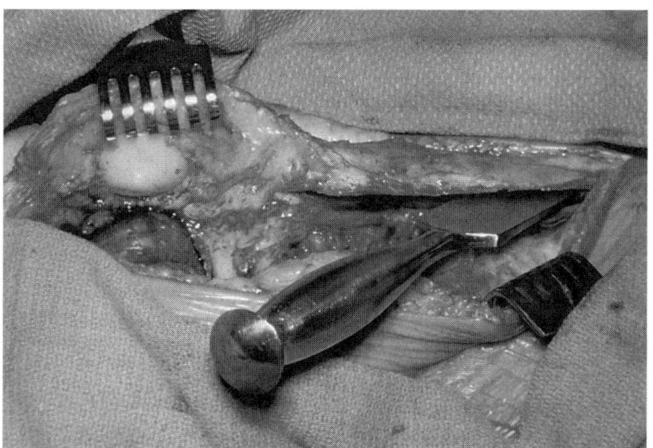

FIGURE 1.—An osteotome is inserted proximomedially toward the lateral side of the tibial crest. The bone fragment is tapered in size from proximal to distal. (Courtesy of Ries MD, Richman JA: Extended tibial tubercle osteotomy in total knee arthroplasty. *J Arthroplasty* 11:964–967, 1996.)

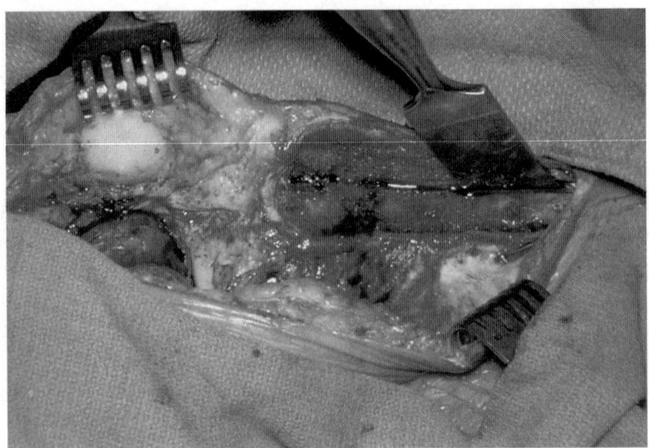

FIGURE 2.—The osteotomized bone fragment in continuity with the anterior compartment muscles and extensor mechanism is everted laterally. A wide area of cancellous bone is exposed to promote healing. (Courtesy of Ries MD, Richman JA: Extended tibial tubercle osteotomy in total knee arthroplasty. *J Arthroplasty* 11:964–967, 1996.)

osteally from the proximal medial tibia to allow external rotation, and scarring was excised from the lateral gutter. If excess tension remained in the extensor mechanism and patellar tendon avulsion was a risk, a tibial tubercle osteotomy was done. A fragment of bone 8–10 cm long in continuity with the anterior compartment muscles was elevated with osteotomes and everted laterally. At the level of the tibial tubercle, the osteotomy was 1–2 cm in depth, and the width of the bone fragment was between 2 and 3 cm, depending on the size of the tibia. The bone fragment was tapered distally (Fig 1 and Fig 2). The tapered shape avoids a sharp stress riser, which can occur with a transverse distal cut. Three or 4 titanium screws were used for fixation.

Results.—In 29 of the 30 cases, the osteotomies healed primarily. Postoperative displacement of the tibial tubercle developed in 1 patient; an additional screw and suture fixation was used.

Discussion.—Tibial tubercle osteotomy allows adequate exposure during difficult total knee arthroplasty. The authors had previously used the quadriceps snip in difficult total knee arthroplasty, but the exposure is not as extensile as that gained with tibial tubercle osteotomy. The quadriceps snip is now used with deficient tibial bone stock, when tibial tubercle osteotomy is contraindicated.

▶ In many revision situations, especially those with limited motion, exposure of the knee may be difficult using standard approaches. The tibial tubercle osteotomy has been recommended by a number of authors and has been shown to improve access for removal of components. This article stresses the importance of operative technique if one is to avoid complications. The authors emphasize that the osteotomy fragment should be tapered toward the distal end so that it emerges gradually and avoids a sharp stress riser that might lead to fracture of the tibial shaft.

C.B. Sledge, M.D.

Tibial Shaft Fracture Following Tibial Tubercle Osteotomy
Ritter MA, Carr K, Keating EM, et al (Ctr for Hip and Knee Surgery, Mooresville, Ind)
J Arthroplasty 11:117–119, 1996   5–17

Introduction.—Tibial tubercle osteotomy is reported to be an excellent means of exposing the knee joint in patients who have limited flexion or are undergoing knee revision requiring a total knee arthroplasty. The Center for Hip and Knee Surgery performed 657 primary and 16 revision total knee arthroplasties in 1993. Tibial tubercle osteotomy was used in 9 cases, and 2 of these later developed tibial shaft fractures. These 2 cases of fracture after total knee arthroplasty were reviewed.

> *Case Report.*—Woman, 73, had revision arthroplasty some 20 years after a McIntosh prosthesis implantation and patellectomy. Examination showed 5-degree flexion contracture, 65 degrees of flexion, and a 14-degree valgus deformity. The patient had a McIntosh loose prosthesis, creating a defect in the medial femoral condyle; lateral joint space narrowing; and no visible patella. Two to 4 weeks after surgery, pain developed in the calf. A callous formation on the proximal aspect of the tibia at the site of the osteotomy indicated a fracture. After 3 months, the patient had less pain. At 1 year, the fracture had healed, motion was limited to 85 degrees of flexion, and the patient had no pain.

Discussion.—These and other findings indicate that the discontinuity created by tibial tubercle osteotomy can weaken the bone and result in stress and a fracture. Because of this, a distal transverse cut is no longer used. Instead, the osteotomy is gradually sloped so that there is a smooth transition from the 5-mm depth to the top of the crest at the distal end of the osteotomy. This revised technique has now been performed 4 times without fracture.

▶ This case report illustrates the importance of avoiding a stress riser at the distal end of the tubercle osteotomy.

C.B. Sledge, M.D.

Allografts in Revision

Impacted Morsellized Allograft and Cement for Revision Total Knee Arthroplasty
Ullmark G, Hovelius L (Gävle Hosp, Sweden)
Acta Orthop Scand 67:10–12, 1996   5–18

Introduction.—Allografts have been used successfully in revision knee arthroplasty. Morsellized allografts have been used with allograft blocks and pieces by Samuelson and de Waal Malefijt et al. Good results have been reported after impaction of morsellized allografts in the femur and

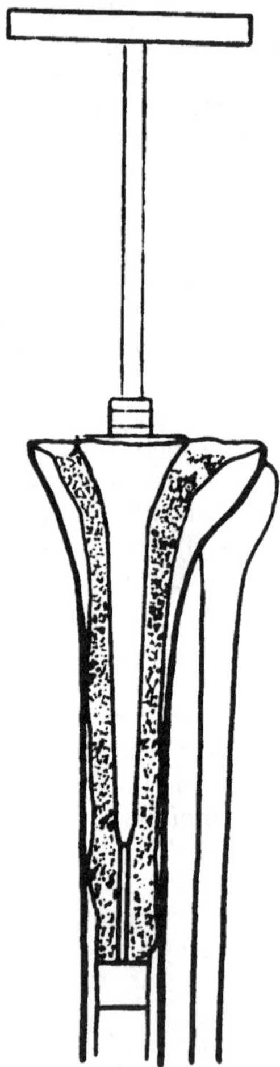

FIGURE.—After filling the total cavity with morsellized grafts, the tibia side impactor is brought down along the centralizer to an appropriate level. (Courtesy of Ullmark G, Hovelius L: Impacted morsellized allograft and cement for revision total knee arthroplasty. *Acta Orthop Scand* 67:10–12, 1996.)

acetabulum in revision hip arthroplasty. A surgical technique and early results of 3 cases of revision total knee arthroplasty with impacted morsellized allografts surrounding the entire stems were reported.

Case Report.—Woman, 61, had had rheumatoid arthritis for more than 50 years. The patient had a unicondylar replacement of the lateral compartment and synovectomy of the right knee in 1977, a revision procedure 6 years later because of mechanical loosening, an ipsilateral hip arthroplasty in 1985, and a second revision of the right knee in 1986. For 5 years, the patient was pain free. However, in 1992, the patient became very disabled; the prosthesis was loose and a third revision was done using the technique described in this report. At 3 months, the patient was walking with 1 stick and knee motion was 5 degrees to 90 degrees. At 28 months, radiographs had not changed from the postoperative examination, and the patient reported no pain.

Technique.—The bone grafts were prepared from frozen femoral heads using a bone mill that osteotomizes the heads into small chips of different sizes, which stabilizes the impaction. The grafts were firmly packed on top of the plug in the revision cavern with a distal impactor until the chips reached several centimeters above the planned level of the tip of the stem. The entire cavern was filled with morsellized grafts that were pressed together with a distal impactor. A tibia impactor was intruded on the centralizer down in the grafted cavern to produce a firm graft impaction (Fig).

Discussion.—This technique is one of several options for revision knee arthroplasties and has shown encouraging results. It may present an alternative in cases of large intramedullary cavities. In these 3 patients, the diagnosis at initial operation was rheumatoid arthritis. New cortical bone formation was seen in case 2 and new trabeculation was seen in case 3. This technique may restore deficient bone stock.

Structural Allografting in Revision Total Knee Arthroplasty

Mow CS, Wiedel JD (Univ of Colorado, Denver)
J Arthroplasty 11:235–241, 1996   5–19

Background.—Managing bone loss observed during revision of failed total knee arthroplasty is challenging. Some authors have recommended the use of large allografts, such as femoral heads, but few recent data are available on the outcomes of such techniques. One experience with structural allografts in the treatment of large bone defects in revision total knee arthroplasty was reported.

Methods.—Fifteen patients with large segmental, cavitary, or combination defects of the femur and/or tibia underwent structural allografting during revision total knee arthroplasty between 1985 and 1991. Allografting was performed in 7 distal femurs and 12 proximal tibias. The mean age at surgery was 63 years. The average length of follow-up was 47 months.

Outcomes.—The mean range of motion preoperatively was 4 to 93 degrees; postoperatively, it was 2 to 104 degrees. Mean knee scores before and after surgery were 47 and 86, respectively. Preoperatively, mean alignment averaged 5 degrees varus, compared with 4 degrees valgus postoperatively. Pain and stability improved in all but 1 patient. All 15 allografts available for follow-up healed to host bone. Thirteen showed evidence of incorporation. No allograft infections or fractures occurred. There was 1 complication directly related to the allograft, occurring in a patient with a tibial component fracture over a proximal tibial allograft 3 years after surgery. In addition, tibial loosening occurred in a patient receiving a distal femoral allograft, and a proximal tibial fracture occurred in a patient receiving a distal femoral allograft. There was also 1 instance of intraoperative patellar tendon avulsion.

Conclusion.—Structural allografting appears to be a satisfactory technique for treating large bone defects in the failed total knee arthroplasty. The rate of complications in this series was acceptably low.

▶ There is often a problem of inadequate bone stock in revision knee arthroplasty, and this inadequacy can be addressed either by additional mass of prosthesis or by bone grafting. Bone grafting is probably preferable in younger patients in whom restoration of bone stock is a long-term goal and in older patients where there may be a reduced incidence of infection using smaller implants.

The paper by Ullmark and Hovelius (see Abstract 5–18) reports the impaction of morsallized grafts in the tibia in a manner analagous to that popularized by Ling for the proximal femur in revision total hip arthroplasty.[1] Although the Ullmark and Hovelius report only involves 3 cases, the early results appear good and the longer results of the technique applied to the hip have been excellent. If there is a major cortical defect in the proximal tibia, impaction morsallized allografts will not provide sufficient mechanical strength. In such instances, structural allografts may be used as reported in the series of 15 patients by Mow and Wiedel.

C.B. Sledge, M.D.

Reference

1. Gie GA, Linder L, Ling RSM, et al: Impacted cancellous allografts and cement for revision total hip arthroplasty. *J Bone Joint Surg Br* 75:14–21, 1993.

The Patella in Total Knee Replacement

The Effects of Patellar Thickness on Patellofemoral Forces After Resurfacing

Star MJ, Kaufman KR, Irby SE, et al (Scripps Clinic and Research Found, La Jolla, Calif; Children's Hosp, San Diego, Calif)
Clin Orthop 322:279–285, 1996   5–20

Background.—Patella and patellar implant complications after total knee arthroplasty are now considered to be the most important reason for arthroplasty failure. The effect of patellar bone and implant thickness on patellofemoral forces after resurfacing in total knee arthroplasty was investigated.

Methods and Findings.—An Oxford Knee Testing Rig was used on 7 cadaver knees, giving the specimens 6 degrees of freedom during dynamic data collection. The knees were assessed from full extension to 95 degrees of knee flexion. Knees were implanted with Press Fit Condylar femoral, tibial, and patellar implants. Custom modular oval-domed polyethylene patellar components with progressive thickness increments of 2 mm were used to determine the effect of varying patellar thickness on patellofemoral forces. A custom-designed uniaxial patellar load cell was used to measure patellofemoral forces. Patellofemoral compression forces were significantly increased from 70 to 95 degrees of flexion with increased patellar bone and implant thickness.

Conclusion.—Patellar thickness differences as low as 10% significantly change patellofemoral forces at higher knee flexion angles. Increased patellar thickness increases patellar forces at greater flexion angles. Clinical studies are now needed to analyze the effect of postoperative patellar thickness on patellofemoral complications.

Component Design Affecting Patellofemoral Complications After Total Knee Arthroplasty

Theiss SM, Kitziger KJ, Lotke PS, et al (Univ of Pennsylvania, Philadelphia)
Clin Orthop 326:183–187, 1996   5–21

Background.—Patellofemoral problems account for an estimated 50% of all complications after total knee arthroplasty. Design differences in the patellofemoral articulation that may result in increased complications were studied.

Methods and Findings.—Two hundred eighty-nine patients underwent 301 primary cemented total knee arthroplasties. In 148 knees, the Miller-Galante I prosthesis was used, and in 153, the Press Fit Condylar prosthesis was used. The patients were followed for at least 2 years. The complication rates in the Miller-Galante I and Press Fit Condylar prostheses groups were 10.1% and 0.7%, respectively. All other parameters were comparable in the 2 groups.

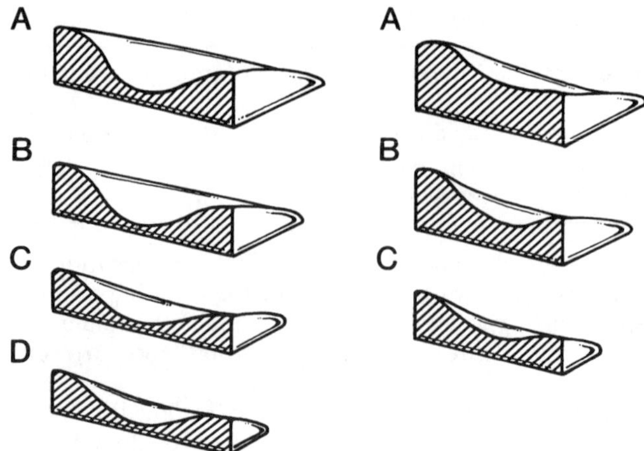

FIGURE 2.—The patellar groove of the Press Fit Condylar prosthesis, seen in a tangential view (**left**), is deeper and wider than the groove of the Miller-Galante I prosthesis (**right**). Note the raised lateral wall on the Miller Galante I. Points *A*, *B*, *C*, and *D* correspond to the indicated distance from the joint line. (Courtesy of Theiss SM, Kitziger KJ, Lotke PS, et al: Component design affecting patellofemoral complications after total knee arthroplasty. *Clin Orthop* 326:183–187, 1996.)

Conclusion.—The pronounced difference in the patellofemoral complication rate between these 2 groups may be explained by design differences in the femoral component. A short, narrow anterior flange; a shallow patellar groove; and an abrupt anterior-to-distal transition with a smaller radius of curvature may have contributed to patellofemoral morbidity (Fig 2). Long-term assessment of new designs should be performed before widespread use.

Patellar Resurfacing Versus Retention in Total Knee Arthroplasty

Feller JA, Bartlett RJ, Lang DM (Austin Hosp, Melbourne, Australia)
J Bone Joint Surg Br 78B:226–228, 1996   5–22

Background.—The necessity of resurfacing the patella as part of total knee arthroplasty is still debated. There are relatively few controlled studies of its potential benefits. The role of patellar resurfacing in a standard total knee arthroplasty for osteoarthritis was further explored.

Methods.—Forty patients without severe patellar deformities undergoing primary total knee arthroplasty for osteoarthritis were randomly assigned to patellar retention or resurfacing with a cemented, all-polyethylene component, regardless of the state of the patellar articular cartilage. One type of prosthesis was used in all patients. Except for osteophyte removal, no surgery was done on the retained patellae. The 38 surviving patients were assessed at 3 years.

Findings.—At follow-up, the mean Hospital for Special Surgery and Patellar scores were 89 and 28, respectively, in the patellar retention group, compared with 83 and 26, respectively, in the resurfacing group.

Women and heavier patients had significantly lower scores on both assessments. The retention group had significantly better stair-climbing scores. No complications were associated with patellar resurfacing.

Conclusion.—Resurfacing the patella during total knee arthroplasty in this patient population has no apparent medium-term benefits. Resurfacing resulted in no complications in this series.

▶ The patella has been 1 of the major sources of complications after total knee arthroplasty. Opinion is divided regarding whether it is better to resurface or not resurface the patella and what steps can be taken to reduce the incidence of complications after patellar resurfacing. The paper by Star et al. (See Abstract 5–20) examines the effect of patellar thickness on patellofemoral forces and concludes that a change in patella thickness by as little as 10% significantly alters forces across the patellofemoral joint. These authors recommend careful measurement of patellar thickness before resurfacing and using that thickness as the goal.

The paper by Theiss (See Abstract 5–21) et al., examining patellar complications with 2 different types of prosthesis, found a striking difference between the 2. One implant had a 10% complication rate ascribed to the patellofemoral joint and the other design had a complication rate of 0.7%. The authors conclude that subtle differences in the length of the anterior flange, depth of the patellar groove and rate of transition from gentle to steep curve in the intercondylar notch may have a profound effect on function of the resurfaced patella and, therefore, the complication rate.

The paper by Feller et al. suggests that in patients with osteoarthritis, there may be no significant benefit from resurfacing the patella, at least at a short-term follow-up of 3 years. In contrast, there is a trend toward more routine resurfacing of the patella, as longer-term follow-up studies have shown deterioration of an unresurfaced patella, leading to revision. With modern designs of patellar implants and attention to surgical technique, the rate of complications after resurfacing has dropped dramatically. Many surgeons now use routine patellar resurfacing.

C.B. Sledge, M.D.

Complications of Total Knee Arthroplasty

Deep Venous Thrombosis After Total Joint Arthroplasty
Garino JP, Lotke PA, Kitziger KJ, et al (Univ of Pennsylvania, Philadelphia)
J Bone Joint Surg Am 78:1359–1365, 1996   5–23

Objective.—Ascending venography, plethysmography, radioactive fibrinogen uptake, and Doppler testing are techniques for detecting deep vein thrombosis after total joint (hip or knee) arthroplasty. All these methods have drawbacks such as discomfort, allergy, or lack of accuracy. Screening results for deep vein thrombosis using ultrasonography were compared with results using ascending venography for accuracy and reliability.

Methods.—Phase I involved venograms and ultrasonograms of 121 patients (126 joints), aged 26–86 years, who had total joint arthroplasty between September 1989 and February 1991. Phase II included venograms and ultrasonograms of 84 patients (87 joints) who had total joint replacements between April 1992 and October 1992. Venograms and ultrasonograms were independently reviewed and compared for the ability to detect deep vein thromboses.

Results.—In phase I, 3 ultrasonograms were considered to be positive. The remaining 123, evaluated as negative, included 7 legs with a clot detected by venography. Venography demonstrated a thrombus in 62 legs. In phase II, 7 ultrasonograms were positive for a thrombus, including 5 wherein venography also confirmed a clot. Venography visualized a thrombus in 43 legs. In phase I, ultrasonography gave false negative results, a sensitivity of 0%, a positive predictive value of 0%, a negative predictive value of 94%, and an accuracy of 92%, primarily as a result of negative readings in 116 legs. Venography had a specificity of 97%. The sensitivity of duplex Doppler ultrasonography was 0%, and the specificity was 98%. In phase II, the sensitivity of ultrasonography was 100% and the specificity was 98%. The accuracy of ultrasonography was 98%. The development of a clot was not related to the type of arthroplasty nor to the type of anticoagulant therapy. Thrombi distal to the knee were found in 30% of total hip arthroplasties and 71% of total knee arthroplasties. Lack of technical experience is suspected to be the primary reason for false negative ultrasonogram results.

Conclusion.—The expertise of the technician performing ultrasonography determined the accuracy and reliability of detection of deep vein thrombosis after total knee or hip arthroplasty.

▶ Ultrasonography is frequently used to detect deep venous thrombosis in the lower extremities after joint replacement surgery. It is useful because it is relatively inexpensive and painless, and it is reported to have good accuracy proximal to the knee. The paper by Garino et al. reports that the technique is extremely sensitive to the experience and skill of the technician. Studies of various prophylactic regimens in which ultrasound is used as the end point are suspect unless technician variability is accounted for.

C.B. Sledge, M.D.

Prevention of Venous Thromboembolism After Knee Arthroplasty: A Randomized, Double-Blind Trial Comparing Enoxaparin With Warfarin
Leclerc JR, Geerts WH, Desjardins L, et al (McGill Univ, Montréal; Université de Montréal; Univ of Toronto; et al)
Ann Intern Med 124:619–626, 1996   5–24

Background.—Venous thromboembolism continues to be a major complication of knee arthroplasty. The efficacy and safety of fixed-dose enoxaparin and adjusted-dose warfarin in preventing venous thromboembolism after knee arthroplasty were investigated.

Methods.—Six hundred seventy consecutive patients undergoing knee arthroplasty were enrolled in the randomized, double-blind, controlled study. Patients received enoxaparin, 30 mg subcutaneously every 12 hours, or adjusted-dose warfarin at the international normalized ratio between 2.0 to 3.0. These regimens were begun after surgery.

Findings.—Four hundred seventeen patients had adequate venograms. Fifty-two percent of the warfarin recipients and 36.9% of the enoxaparin recipients had deep venous thrombosis. The absolute risk difference was 14.8%. Proximal venous thrombosis developed in 10.4% of the warfarin group and in 11.7% of the enoxaparin group, with an absolute risk difference of 1.2%. The incidences of major bleeding were 1.8% and 2.1% in the warfarin and enoxaparin groups, respectively, with an absolute risk difference of 0.3%.

Conclusion.—In patients undergoing knee arthroplasty, a postoperative fixed-dose enoxaparin regimen prevents total deep venous thrombosis more effectively than adjusted-dose warfarin. The incidences of proximal venous thrombosis and clinically overt bleeding did not differ between groups.

▶ Adjusted-dose warfarin has become the gold standard for prophylaxis of thromboembolic complications after joint arthroplasty. It is expensive to administer because of the need for frequent determinations of prothrombin time and the need to have a physician or physician assistant regulate the dose in response to those laboratory results. Enoxaparin is an attractive alternative because it can be administered in a fixed-dose regimen. This paper studied 670 consecutive patients undergoing knee arthroplasty and concluded that enoxaparin was more effective than warfarin and caused no greater incidence of complications, including bleeding.

C.B. Sledge, M.D.

Risk of Deep-Venous Thrombosis After Hospital Discharge in Patients Having Undergone Total Hip Replacement: Double-blind Randomised Comparison of Enoxaparin Versus Placebo
Planes A, Vochelle N, Darmon J-Y, et al (Clinique Radio-Chirurgicale du Mail, La Rochelle, France; Rhône-Poulenc Rorer Pharma Inc, Neuilly sur Seine, France)
Lancet 348:224–228, 1996   5–25

Purpose.—Patients who have undergone total hip replacement (THR) are at risk of deep vein thrombosis (DVT) and pulmonary embolism, for which they receive antithrombotic prophylaxis. Although prophylaxis is generally stopped when the patient leaves the hospital, there is evidence that the risk of postoperative venous thromboembolism persists after discharge. The extent of this continued risk and the efficacy of continuing prophylactic therapy were evaluated in a prospective, double-blind trial.

Methods.—The study included 179 consecutive patients who were being discharged from the hospital 2 weeks after THR. All were free of DVT, as assessed by bilateral ascending venography of the legs. They were randomly assigned to receive further prophylaxis with enoxaprin, 40 mg subcutaneously once a day for 21 days, or placebo. The patients were then studied for DVT or pulmonary embolism, with venography repeated after 21 days or as indicated.

Results.—None of the patients died or had pulmonary embolism. On intention-to-treat analysis, the rate of venogram-detected DVT was 7% in the patients treated with enoxaprin vs. 19% in the placebo group. The rate of distal DVT was 1% in the enoxaprin group vs. 11% in the placebo group. The corresponding rates of proximal DVT were 6% and 8%. The advantage of continued prophylaxis was confirmed on efficacy analysis in 155 patients. Three patients in the enoxaprin group and 1 in the placebo group had minor bleeding episodes, none of which required withdrawal from the trial.

Conclusions.—The risk of late DVT continues for at least 1 month after THR in patients who are free of DVT at discharge and who do not receive continued antithrombotic prophylaxis. The results suggest that enoxaprin prophylaxis should continue after hospital discharge. Prophylaxis should be continued for at least 35 days after THR.

▶ Planes and colleagues evaluated the risk of late DVT in THR patients after discharge from the hospital. Patients in this study had venograms performed before discharge to exclude those with DVT. Those with negative screening results were sent home either without prophylaxis (placebo group) or with enoxaparin prophylaxis. The placebo group showed a significantly higher rate of DVT occurring as late as 35 days after surgery, whereas the enoxaparin group showed a lower incidence. The authors conclude that patients should receive some type of prophylaxis for several weeks after discharge.

C.B. Sledge, M.D.

Supracondylar Femoral Fracture Following Total Knee Arthroplasty
Moran MC, Brick GW, Sledge CB, et al (Harvard Med School, Boston; Marietta Orthopaedic Associates, Ga; Queen Mary Hosp, Hong Kong)
Clin Orthop 324:196–209, 1996   5–26

Background.—A variety of methods have been proposed for the treatment of supracondylar femoral fractures above total knee arthroplasties. Closed treatment was compared with open reduction and internal fixation using plates.

Methods and Findings.—This retrospective study included 29 supracondylar femoral fractures above total knee arthroplasties. The outcomes of 5 nondisplaced fractures managed with closed treatment were satisfactory.

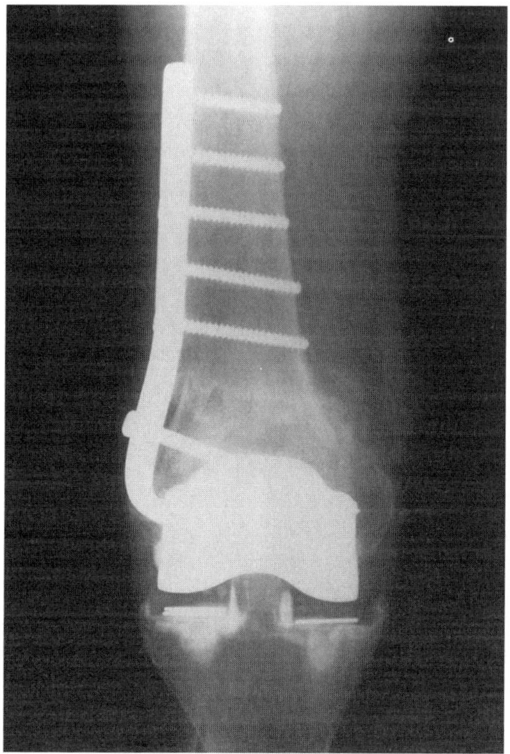

FIGURE 4.—Imaging in a 68 year old woman with rheumatoid arthritis. Anteroposterior radiograph 6 months after open reduction and internal fixation using a blade plate, shows a satisfactory result. (Courtesy of Moran MC, Brick GW, Sledge CB, et al: Supracondylar femoral fracture following total knee arthroplasty. *Clin Orthop* 324:196–209, 1996.)

However, none of the 9 displaced fractures managed by the closed technique had satisfactory results. Eight malunions occurred, and 2 knees required revision. Among the 15 displaced fractures managed with open reduction and internal fixation, 10 outcomes were satisfactory, 3 knees needed revision or repeat fixation, and 2 malunions occurred (Figs 4 and 6).

Conclusion.—Closed treatment is recommended for nondisplaced fractures above total knee arthroplasties. For displaced fractures, early open reduction and internal fixation offers the best chance for a satisfactory outcome, although the complication rate is significant.

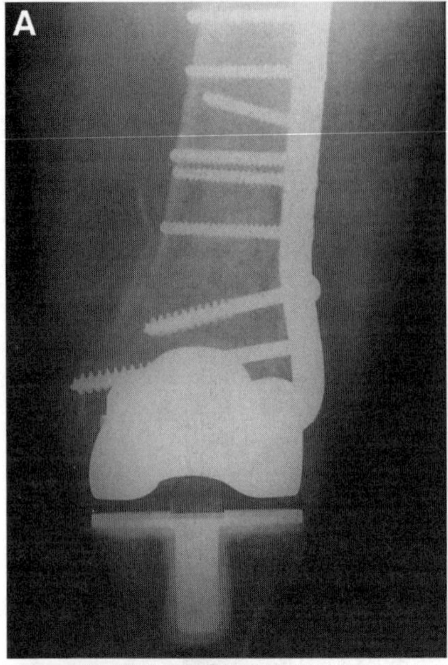
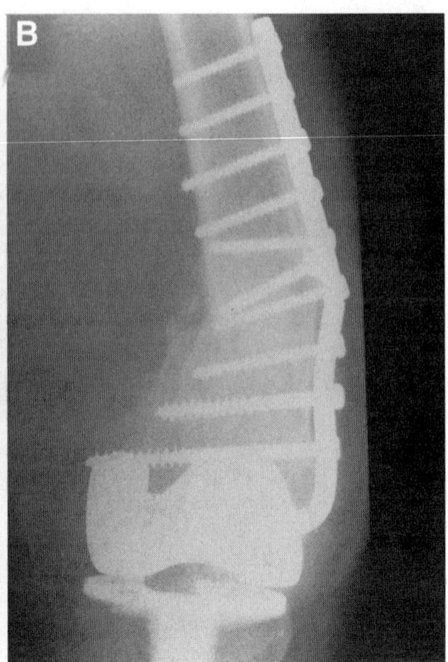
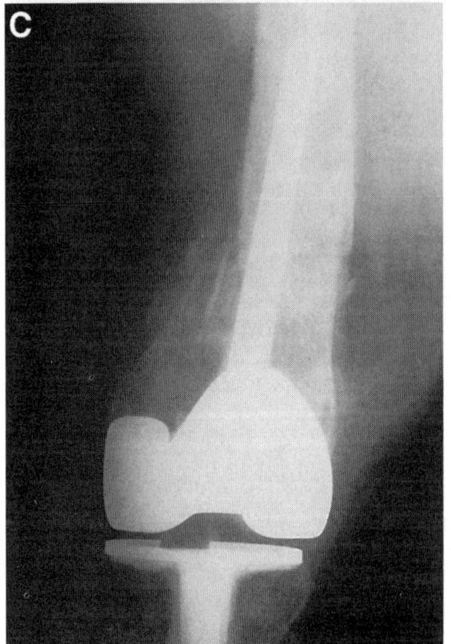

FIGURE 6.—Imaging in a 64-year-old woman with rheumatoid arthritis. **A,** anteroposterior radiograph immediately after open reduction and internal fixation. **B,** eight months postoperatively, plate fracture occurred secondary to nonunion and absence of medial support. **C,** the fracture healed after revision with a long-stemmed prosthesis and bone grafting. (Courtesy of Moran MC, Brick GW, Sledge CB, et al: Supracondylar femoral fracture following total knee arthroplasty. *Clin Orthop* 324:196–209, 1996.)

Use of a Supracondylar Nail for Treatment of a Supracondylar Fracture of the Femur Following Total Knee Arthroplasty

Smith WJ, Martin SL, Mabrey JD (Brooke Army Med Ctr, Fort Sam Houston, Texas; Univ of Texas, San Antonio)
J Arthroplasty 11:210–213, 1996   5–27

Background.—Treating a supracondylar fracture proximal to total knee arthroplasty is difficult. The use of a supracondylar nail for this purpose was illustrated.

Case Report.—Man, 78, sustained a displaced, comminuted supracondylar fracture when he fell on his left knee. He had had a total knee arthroplasty 2.5 years earlier, with good results. However, he had multiple medical problems. During an initial attempt at closed reduction for the fracture, adequate reduction could not be obtained. On the third day of hospitalization, a supracondylar nail was placed. Preoperative planning included checking the clearance of the nail through a sample femoral total knee component of the same size and type as the patient's. Sufficient access to the intercondylar notch was achieved by a standard medial parapatellar arthrotomy. With an 8 mm drill, access was gained to the medullary canal, and a beaded guidewire was inserted and passed proximal to the fracture site. Flexible reamers were passed over the guide rod, and the nail was fixed rigidly to an outrigger and passed retrograde over the rod under fluoroscopic guidance. Accurate placement of the transverse fixation screws was achieved by alignment holes on the outrigger.

Postoperatively, the patient was placed in a knee immobilizer. Rehabilitation included home therapy. The patient was instructed to keep weight off the knee for 6 weeks after surgery. Six weeks postoperatively, radiographic evidence of healing was apparent. A hinged knee brace replaced the knee immobilizer. Bony healing was shown on the 3-month radiographs. The patient now has a pain-free range of motion of 7 to 75 degrees and a Hospital for Special Surgery knee score of 75.

Conclusion.—The supracondylar nail is a new implant with theoretical advantages over the traditional open surgery for patients with supracondylar fracture proximal to total knee arthroplasty. The outcomes of the supracondylar nail should now be compared with those of traditional open surgical techniques in a well-designed, prospective study.

▶ Moran et al. (See Abstract 5–26) report 29 supracondylar femoral fractures above total knee arthroplasties and suggest that closed treatment is satisfactory for undisplaced fractures but that displaced fractures require early open reduction and internal fixation. A variety of fixation techniques were used. Several fractures of supracondylar blade plates were noted. A dynamic condylar screw was found to be stronger and to provide more reliable fixation.

Smith et al. report that an intramedullary nail, inserted retrograde through the intercondylar notch of the femoral component and used in an interlocked fashion, provided good fixation of the supracondylar fracture. Before undertaking this treatment, it is important to know the dimensions of the intercondylar space both anteroposteriorly and laterally to ensure that the intramedullary device chosen can be inserted. In patients with posterior stabilized prostheses, there may not be enough space for this method.

C.B. Sledge, M.D.

Arthroscopy of Symptomatic Total Knee Replacements
Bae DK, Lee HK, Cho JH (Kyung Hee Univ, Seoul, Korea)
Arthroscopy 11:664–671, 1995   5–28

Background.—Complications have been reported after total knee replacement. The role of arthroscopic diagnosis and treatment of symptomatic total knee replacements was investigated.

Methods.—Arthroscopy was performed on 21 knees in 19 patients with primary total knee replacements between 1983 and 1992. The mean interval between total knee replacement and arthroscopy was 20 months. Metal bars of 5 and 8 mm in diameter and 40 cm long were designed for arthroscopic treatment of fibroarthrosis.

Findings.—Eleven patients with 13 knees affected by arthrofibrosis had a mean improvement of 42 degrees arc of motion 1 year after arthroscopic surgery. Three knees had a mean 15-degree increase in motion and were considered failures. In 2 patients undergoing arthroscopic resection of fibrous bands, complete relief of patella pain was achieved. Four of 6 patients undergoing revision of total knee replacements after arthroscopic diagnosis had wear in the metal-backed patella components. Another 2 had wear in the tibial insert and loosening of the cementless patella component.

Conclusion.—In these patients, an early diagnosis of implant failure under arthroscopic control was made, allowing revision of the metal-backed patellar button before metallosis and massive osteolysis developed from the marked wear of polyethylene. The specially designed metal bars permitted an easier release of the adhesion, thereby avoiding damage to valuable arthroscopic instruments.

Arthroscopic Treatment of Peripatellar Fibrosis After Total Knee Arthroplasty

Markel DC, Luessenhop CP, Windsor RE, et al (Wayne State Univ, Southfield, Mich; Orthopedic Sports and Rehabilitation Ctr, Claremore, Okla)
J Arthroplasty 11:293–297, 1996   5–29

Purpose.—Patients who have undergone total knee arthroplasty are at risk for patellofemoral complications. One unusual complication of this type is peripatellar fibrosis forming intra-articular bands or nodules. Manifestations include pain or impingement in the patellofemoral joint or abnormal tracking of the patella accompanied by other signs. The arthroscopic treatment of post–total knee arthroplasty peripatellar fibrosis was reported.

Methods.—The experience included 42 patients with symptomatic peripatellar fibrosis after total knee arthroplasty. All patients had pain in the knee and 98% had clicking or clunking. Seventy-three percent had problems climbing stairs, and 19% had motion problems. Arthroscopic surgery was performed in 48 symptomatic knees. The fibrous tissue was debrided by a standard 3-portal arthroscopic technique, with a fourth portal added as necessary.

Results.—At a mean follow-up of 33 months, the results were rated as good in 42% of patients, fair in 19%, and poor in 40%. Debridement was complicated and difficult; 42% of knees required a fourth arthroscopic portal. None of the total knee components was found to be loose at arthroscopy. The results of arthroscopic treatment were unrelated to pattern of fibrosis or any other variable analyzed.

Conclusion.—In contrast to previous reports, this study finds that the results of arthroscopic surgery for post–total knee arthroplasty peripatellar fibrosis are unpredictable. The procedure is tedious and technically difficult. Although the authors do recommend arthroscopic treatment for this indication, they are careful to set limited and specific surgical goals.

Clinical Symptoms Caused by Intra-articular Fibrous Plicae After Knee Replacement: Arthroscopic Diagnosis and Therapy

Jerosch J, Schröder M (Westfälische-Wilhelms-Univ, Münster, Germany)
Arch Orthop Trauma Surg 115:195–198, 1996   5–30

Background.—Patients with total knee replacements are at risk of ongoing clinical problems, more so than patients with total hip replacements. The patellofemoral joint is a common source of problems. There has been little attention to problems caused by peripatellar fibrous hyperplasia or other fibrous bands. The arthroscopic diagnosis and treatment of clinical problems related to intra-articular plicae after knee replacement were reported.

Patients.—In 29 of 45 patients undergoing arthroscopy after knee replacement, subsequent surgery was needed for clinical complaints related to intra-articular fibrous plicae. In 26 patients, diagnosis and resection were performed during the same arthroscopic procedure. Although clinical complaints varied, all patients had pain during activity that did not respond to conservative therapy. After careful arthroscopic evaluation, the patients underwent excision of all synovial adhesions and fibrous plicae showing mechanical impingement or other signs of mechanical alteration. Follow-up data were available on 23 patients.

Findings.—Five patients were found to have a transverse suprapatellar band causing snapping during active knee extension and painful passive translation of the patella in extension. Seven patients had a lateral plica stretching from the superolateral patellar border to the infrapatellar fat pad. This caused tenderness at the lateral patella and knee snapping during flexion. Four patients had a fibrous, very dense plica at the distal patellar pole, which tethered the patella to the intercondylar notch. Six patients had a discrete fibrous nodule at the proximal patellar pole, causing a painful clunk in extension. Finally, 7 patients had a meniscoid plica in the femorotibial area, with local tenderness over the joint line and signs similar to those of a meniscoid lesion in rotation.

Arthroscopic resection was possible in 26 patients. Three required arthrotomy for resection. The symptoms resolved after arthroscopic resection in 25 of 26 patients. At follow-up, all prostheses were in place and no further surgical revisions were necessary.

Conclusion.—Arthroscopy assists in the diagnosis and treatment of intra-articular fibrous plicae after knee replacement surgery. The causes of these fibrous plicae or nodules are unclear; multiple factors are probably involved.

▶ Severely limited range of motion after total knee arthroplasty is a perplexing complication. No obvious cause is usually evident, and patients respond poorly to manipulation, intra-articular steroid injection, and physical therapy. The paper by Bae et al. (See Abstract 5–28) reports the results of arthroscopic evaluation of 21 knees with symptomatic total knee replacement. Thirteen of those knees had a diagnosis of arthrofibrosis and were successfully treated by arthroscopic lysis of adhesions. Similar results are reported by Markel et al. (See Abstract 5–29) in 48 knees with symptomatic peripatellar fibrosis. Multiple arthroscopic portals were needed. The authors stress the difficulty of the procedure but report satisfactory increase in motion and decrease in pain after the procedure. Jerosch and Schröder report their experience with 26 patients treated by athroscopic resection of scar tissue whom they classified according to 5 types of plicae. Of the 26 patients who underwent arthroscopic resection of this fibrous tissue, 22 were relieved and 4 had persistent complaints.

These 3 papers suggest that arthroscopic lysis of adhesions will be a useful procedure in certain patients with limited range of motion after total knee arthroplasty and in whom the limited motion can be shown to be related to intra-articular adhesions rather than to contracture of the quadriceps muscle. Because contracture of the quadriceps may be the result of long-standing limitation of motion, arthroscopic intervention should be carried out sooner rather than later, but only with a clear understanding of the potential complications of the arthroscopic procedure, including infection.

C.B. Sledge, M.D.

Arthroscopic Release of the Posterior Cruciate Ligament for Stiff Total Knee Arthroplasty
Williams RJ III, Westrich GH, Siegel J, et al (Cornell Med Ctr, New York; Long Island Jewish Med Ctr, New Hyde Park, NY)
Clin Orthop 331:185–191, 1996   5–31

Introduction.—Patients who have undergone total knee arthroplasty sometimes experience loss of knee flexion and/or extension. Knee stiffness can lead to long-term disability and pain. Manipulation under anesthesia is the first treatment option in this situation, but some patients are not seen until after the optimal time for benefit from manipulation. The value of arthroscopic release of the posterior cruciate ligament for patients in this situation was evaluated.

Methods.—The experience included 9 patients with 10 posterior cruciate ligament–sparing total knee arthroplasties. All had postoperative knee stiffness and pain. The problem persisted despite manipulation under anesthesia in 6 knees. The patients' mean knee extension was 4 degrees and mean knee flexion was 73.9 degrees. All underwent arthroscopic release of the posterior cruciate ligament, performed at a mean of 29 months after total knee arthroplasty. The effects of this procedure on knee range of motion and pain were analyzed. The mean follow-up was 20 months.

Results.—Immediately after posterior cruciate ligament release with manipulation, mean extension was 1.3 degree and mean flexion was 112 degrees. In the immediate postoperative period, flexion increased by an average of 40.1 degrees. At follow-up, the knees had a mean extension of 1.5 degrees and a mean flexion of 104.5 degrees. Flexion had increased by an average of 30.5 degrees by follow-up. The average Knee Society knee score improved from 70.9 to 86.4 after arthroscopic posterior cruciate ligament release. The average Knee Society function score improved from 71 to 88, and the pain score improved from 33.5 to 42. All patients reported improvements in pain and stiffness, and 88% were satisfied with the procedure. The total knee arthroplasty had to be revised in 22% of patients.

Conclusion.—Arthroscopic posterior cruciate ligament release provides good results for most patients with persistent knee pain and stiffness after posterior cruciate ligament–sparing total knee replacement. This procedure may provide a new alternative for patients who do not improve with manipulation alone. The procedure is safe, convenient, and cost effective, providing good improvement for 88% of patients. It should be performed only in knees that are well aligned and well balanced.

▶ Another cause of limited flexion and pain is excessive tightness of the posterior cruciate ligament in posterior cruciate ligament–retaining implants. These authors report arthroscopic release of the posterior cruciate ligament in 10 knees. There were 8 satisfactory results; 2 patients required revision total knee arthroplasty for persistent symptoms.

C.B. Sledge, M.D.

Recurrent Hemarthrosis After Total Knee Arthroplasty

Kindsfater K, Scott R (Brigham & Women's Hosp, Boston; New England Baptist Hosp, Boston)
J Arthroplasty 10:52S–55S, 1995   5–32

Objective.—Spontaneous hemarthrosis of the knee is a rare problem in patients who have had total knee arthroplasty. When it happens, it can be a recurrent, disabling problem. A large group of patients with recurrent hemarthrosis after TKA were evaluated.

Patients.—Thirty patients with recurrent hemarthrosis after total knee arthroplasty were identified through a questionnaire sent to members of the Knee Society. The 17 women and 13 men, had an average age of 70 years. The patients were followed for 28 months. The initial episode of bleeding occurred an average of 24 months after prosthesis implantation, and the average number of recurrences was 5.5. Nine patients responded to initial aspiration and conservative care. Surgical treatment was needed in the remaining 21 knees. Open synovectomy was curative in 14 of 15 knees, including 2 knees in which arthroscopic synovectomy failed. Arthroscopic synovectomy succeeded in another 2 knees. The remaining 4 knees were successfully treated by revision of the total knee arthroplasty components, with no need for synovectomy.

Of 21 surgically treated knees, just 9 had an identifiable cause of hemarthrosis. In these cases, there was entrapment of proliferative synovial tissue or of the fat pad between components of the knee prosthesis. The histologic findings included focal synovial hyperplasia with significant hemosiderin deposition.

Conclusion.—Recurrent hemarthrosis of the knee can cause significant problems for patients with total knee arthroplasty. It may result from a proliferative synovitis that becomes entrapped between the prosthetic components. If aspiration and other conservative treatments fail to prevent recurrent episodes, open synovectomy is needed. The histologic findings are similar to, but should not be confused with, those of pigmented villonodular synovitis.

▶ Recurrent hemarthrosis is a rare complication of total knee arthroplasty. To find the 30 patients that are the subject of this report, Kindsfater and

Scott surveyed members of the Knee Society and identified 21 patients, whom they added to their own personal series of 9 cases. In 21 patients, symptoms were sufficiently severe to warrant surgical intervention. In 15 of those patients, synovectomy was carried out and appeared to be curative in 14. Nine patients had an identifiable piece of synovium that appeared to be trapped between the components. In the remaining patients, there was no identifiable source of the hemorrhage but synovectomy was curative. The authors point out that in diagnosing the condition, all other causes for pain and recurrent bleeding should be excluded, including loose components. This must remain a diagnosis of exclusion.

C.B. Sledge, M.D.

Arterial Complications After Knee Arthroplasty: 4 Cases and a Review of the Literature
Holmberg A, Milbrink J, Bergqvist D (Univ Hosp Uppsala, Sweden)
Acta Orthop Scand 67:75–78, 1996   5–33

Purpose.—Rarely, a patient will experience arterial complications after total knee replacement. Severe ischemia can lead to amputation if the problem is not recognized and treated in time. Forty-four cases of arterial complications after total knee replacement were reviewed and analyzed, including 4 new cases.

Findings.—The estimated incidence of arterial problems after total knee arthroplasty is 0.2% to 0.03%. When the problems occur, however, these complications are serious. Eleven of the 44 patients required amputation from the midtarsal level to above the knee, and 1 died. The most common complication of this type is thrombotic occlusion; others include severed popliteal artery, arteriovenous fistula and false aneurysm, and accelerated arteriosclerotic disease. The postoperative evaluation must include signs of acute ischemia in the lower limb: pulselessness, pallor, pain, paresthesia, and paralysis (the 5 P's). Immediate treatment, usually including treatment by a vascular surgeon, is needed whenever an arterial complication is suspected or recognized. Delay reduces the chances of limb salvage. Surgical procedures may include thrombectomy, arterial patching, bypass, or direct anastomosis. In some cases, fasciotomy may be indicated; such cases include delayed reconstruction, extensive swelling, paresthesia and paralysis, and pain on passive muscle extension. Prevention starts with evaluation of the risk factors for arterial injury (Table 4). Patients with any risk factor should have measurement of ankle pressures.

Discussion.—Arterial complications are a rare but dangerous occurrence in patients who have had total knee arthroplasty. This article includes a review of the potential risk factors and prevention of complications. The need for a tourniquet may be questioned in patients with extensive arterial calcifications. For patients with any of the preoperative

---

TABLE 4.—Preoperative Risk Factors for Arterial Injury in Connection
With Total Knee Arthroplasty

Intermittent claudication
Ischemic rest pain
Arterial ulcers
Limb pulses not palpable
Popliteal aneurysm suspected
Previous arterial reconstruction
Arterial calcification on plain radiographs

(Courtesy of Holmberg A, Milbrink J, Bergqvist D: Arterial complications after knee arthroplasty:
4 cases and a review of the literature *Acta Orthop Scand* 67:75–78, 1996.)

---

risk factors, intraoperative manipulation of the knee should be kept to a
minimum.

▶ Arterial problems are rare complications of total knee replacement but
may have disastrous consequences unless recognized and dealt with immediately. In this review of 44 cases, amputation or death occurred in one
fourth of the cases. In patients with pre-existing peripheral vascular
disease—especially those with absent pedal pulses or significant arterial
calcification—extreme caution should be exercised and a very low index of
suspicion maintained.

C.B. Sledge, M.D.

Peroneal Nerve Palsy After Total Knee Arthroplasty: Assessment of Predisposing and Prognostic Factors

Idusuyi OB, Morrey BF (Mayo Clinic and Mayo Found, Rochester, Minn)
J Bone Joint Surg Am 78:177–184, 1996   5–34

Background.—Peroneal nerve injury may occur in patients who have
had total knee arthroplasty and may be associated with preoperative
flexion or valgus deformity. However, some patients have neither of these
deformities and no identifiable cause of injury. A large group of patients
with peroneal nerve palsy after total knee arthroplasty was reviewed to
gain insight into the risk factors for this complication.

Methods.—In a series of 10,361 consecutive total knee arthroplasties,
there were 32 cases of postoperative peroneal nerve palsy. Two patients
had the bilateral form. The 18 men and 15 women had a mean age of 65
years. The diagnosis was usually made in the first 3 postoperative days.
Proximal tibial osteotomy had been performed previously in 4 patients,
and lumbar laminectomy had been done in 5. Ten patients had 12 degrees
or more of valgus alignment before surgery. The patients were matched to
a group of 100 patients who had total knee arthroplasty during the same
period but did not have peroneal nerve palsy. The data were analyzed in an
attempt to clarify which patients are at risk of peroneal nerve palsy and to
identify avoidable risk factors.

Results.—Three factors were significantly associated with peroneal nerve palsy: epidural anesthesia for postoperative pain control, previous laminectomy, and preoperative valgus deformity. Although patients with previous tibial osteotomy were more likely to have peroneal nerve palsy, this factor was not significant. On subgroup analysis of 4,388 total knee arthroplasties performed from 1988 through 1992, 25 cases of peroneal nerve palsy were identified. Of these, 18 occurred in patients who had received epidural anesthesia.

Conclusion.—Patients who receive epidural anesthesia for postoperative pain control after total knee arthroplasty have decreased proprioception and sensation. Under these conditions, limb positioning could be an important factor in the development of palsy. This type of "double-crush" injury could account for the cases of peroneal nerve palsy observed in patients having lumbar laminectomy and asymptomatic peripheral neuropathy.

▶ Thirty-two cases of peroneal nerve palsy detected after total knee arthroplasty are the subject of this report. Epidural anesthesia was identified as a risk factor, with an incidence 2.8 times greater in those patients than in those who received general or spinal anesthesia. The authors attribute the increased risk in patients with epidural anesthesia to the period of diminished sensation in the postoperative period, leading to failure of the patients to report pressure on the peroneal nerve from positioning of the extremity and pressure against external devices such as continuous passive motion machines.

C.B. Sledge, M.D.

Fracture of the Metal Tibial Tray After Kinematic Total Knee Replacement

Abernethy PJ, Robinson CM, Fowler RM (Princess Margaret Rose Orthopaedic Hosp, Edinburgh, Scotland)
J Bone Joint Surg Br 78:220–225, 1996   5–35

Objective.—Fracture of the baseplate is a rare complication in total knee replacement, at least since the introduction of metal-backed tibial components. In 1983, the authors switched from the Total Condylar prosthesis, which has an all-plastic tibial component, to the Kinematic Condylar prosthesis, which has a metal tibial tray. Their experience with these 2 prostheses was reviewed to assess the effects of a metal-backed tibial component on implant survival.

Methods.—From 1980 to 1990, Total Condylar replacements were placed in 550 patients and Kinematic Condylar prostheses were placed in 1,017 patients. Implant survival was compared in these 2 groups. The analysis also investigated factors affecting fracture of the metal tibial tray and the results of revision surgery.

Results.—The 10-year survival rate was 88% for the Kinematic Condylar prosthesis vs. 92% for the Total Condylar prosthesis. The advantage of the Total Condylar design arose mainly from 16 revisions performed for fracture of the metal baseplate in the Kinematic group. There were no fatigue fractures of the tibial component in patients with the Total Condylar prosthesis. Also, despite their longer follow-up, fewer patients in the Total Condylar group required surgical revision for aseptic complications.

For patients with Kinematic prostheses, baseplate fracture was the major cause of aseptic failure. The main factor associated with baseplate fracture in Kinematic prostheses was preoperative varus deformity, with a hazard ratio (HR) of 8.8. Hazard ratios were somewhat elevated for male patients and osteoarthritic knees (HR, 1.9 and 1.8, respectively). Nine fractures occurred within 4 years after implantation of the Kinematic prosthesis. In this group, fracture was strongly associated with failure to correct preoperative varus deformity (HR, 13.9) and with the use of a bone graft to correct varus deformity (HR, 15.8). Neither these nor any other factors were identified in the 8 fractures occurring more than 5 years after implant placement. Sixteen revision procedures were done for patients with tray fracture. There were 2 complications in this group—1 deep infection and 1 case of refracture.

Conclusion.—This experience suggests that deformation of all-plastic tibial components is less frequent than previously thought. Fracture of the metal tibial baseplate is a relatively common cause of failure with the Kinematic Condylar knee replacement. The authors are conducting a randomized trial to compare all-plastic vs. metal-backed tibial component designs.

▶ The authors report 16 revisions required for fracture of the metal baseplate in 853 total knee arthroplasties. Contributing factors were persistent axial malalignment in the 9 fractures that occurred in the first 4 postoperative years. In the 8 fractures that occurred more than 5 years after replacement, the authors could detect no significant risk factors and suggest that the tibial plate was not sufficiently strong.

C.B. Sledge, M.D.

Infections

Multiple Prosthetic Infections After Total Joint Arthroplasty: Risk Factor Analysis
Luessenhop CP, Higgins LD, Brause BD, et al (Hosp for Special Surgery, New York)
J Arthroplasty 11:862–868, 1996   5–36

Purpose.—In patients with total joint arthroplasties, infection is an uncommon but devastating complication. Various host factors have been evaluated for their role in prosthetic sepsis. However, few studies have investigated the risk associated with hematogenous spread of infection from 1 arthroplasty to another in patients with multiple arthroplasties.

Risk factors for the development of multiple prosthetic infections in patients with more than 1 joint arthroplasty were analyzed.

Methods.—The retrospective study included 145 patients with multiple prostheses who had infection of at least 1 of the joints. The patients had a total of 360 replacement arthroplasties and 174 deep infections of total arthroplasties: 103 in the knee, 69 in the hip, and 2 in the shoulder. Risk factors for multiple infections were analyzed, including diagnosis, age, sex, corticosteroid use, diabetes, and other major infections not involving a joint arthroplasty.

Results.—Twenty-seven patients had infection of more than 1 arthroplasty, for an incidence of 19%. Nineteen of these 27 patients had rheumatoid arthritis (RA). Seventeen had an associated major nonprosthetic infection; 6 of these had septicemia with no other primary source of infection identified, and 4 had an infected decubitus ulcer. According to American Rheumatism Association classification, patients with RA with multiple infections had poorer overall function than those with a single infection. In more than half of cases, a patient's multiple infections came to clinical attention within 1 month of each other; most multiple infections were associated with a nonprosthetic infection.

Conclusion.—In patients with multiple joint arthroplasties, RA and major nonprosthetic infection are significant risk factors for infection of more than 1 arthroplasty. It is impossible to predict the risk of further infection in patients with 1 infected arthroplasty. In many cases, the infected arthroplasties may be seeded simultaneously during a period of septicemia.

▶ Infection of a total joint arthroplasty is a major life-threatening complication; infection of multiple joints in a patient with multiple arthroplasties is truly disastrous. This paper confirms earlier studies showing that RA is a significant risk factor for the development of a postoperative infection and for those with multiple prosthetic infections, it is the *major* risk factor. Most of these patients also had nonprosthetic infections that often preceded the first prosthetic infection. This would suggest that extreme diligence in preventing soft-tissue infections or infections of the urinary tract etc., should be in place. In addition, such soft-tissue infections in patients with joint replacements should be treated early and aggressively. Although the literature is ambiguous, I believe such patients should receive prophylactic antiobiotic treatment for soft-tissue procedures, such as dental treatment in the face of gingivitis and for manipulations of the gastrointestinal and genitourinary tracts.

C.B. Sledge, M.D.

Serum C-Reactive Protein Levels After Total Hip and Knee Arthroplasty

Niskanen RO, Korkala O, Pammo H (Lahti City Hosp, Finland)
J Bone Joint Surg Br 78:431–433, 1996   5–37

Background.—The tissue damage caused by any surgery produces an elevation in serum C-reactive protein (CRP). The elevation persists for only 2 or 3 days, if there are no complications. It is unknown what happens to the CRP level if complications occur. Changes in the CRP level associated with complications of joint replacement arthroplasty were analyzed, including the possible impact of cemented vs. uncemented prostheses.

Methods.—The study included 100 patients with minor or major complications after primary total hip or knee arthroplasty. "Various medical problems" was the most common category of complications, followed by prolonged wound exudates and hematomas. Two hundred seventy-three patients without complications were studied for comparison. Serum CRP levels after surgery were monitored. All patients had normal CRP levels of less than 10 mg/L before surgery.

Results.—The complication rate was slightly higher for patients with cemented prostheses. For patients without complications, the CRP level peaked at 2 or 3 days after surgery. For patients with complications, the 75th percentile CRP curve was different; the descending part of the curve occurred later, with peaks at 1 and 2 weeks postoperatively. Both groups had a slight increase in body temperature in the first few postoperative days. None had any deep prosthetic infections.

Conclusion.—The serum CRP level may be a useful indicator of infections after total hip and knee arthroplasty. A peak CRP level on the second or third postoperative day is normal. A further increase at 1 or 2 weeks suggests a serious complication.

▶ The erythrocyte sedimentation rate (ESR) is an insensitive test for infection after total joint arthroplasty. In the absence of infection, the ESR may remain elevated for 6 months or more and, in the presence of infection, it may respond slowly. The study reported by Niskanen and colleagues shows that the CRP produces a much more responsive and sensitive test, with the CRP falling to normal within 8–12 days in uncomplicated cases. This makes for a much more reliable test if infection is suspected in the first 6 months after joint arthroplasty.

C.B. Sledge, M.D.

Aspiration of the Knee Joint Before Revision Arthroplasty

Duff GP, Lachiewicz PF, Kelley SS (Univ of North Carolina, Chapel Hill)
Clin Orthop 331:132–139, 1996   5–38

Introduction.—Acute infection of a replacement knee joint is usually obvious, but subacute or low-grade infections can be difficult to recognize.

Preoperative aspiration of the prosthetic knee joint would seem to be an important procedure, yet there have been no studies of its accuracy. The sensitivity, specificity, and accuracy of preoperative aspiration was studied in patients undergoing revision arthroplasty.

Methods.—The retrospective study included 64 revision arthroplasties performed in 55 patients with prosthetic knees. The indications for revision were pain, loosening, instability, or suspected infection. Preoperative aspiration was performed in 43 knees, and the ability of this procedure to recognize infection was analyzed. The clinical, laboratory, and radiographic variables were analyzed for their ability to predict which knees are likely to be infected and should be aspirated.

Results.—In 19 of 43 knees, the aspirate showed growth on solid media. Intraoperative cultures confirmed the presence of infection in 18 of these knees. The remaining patient was receiving an IV antibiotic at the time of arthroscopic irrigation and debridement. Of the 24 knees with negative preoperative aspiration results, only 1 had a positive intraoperative culture. This patient had a single intraoperative culture growing *Staphylococcus epidermidis*, and the clinical and radiographic findings all pointed to aseptic loosening of a cemented total knee arthroplasty. The sensitivity, specificity, and accuracy of preoperative aspiration were, thus, considered to be 100%. Other variables—including Westergren erythrocyte sedimentation rate, peripheral leukocyte count, and presenting symptoms—were not good indicators of infection. Radiographs showed component loosening, periostitis, focal osteolysis, and radiolucent lines in infected and noninfected knees alike.

Conclusion.—In patients undergoing revision of a total knee arthroplasty, preoperative aspiration of the knee is the most helpful diagnostic technique for recognition or exclusion of infection. As suggested in previous reports, all painful knee arthroplasties should be considered infected until proven otherwise. Aspiration should be routinely performed in any painful or otherwise problematic total knee arthroplasty before open or arthroscopic examination or revision.

▶ Analysis of 55 patients undergoing revision knee arthroplasty revealed that aspiration of the knee was the most helpful study for the diagnosis or exclusion of infection. In 19 knees, the aspirate showed growth on solid media, and in 18 of those knees, the diagnosis of infection was confirmed by the intraoperative cultures. In the 1 case in which intraoperative cultures did not confirm the preoperative aspiration, the patient was receiving antibiotics at the time of the intraoperative culture. In 23 of 24 knees with negative preoperative aspiration results, the intraoperative cultures were also negative; the 1 exception showed a single colony of *Staphylococcus*. In the hands of these authors, preoperative aspiration of a failed total knee arthroplasty is an extremely important and reliable test.

C.B. Sledge, M.D.

The Role of Intraoperative Frozen Sections in Revision Total Joint Arthroplasty

Feldman DS, Lonner JH, Desai P, et al (Hosp for Joint Diseases, New York City)
J Bone Joint Surg Am 77:1807–1813, 1995   5–39

Objective.—Various approaches have been tried, with limited success, for preoperative and intraoperative identification of loose, painful total hip and knee replacements. Previous reports have suggested histologic analysis of frozen sections of intraoperative specimens as an approach to identifying infection. The sensitivity, specificity, and accuracy of this approach were retrospectively analyzed.

Methods.—Thirty-three consecutive patients undergoing total hip or knee revision arthroplasty were studied. During surgery, frozen sections were taken of periprosthetic tissue at the bone-cement interface or the pseudocapsule and examined microscopically for signs of infection. Those with more than 5 polymorphonuclear leukocytes per high-power field in at least 5 distinct microscopic fields were classified as positive for active infection. The patients were followed for an average of 36 months.

Results.—Frozen sections were positive in 10 patients and negative in 23. The findings on frozen section correlated 100% with those of the permanent histologic sections. Nine of 9 patients with positive intraoperative sections also had positive frozen sections; 23 of 24 patients with negative intraoperative sections had negative frozen sections. Just 2 of 9 patients with positive intraoperative cultures had a positive intraoperative Gram's stain. Compared with the final pathologic diagnosis, the surgeon's operative prediction regarding the presence or absence of infection was 70% sensitive, 87% specific, and 82% accurate. All 10 patients with positive frozen sections underwent excision arthroplasty; 6 later had reimplantation. Most of the patients with negative frozen sections had primary exchange revision arthroplasty. No patient in either group had later evidence of infection.

Conclusion.—Intraoperative frozen sections of periprosthetic tissue provide a reliable indicator of active infection in patients undergoing revision joint arthroplasty. Even in patients with negative or equivocal workup results, signs of acute tissue inflammation in frozen sections should be regarded as presumptive evidence of infection. Together with other standard tests, intraoperative frozen sections can help to differentiate between aseptic and septic loosening.

▶ By the time the intraoperative culture reports are back, the revision hip or knee arthroplasty is over. In some instances, there will be no preoperative aspiration and culture; in other instances, the results of that aspiration will be ambiguous. This paper shows that intraoperative frozen sections can be a very useful guide. If there are more than 5 polymorphonuclear leukocytes per high power field in at least 5 distinct microscopic fields, the patient can be assumed, with 100% accuracy, to be infected. Conversely, if the frozen section does not meet those criteria, the specificity is 96%.

C.B. Sledge, M.D.

Removal of Surface Bacteria by Irrigation
Anglen J, Apostoles PS, Christensen G, et al (Univ of Missouri, Columbia)
J Orthop Res 14:251–254, 1996   5–40

Introduction.—Power irrigation of contaminated wounds is an accepted practice in orthopedic procedures. Various antibiotics are commonly added to the irrigation solution to reduce the risk of subsequent infection. By using a laboratory model, 4 irrigation solutions were tested for their efficacy in removing bacteria from 3 different surfaces.

Methods.—Titanium, stainless-steel, and cortical bone surfaces were coated with 3 bacterial species (*Staphylococcus aureus, Pseudomonas aeruginosa,* and *Staphylococcus epidermidis*), then irrigated with 1 L of fluid delivered by jet lavage. The 4 fluids tested were normal saline and solutions of bacitracin, neomycin, and Castile soap (Triad Medical, Franklin, Wis). One set of specimens served as a control and was not irrigated. To remove residual bacteria, the specimens were sonicated after irrigation. Sonicates were then quantitatively cultured so that the amount of residual bacteria on the surfaces could be evaluated.

Results.—Compared with control specimens, all irrigation solutions resulted in significantly less mean bacterial growth. For all 3 surfaces coated with *S. epidermidis*, the 4 treatments did not differ significantly overall in removal of bacteria; soap, however, removed significantly more of this bacteria from steel and titanium surfaces. Neomycin solution showed a significant advantage in the removal of *P. aeruginosa* from bone.

Conclusions.—Although all irrigation groups were superior to the no-irrigation control, soap solution was as good or better than saline or antibiotic solutions at removing all types of bacteria from all surfaces. Thus, soap solution may prove to be the preferred irrigation additive.

▶ It is accepted dogma that tissue irrigation is effective in reducing contamination of wounds. The effectiveness, however, has not been subject to rigorous investigation. The authors of this article show that jet lavage with 1 L of fluid was effective in reducing bacterial contamination of both metallic implants and cortical bone. When the usefulness of normal saline, antibiotic solutions, and soap was compared, soap emerged as the most effective. This is probably because of its detergent effect on the glycoprotein coating in which the bacteria are sequestered on such surfaces.

C.B. Sledge, M.D.

Risk Factors for Septic Arthritis in Patients With Joint Disease: A Prospective Study

Kaandorp CJE, van Schaardenburg D, Krijnen P, et al (Jan van Breemen Inst, Amsterdam; Erasmus Univ, Rotterdam, The Netherlands; Med Spectrum, Twente, The Netherlands)

Arthritis Rheum 38:1819–1825, 1995   5–41

Introduction.—Septic arthritis is associated with a high rate of mortality, and surviving patients often experience a permanent loss of joint function. Various risk factors have been identified, including diseases and medications that reduce immunocompetence, joint prostheses, and joint surgery. To quantify potential risk factors for septic arthritis so that preventive strategies might be adopted, a prospective study was conducted.

Methods.—Study participants were adult patients attending a rheumatic disease clinic in The Netherlands between 1990 and 1992. Disease categories included rheumatoid arthritis (RA), undifferentiated oligoarthritis or polyarthritis, juvenile chronic arthritis, ankylosing spondylitis, and osteoarthritis. Questionnaires were sent every 3 months to patients who gave informed consent. The occurrence of septic arthritis between October 1990 and October 1993 was recorded in all patients who attended the clinic network. Those with septic arthritis were interviewed by an investigator. Risk factors for septic arthritis were identified by comparing data on patients in whom septic arthritis developed with data on those without septic arthritis.

Results.—During the study period, septic arthritis developed in 37 of the 4,907 patients with joint disease. Diagnoses were made in 24 cases during the 2 years of questionnaire mailing and in 13 cases during the third year of case finding. Bacteria were cultured from joint fluid or tissue in 32 patients, 15 of whom were found to be infected with *Staphylococcus aureus*. Patients with septic arthritis had a mean age of 65 years; 23 were women and 14 were men. Twenty-five had RA, and the mean duration of their disease was 22 years. Twelve patients, all with RA, were treated with immunosuppressive agents. The 37 patients had 46 infected joints; in 27 patients the infected joint contained foreign material. The most frequent probable cause of septic arthritis was direct inoculation of bacteria into the joint, which occurred in 15 patients. Multivariate analysis identified 7 risk factors for septic arthritis and their odds ratios (ORs): age 80 years or older (OR, 3.5); diabetes mellitus (OR, 3.3); RA (OR, 4.0); recent joint surgery (OR, 5.1); hip or knee prosthesis without skin infection (OR, 15.0); no hip or knee prosthesis, with skin infection (27.2); and hip or knee prosthesis and skin infection (OR, 72.7).

Discussion.—Most patients with septic arthritis had RA of long duration and with considerable joint destruction. Another important risk factor is skin infection, and all patients with a skin infection as the cause of septic arthritis had RA. With a knowledge of significant risk factors, preventive measures can be directed toward patients at highest risk for septic arthritis.

▶ In this study of nearly 5,000 patients seen in a rheumatic disease clinic, risk factors for the development of septic arthritis were identified. The major risk factors were the presence of a joint prosthesis or skin infection. In addition, patients older than 80 years, and those with diabetes or RA were at increased risk. Prophylactic measures in these patients must be rigorous and continuous because many of the infections show up late.

C.B. Sledge, M.D.

Retroviral Transmission in Bone Allotransplantation: The Effects of Tissue Processing

Nemzek JA, Arnoczky SP, Swenson CL (Michigan State Univ, East Lansing)
Clin Orthop 324:275–282, 1996
5–42

Introduction.—Transmission of HIV through transplantation of cancellous bone has been reported, and it is theorized that bone marrow is responsible for the viral transmission. Methods suggested for reducing the risk of viral transmission include removal of bone marrow from bone allografts and freezing of bone. To determine whether a retrovirus could be transmitted through transplantation of cortical and corticocancellous bone allografts that had been processed by various techniques, a study using the feline leukemia virus was conducted.

Methods.—Three techniques for processing bone grafts were studied: a single freeze/thaw cycle, a double freeze/thaw cycle, and a double freeze/thaw cycle with a water flush. The retrovirus used in the study, feline leukemia virus, had biological similarities to HIV. Four cats, 8 weeks of age, were inoculated with the virus. Eight weeks later, the femurs and humeri of the animals were harvested. Three long bones from each of the donor cats were used for transplantation into specific-pathogen-free cats, also 8 weeks of age. Seven recipients had frozen allografts, 8 had double frozen allografts, and 8 had water-flushed allografts. One cat underwent identical surgical handling but did not receive an allograft. Plasma samples were obtained weekly and tested for viral antigen with an enzyme-linked immunosorbent assay.

Results.—All donor animals tested positive for viral antigen at the time of harvest. Highly cellular bone marrow was found to be present in the metaphyseal portion of the bone at histologic examination of the bone adjacent to the graft donor sites in the single freeze/thaw and double freeze/thaw groups. Few bone marrow cells were present at the graft donor site in the double/freeze, water-flushed bones, but groups of lacunae in the bone still contained pyknotic nuclei. Antigen and antibody testing revealed transmission of virus in all cortical and cancellous bone allografts in each of the 3 treatment groups.

Conclusions.—Despite routine processing and removal of bone marrow, feline leukemia virus was transmitted by bone allografts. Thus, HIV, with a structure and replication cycle similar to feline leukemia virus, may be transmitted through transplantation of bone allografts treated by freeze/thaw methods.

▶ Musculoskeletal allograft tissue has become increasingly important in orthopedic surgery, whether it be for anterior cruciate ligament grafts cartilage, menisci, or bone. Unfortunately, the usefulness of such tissues is limited by the risk of viral transmission such as HIV. The authors of this study report that bone grafts subjected to freezing and thawing with water flushing to remove bone marrow still transmitted virus. They appropriately conclude that other methods of sterilization of allograft tissue should be done before their clinical use.

C.B. Sledge, M.D.

Anterior Cruciate Ligament

Non-operative Management of Anterior Cruciate Ligament Injuries in the General Population
Casteleyn P-P, Handelberg F (Vrije Universiteit Brussel, Belgium)
J Bone Joint Surg Br 78:446–451, 1996   5–43

Introduction.—Operative treatment using grafts is commonly recommended for athletes with lesions of the anterior cruciate ligament (ACL). However, many of these injuries occur in nonathletes—the result of accidents or less-demanding recreational activities. The status of a group of patients who were not professional or high-level athletes was followed for long-term outcome after conservative treatment of ACL lesions.

Methods.—The conservatively managed group included 228 of the 274 (83%) patients treated over 12 years. Among the 46 patients treated by ACL reconstruction were those with gross or multidirectional joint laxity and all high-level or professional athletes. The patients who had nonoperative management had a mean age of 33.2 years at the time of injury. Most had been injured during recreational or daily living activities. No reconstructive ACL surgery was done during the initial arthroscopy; meniscal surgery was undertaken if indicated and feasible. Partial arthroscopic meniscectomy was used to treat 77.1% of the medial and 85.2% of the lateral meniscal lesions. All patients took part in a 6- to 8-week comprehensive rehabilitation program. Follow-up ranged from 2 to 12 years.

Results.—Of the 203 patients followed up for at least 2 years, only 11 (5.4%) needed secondary ACL surgery and 7 (3.5%) had secondary meniscal surgery—all during the first 3 years after injury. Slightly more than half (55%) of the patients reported no modification of their activity level after ACL injury; 87 reported some decrease in activity level, but 30 said that their reduced activity level was unrelated to the ACL injury. A subgroup of 109 patients was followed up for at least 5 years (mean, 8.5 years) and evaluated with the IKDC score. Outcome was reasonably satisfactory in these patients, with 83% achieving grades A or B. The final evaluation grade showed no correlation with age at time of injury, associated lesions, or activity levels.

Conclusions.—Nonoperative treatment can yield acceptable functional results in patients who do not participate in sports activities at a high level. Long-term follow-up showed no deterioration with time and only very limited osteoarthritic changes.

▶ The treatment of rupture of the ACL remains controversial: who should have surgical repair, who can function adequately with conservative treatment, what surgical repair is best, and what is the optimal time for surgical repair. This article reports the nonoperative management of ACL tears in a group of recreational athletes, as contrasted with the usual report of results in the competitive athlete. For the 228 patients studied (all with arthroscopically proven rupture of the ACL), only 5.4% needed secondary ACL surgery and 3.5% had meniscal surgery, all within the first 3 years after the injury.

These findings emphasize the importance of determining the level of athletic activity that the patient wishes to pursue after the injury; for those patients who wish only to return to occasional recreational athletics not involving sudden shift in direction, conservative management can produce satisfactory results. These results parallel those reported by Daniel and Fithian.[1]

C.B. Sledge, M.D.

Reference

1. Daniel DM, Fithian DC: Indications for ACL surgery. *Arthroscopy* 10:434–441, 1994.

Reconstruction of the Chronically Insufficient Anterior Cruciate Ligament: Long-term Results of the Eriksson Procedure

Natri A, Järvinen M, Lehto M, et al (Univ of Tampere, Finland; UKK Inst, Tampere, Finland)
Int Orthop 20:28–31, 1996   5–44

Introduction.—Chronic anterior cruciate ligament (ACL) insufficiency eventually develops in most patients who are treated conservatively for a torn ACL. Instability also occurs frequently after primary suture of the torn ACL without augmentation or reconstruction. Long-term results are reported for patients with chronic insufficiency of the ACL treated by reconstruction using the medial one third of the patellar tendon.

Methods.—Between 1981 and 1987, 42 patients operated on at the study institution for unilateral chronic ACL insufficiency had the medial one third of the patellar tendon as the graft. Thirty-five of these patients were re-examined at follow-up; 3 were excluded from analysis because they had a second reconstruction of the ACL during the follow-up period. Patients whose outcome is reported were 26 men and 6 women with an average age of 30 years at the time of reconstruction. Most were injured during sports activities (56%) or at work (25%). The knee injury had occurred at a mean of 4.8 years before reconstruction, during which time 28 operations had been done in 20 patients. All had symptoms of instability with giving way. Surgery revealed the ACL to be completely atrophied and functionless in all cases.

Results.—Follow-up examinations were done an average of 6.6 years after reconstruction, with normal healthy knee used as a control. The Lysholm knee scores, calculated from subjective, functional, and clinical evaluations, showed results to be excellent or good in 58% of patients. Twenty reported little or no anterior knee pain, 7 had moderate pain, and 5 had marked pain. Of 29 patients who were active in sports before injury, 21 could continue at the same or a reduced level of activity. The Lachman test showed that 50% of the knees were completely stable and none had severe laxity. Results from the anterior drawer test were negative in 59% and from the pivot shift, in 69%.

Conclusions.—Reconstruction of the chronically insufficient ACL using the medial one third of the patellar tendon restored stability and relieved pain in most patients. Although only 50% of patients were subjectively satisfied with the end result, two thirds of those who had been active in sports before injury were able to continue with their activity.

▶ In patients with ACL rupture in whom acute repair is not undertaken, a certain percentage will come to late reconstruction. There has been concern that the results of this late reconstruction would be so inferior to primary reconstruction that the former was to be routinely used. This article would tend to confirm those suspicions. The average delay before operation was nearly 5 years, and only 50% of patients were satisfied with the outcome even though most had good restoration of stability. Major causes of failure were inadequate range of motion and decreased quadriceps strength as well as patellar pain.

The authors point out that the surgical technique used, which used the medial third of the patellar tendon, probably produced a graft that was too short to allow an adequate range of motion and increased patellofemoral pressure. A subsequent group using bone-patellar tendon-bone autograft for reconstruction produced a 93% satisfactory outcome. My interpretation of this article is that, using modern techniques of ACL reconstruction with adequate length of the autograft and contemporary rehabilitation techniques, extremely satisfactory results can be expected with late reconstruction of the ACL. This would bring into question the philosophy of immediate repair of *all* ACL ruptures.

C.B. Sledge, M.D.

Graft Selection in Anterior Cruciate Ligament Revision Surgery

Ritchie JR, Parker RD (Cleveland Clinic Found, Ohio)
Clin Orthop 325:65–77, 1996

5–45

Background.—Reconstruction of the anterior cruciate ligament is reported to have a failure rate of 10% to 25%, and revision procedures are becoming more commonplace. Patients must understand that the expected outcome of revision surgery differs from that of primary anterior cruciate ligament reconstruction. It is also important to determine why the original procedure failed, because reason for failure may affect the choice of graft. Various options for tissue use for revision anterior cruciate ligament surgery were described. Three types of replacements are available: autografts, allografts, and synthetic materials.

Autografts.—Autogenous tissue has several advantages, including elimination of the potential for disease transmission and of an immune reaction to the graft tissue. Disadvantages include increased operative time and donor site morbidity. An optimal source of graft material is the bone-patellar tendon-bone (patellar tendon) autograft. The strength of the patellar tendon complex makes early graft failure less likely and restoration of stability more predictable. Some studies, however, suggest that patellofemoral pain may develop and quadriceps strength may be reduced. The contralateral patellar tendon autograft has the potential to create a symptomatic problem in the previously normal knee, but a study of 20 patients followed up for an average of 2 years reported graft site morbidity to be of short duration. Semitendinosus/gracilis autografts appear to have minimal donor site morbidity and should be comparable in many ways to patellar tendon grafts. A potential disadvantage of hamstrings in revision surgery is their inability to fill large bony defects.

Allografts.—Animal studies found allografts to lag histologically behind autografts at 8 weeks, but the 2 materials were comparable in biomechanical strength. Advantages of allograft tissue include ready availability and decreased operative time; disadvantages are a risk of viral disease transmission, a longer time for graft incorporation, and potential for immune reactions. Patellar tendon, Achilles' tendon, and fascia lata allografts may be selected for anterior cruciate ligament revision surgery; the latter type appears to be the least useful.

Synthetic Grafts.—Three types of prosthetics are available: permanent, stent, and ingrowth. The permanent prosthesis has limited potential for ingrowth; the stent is used to augment autogenous tissue and protects the graft as it matures; the ingrowth type is designed to rely on ingrowth of host tissue. The permanent Gore-Tex (polytetrafluorothylene) prosthetic ligament is now approved only for failed autogenous reconstructions, and no synthetic graft is indicated for routine use.

Conclusions.—The surgeon and the patient must decide on a graft source in anterior cruciate ligament revision surgery. At present, the choice is either autograft or allograft. Because no long-term studies have yielded clear recommendations, the decision must be determined individually by patient need and expectations.

▶ If the initial surgery for repair of a ruptured anterior cruciate ligament fails, graft sources for the revision may be limited. The authors examine the advantages and disadvantages of other tissue sources. Because the patellar tendon usually will have been used in the primary procedure, it is probably not available for the revision. The contralateral patellar tendon is available, as are the ipsilateral hamstring tendons. These probably represent the best alternative when compared with the contralateral quadriceps tendon, allografts of various sorts, the fascia lata, and synthetic grafts.

C.B. Sledge, M.D.

Biomechanical Consequences of Replacement of the Anterior Cruciate Ligament With a Patellar Ligament Allograft: II. Forces in the Graft Compared With Forces in the Intact Ligament
Markolf KL, Burchfield DM, Shapiro MM, et al (Univ of California, Los Angeles)
J Bone Joint Surg Am 78:1728–1734, 1996 5–46

Introduction.—During the early postoperative period after reconstruction of the anterior cruciate ligament, full activity may produce forces that jeopardize the future of the graft. Most studies related to forces in these grafts have involved synthetic ligaments implanted in specimens from cadavers and have measured forces during straight extension of the knee or application of a straight anterior tibial force. A cruciate load-cell technique was developed that allows the force in the graft to be compared with that in the intact anterior cruciate ligament for a variety of loading experiments.

Methods.—Seventeen fresh frozen knee specimens from cadavers were used in the study; 4 were analyzed separately because of unacceptable placement of the graft. Specimens were instrumented with a load-cell attached to a mechanically isolated cylinder of subchondral bone containing the tibial insertion of the anterior cruciate ligament. Forces in the intact ligament were recorded as the knee was passively extended from 90 degrees of flexion to 5 degrees of hyperextension, without and with 3 tibial loads: 100 newtons of anterior tibial force, 10 newton meters of internal and external tibial torque, and 10 newton meters of varus and valgus moment. After the resected ligament received a bone-patellar ligament-bone graft, the knee was flexed to 30 degrees and the graft pretensioned to restore normal anterior-posterior laxity. Knee-loading experiments were repeated at this level of pretension and at a level 45 newtons greater than the laxity-matched pre-tension.

Results.—With passive extension of the knee, forces in the graft were always greater than corresponding forces in the intact ligament. At all positions of flexion, the mean force in the graft at laxity-matched pretension was significantly greater than the corresponding mean force in the intact ligament. Similar results were noted in the overtensioned graft condition. The mean force in the intact ligament was 56 newtons at full extension. In contrast, full extension resulted in a mean force of 168 newtons in the graft at laxity-matched pretension and a mean force of 286 newtons with overtension. Mean forces in the graft generated during all constant loading tests exceeded those for the intact ligament. The forces generated by the anterior tibial force and by varus and valgus moment increased when the graft was overtensioned.

Conclusions.—Pretensioning of a patellar ligament allograft restores anterior-posterior laxity but increases forces in the graft. Internal torque applied to the extended knee may be the most dangerous loading state after anterior cruciate ligament reconstruction. Because of the large forces generated in the graft, it may be advisable to delay a return to full activity.

▶ The authors examined the forces seen in a bone–patellar–bone graft used for replacement of the anterior cruciate ligament in a cadaver model. They point out that the forces seen in the graft were much higher than those seen in the normal anterior cruciate ligament and suggest that this should have an influence on the postoperative rehabilitation effort. They suggest that strenuous rehabilitation be limited until full biological maturation of the graft. Unfortunately, it was not known how long the process of biological maturation takes.

C.B. Sledge, M.D.

A Prospective, Randomized Study of Three Operations for Acute Rupture of the Anterior Cruciate Ligament: Five-Year Follow-up of One Hundred and Thirty-one Patients

Grøntvedt T, Engebretsen L, Benum P, et al (Trondheim Univ, Norway; Univ of Oslo, Norway; Univ of Bergen, Norway)
J Bone Joint Surg Am 78:159–168, 1996,   5–47

Introduction.—A 5-year prospective, randomized study of patients with an acute rupture of the anterior cruciate ligament was conducted. It sought to compare the results after acute primary repair, acute repair with synthetic augmentation, and acute repair augmented with an autologous bone-patellar ligament-bone graft. Although acute primary repair has been a common method of management, some long-term follow-up studies have reported deterioration of results with time.

Methods.—The 150 patients included in the study were treated at 3 hospitals in Norway from May 1986 to April 1988. Patients had a mean age of 29 years, and 83% sustained the rupture during sports activities. Excluded were those with a concomitant rupture of the posterior cruciate or lateral collateral ligament. Randomization was to nonaugmented repair (group 1), repair with a synthetic ligament-augmentation device (group 2), and repair with bone-patellar ligament-bone augmentation (group 3). The

3 groups were comparable in age, sex, and preinjury level of activity. All were operated on within 10 days after the injury and had the repair procedures performed through a medial arthrotomy. Rehabilitation consisted of a cast for 2 weeks, a brace for 6 more weeks, and no weight-bearing on the extremity until 8 weeks after surgery. Participation in contact sports was prohibited for 1 year. Follow-up data were available for 141 patients.

Results.—All 3 operative groups had a lower level of activity at 5-year follow-up than they had before the injury. At 2-year follow-up, group 3 patients had a significantly higher mean level of activity and a significantly higher mean level of function than patients in groups 1 and 2. The mean level of function in group 3 patients was significantly higher at 5 years than that of group 1 patients. All 3 treatment groups showed significant improvement in the ability to attain full extension. The ability to extend the knee showed the greatest gains in Group 3. Patients in all 3 groups improved in their ability to attain full flexion, although a few patients in each group showed a flexion deficit of between 10 and 30 degrees at 5 years. Rotatory and anterior instability progressively increased in all treatment groups. Knees that were repaired with a patellar-ligament graft were significantly more stable, however, than those with nonaugmented repair and those repaired with a ligament-augmentation device. At 2 and 5 years, knees in group 2 were significantly more stable than those in group 1.

Discussion.—This 5-year follow-up study confirms earlier findings of poor outcome after acute primary repair of rupture of the anterior cruciate ligament. Although results were better after acute repair with a synthetic ligament-augmentation device, the failure rate was high. Only repairs that included augmentation with the patellar-ligament graft yielded excellent results.

▶ Three different operative treatments of ruptured anterior cruciate ligament were studied: acute primary repair, acute repair with a ligament augmentation device, and acute repair with autologous patellar tendon graft. Poor results were found with both of the first 2 treatment methods—only repair with patellar tendon autograft produced satisfactory results.

C.B. Sledge, M.D.

Patellofemoral Problems

Pain Reduction After Anteromedial Displacement of the Tibial Tuberosity: 5-Year Follow-up in 21 Knees With Patellofemoral Arthrosis
Sakai N, Koshino T, Okamoto R (Yokohama City Univ, Japan)
Acta Orthop Scand 67:13–15, 1996   5–48

Introduction.—Sixteen patients with painful patellofemoral arthrosis and lateral subluxation of the patella underwent anteromedial displacement of the tibial tuberosity. Their clinical and radiographic outcomes were reviewed.

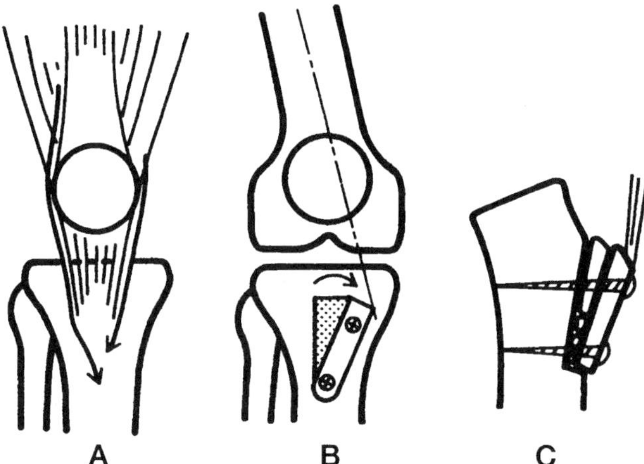

FIGURE 2.—Anteromedial displacement of the tibial tuberosity. **A,** medial and lateral release of the patellar retinaculum. **B,** after osteotomy, the tip of the fragment is rotated medially so that the center of tuberosity reaches the extension of the femoral axis. **C,** the anterior displacement (0.5–1.0 cm) is done by elevating the tibial tuberosity with an iliac bone graft. (Courtesy of Sakai N, Koshino T, Okamoto R: Pain reduction after anteromedial displacement of the tibial tuberosity. *Acta Orthop Scand* 67:13–15, 1996.)

Patients and Methods.—Five patients were affected bilaterally; 21 knees were involved. The mean age at operation was 50 years and the mean follow-up was 5 years. All patients had patellar pain on walking or while ascending or descending stairs. In a standing skyline view of the patella, the patellar joint space was narrowed to less than 3 mm, and there was lateral deviation of more than 5 mm with 30 degrees of knee flexion or more than 15 degrees of lateral tilt. None had varus deformity. The operative procedure involves medial and lateral release of the patellar retinaculum, rotation of the tip of the fragment, and elevation of the tibial tuberosity with an iliac bone graft (Fig 2). The fragment is fixed with 2 screws that are removed after radiographic union. Active motion exercises start 1 week after operation, partial weight-bearing after 4 weeks, and full weight-bearing at 8 weeks.

Results.—Pain on descending or ascending stairs was improved after surgery in 20 of 21 knees, but retropatellar crepitation improved in only 2 of 20 affected knees. Retropatellar pain when squeezing the patella against the femur was present in 17 knees preoperatively; relief was obtained in 16. The smallest width of the patellar joint space line increased from a mean of 0.7 mm to a mean of 3.5 mm; the mean lateral deviation of the patella was reduced from 7.6 mm to 4.4 mm. Screw removal, done an average of 1.6 years after surgery, revealed regenerated cartilage at the site of the previous ulcer in all 21 knees.

Discussion.—The distance of medial displacement was measured pre-operatively on anteroposterior radiographs and medial displacement of the tibial tuberosity done so that the center of the tuberosity reached the extension of the femoral axis. Both patellar deviation and tilt were improved after operation and pain was relieved, despite persistence of retropatellar crepitation in 18 of 20 knees.

▶ Osteoarthritis of the patellofemoral joint is an unusual but disabling condition. A number of conservative and surgical treatments have been advocated but, in the absence of an underlying cause for the degenerative changes, therapy often is poorly directed. This report suggests that if there is radiographically demonstrable lateral displacement of the patella with an abnormal Q-angle and arthritic changes in the patellar cartilage, symptomatic relief can be obtained by anteromedial displacement of the tibial tuberosity combining the techniques of Trillat and Maquet. Twenty of 21 patients treated by this technique showed improvement. It must be stressed, however, that an accurate diagnosis of an abnormality in patellar mechanics must precede application of this or any other treatment that aims to alter patellar mechanics.

C.B. Sledge, M.D.

Acute Dislocation of the Patella: A Correlative Pathoanatomic Study
Sallay PI, Poggi J, Speer KP, et al (Methodist Sports Medicine Ctr, Indianapolis, Ind; OFFUTT Airforce Base, Omaha, Neb; Duke Univ, Durham, NC)
Am J Sports Med 24:52–60, 1996   5–49

Introduction.—A significant number of patients who are treated nonoperatively for acute patellar dislocation have recurrences. A number of operations have failed to reliably restore a stable patella. The pathology of patellar dislocation remains incompletely understood.

Objective.—The mechanisms underlying patellar dislocation and the results of early operative repair were studied in 23 patients with clinical findings of acute dislocation who underwent MR imaging as well as standard radiography. The patients were 20 males and 3 females 14–46 years of age. Nineteen patients were examined with the use of anesthesia and underwent arthroscopic treatment of any intra-articular lesions. Sixteen patients had open exploration of the medial aspect of the knee, and 12 were studied for 2 years or longer.

Pathoanatomy.—A substantial majority of patients had a moderate-to-large effusion and significant tenderness over the posteromedial soft tissues and the adductor tubercle (Fig 5). Radiographs demonstrated patellar fractures in 4 patients and a single lateral femoral condylar fracture. The MR findings included increased signal adjacent to the adductor tubercle on T2-weighted images, and a tear of the femoral insertion of the medial patellofemoral ligament (MPFL) in 20 patients, most evident on axial T2-weighted images. Ten patients had some increased signal in the parapatellar part of the medial capsule, but there was only 1 frank tear at this site. Osseous changes were prevalent. Exploration revealed gross lateral laxity of the patellofemoral articulation. Five patients had tears in the

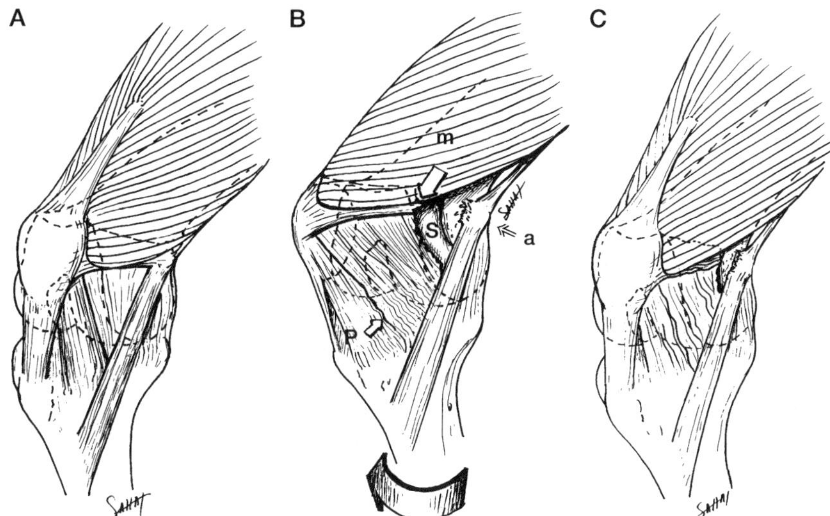

FIGURE 5.—**A,** an artist's rendering of the normal medial ligamentous anatomy; **B,** during patellar dislocation, the vastus medialis obliquus muscle is stripped away from the adductor magnus tendon, the medial patellofemoral ligament (MPFL) is torn completely, and the capsule with the patelloligament is damaged (*m,* MPFL; *a;* adductor tubercle; *p,* patellotibial ligament; *s,* synovium). C, after reduction, the MPFL and vastus medialis obliquus muscle remain displaced and obliquely oriented as a result of the dynamic action of the muscle. (Courtesy of Sallay PI, Poggi J, Speer KP, et al: Acute dislocation of the patella: A correlative pathoanatomic study. *Am J Sports Med* 24:52–60, 1996.)

medial soft tissues. Osteochondral lesions were frequent. A tear of the MPFL was documented in all but 1 of the 16 patients evaluated.

Outcome.—None of the patients had recurrent dislocation after repair of the MPFL. Good to excellent results were achieved in 58% of patients, and fair results in the remainder. Nearly 60% of patients were able to return to their previous sports activity with no major limitations. Three patients had surgical complications.

Implications.—Many operations for acute and chronic patellar instability have failed because they fail to confront the major pathologic condition, posterior rupture of the MPFL. Repairing this structure restores stability in a majority of patients. Lateral release may be indicated in addition if the lateral retinaculum is abnormally tight.

▶ Recurrent subluxation or dislocation of the patella after a single acute episode is quite common. The reported rate varies from 20% to 40% and suggested to the authors of this paper that a thorough understanding of the pathoanatomy might lead to more satisfactory surgical treatment. Both MRI and surgical exploration revealed tears of the MPFL in 15 of the 16 patients. Early surgical repair produced a satisfactory result in most patients with no recurrent dislocations. The paper points out that the usual lesion in this series was a tear of the MPFL from its femoral origin near the adductor tubercle. The usual parapatellar incision might not reveal the lesion unless carried back to the adductor tubercle.

C.B. Sledge, M.D.

Chronic Patellofemoral Instability

Dandy DJ (Addenbrooke's Hosp, Cambridge, England)
J Bone Joint Surg (Br) 78B:328–335, 1996   5–50

Introduction.—Because there are many causes of patellofemoral instability, the choice of a procedure to stabilize the joint should be an individualized one. The causes of patellar instability, methods of assessment, operative choices, patterns of dislocation, special situations, complications, and evaluation of results were studied.

Causes and Assessment of Instability.—The patella will slip laterally if it fails to engage securely in the trochlea at the start of flexion, and complete dislocation may follow. Failure to engage may result from an abnormally high patella, patella dysplasia, or a poorly developed trochlea. In some cases, the patella engages correctly at the start of flexion but then subluxes or dislocates; potential causes are a defective lateral trochlear margin and an unusually shallow trochlear groove. Assessment should include a clinical history, clinical examination, and investigation (radiologic measurements, anatomical details, arthroscopy).

Operative Choices.—In general, procedures designed for stabilizing the patella can be classified as distal re-alignments to transpose the tibial tubercle or proximal re-alignments to alter the tension of the tissues attached to the patella. Distal realignment is required if the patella is abnormally high and the trochlea normal and may be needed if the trochlea is deficient at its upper end. Medial transposition is indicated if the tubercle lies too far laterally; in such cases a distal transposition also is done. Medial transposition alone is suitable when the trochlea is dysplastic and the patella, although of normal size and height, engages poorly in the trochlea. Other procedures that may be appropriate involve adjustment of tissue tension, reconstruction of the lateral condyle, and deepening of the trochlea.

Patterns of Dislocation and Special Disorders.—Dislocations can be recurrent (the most common form), habitual (may occur voluntarily), permanent, and congenital; recurrent subluxation (less drastic than a dislocation) may be similar to dislocation in patients with lax joints. Special situations that are discussed include dislocation in the immature skeleton, pathologic ligament laxity, subluxation in extension, dislocation after patellectomy (Fig 15), and instability in the presence of patellofemoral osteoarthritis.

Complications and Assessment.—Patellofemoral osteoarthritis is common in cases of patellar instability and may be aggravated by inappropriate transfer of the tubercle. Medial dislocation of the patella may follow excessive medial transposition of the tubercle, which should never be moved medial to the center of the tubercle. Loss of flexion can occur in cases with distal transposition or relocation of a permanently dislocated patella. If dislocation recurs after stabilization, the cause of failure should be determined and corrective surgery done. Assessment can be complicated if some patients experience an occasional dislocation during the immediate

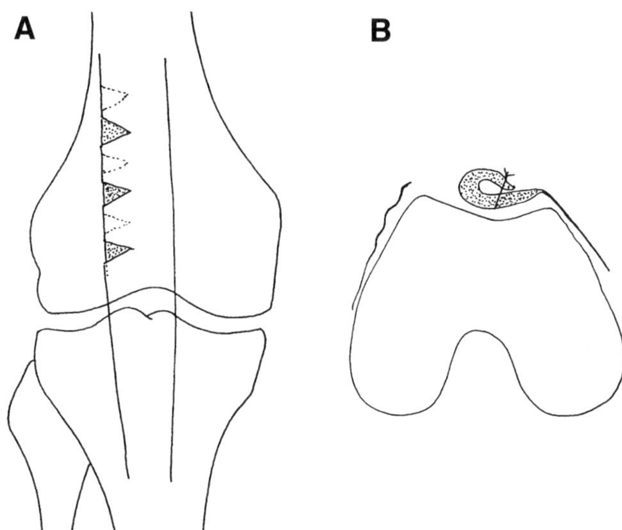

FIGURE 15.—Techniques for stabilization after patellectomy: (**A**) the lateral margin of the tendon is lengthened by transverse incisions; and (**B**) the tendon is rolled into a tube to create a convex undersurface. (Courtesy of Dandy DD: Chronic patellofemoral instability. *J Bone Joint Surg Br* 78:328–335, 1996.)

postoperative period; symptoms of osteoarthritis also may interfere with assessment of stability.

▶ This excellent review article of the multiple causes of patellar instability emphasizes the importance of diagnosis of specific deficiency before undertaking surgical treatment. Included in the discussion are patella alta, hypoplasia of the femoral trochlea, and abnormal Q-angle. On the basis of an understanding of the abnormality, the various surgical approaches are discussed and illustrated. A particularly useful technique for stabilization of the quadriceps mechanism after patellectomy is described. This is a variation of the quadriceps "tubing" operation described by Compere et al[1].

C.B. Sledge, M.D.

Reference

1. Compere CL, Hill JA, Lewinnek GE, et al: A new method of patellectomy for patellofemoral arthritis. *J Bone Joint Surg Am* 61:714–718, 1979.

Patellectomy With Vastus Medialis Obliquus Advancement for Comminuted Patellar Fractures: A Prospective Randomised Trial
Günal I, Taymaz A, Köse N, et al (Osmangazi Univ, Eskisehir, Turkey)
J Bone Joint Surg Br 78:13–16, 1996   5–51

Objective.—Patellectomy may result in knee extension and tibiofemoral joint loading problems. None of the numerous patellectomy techniques

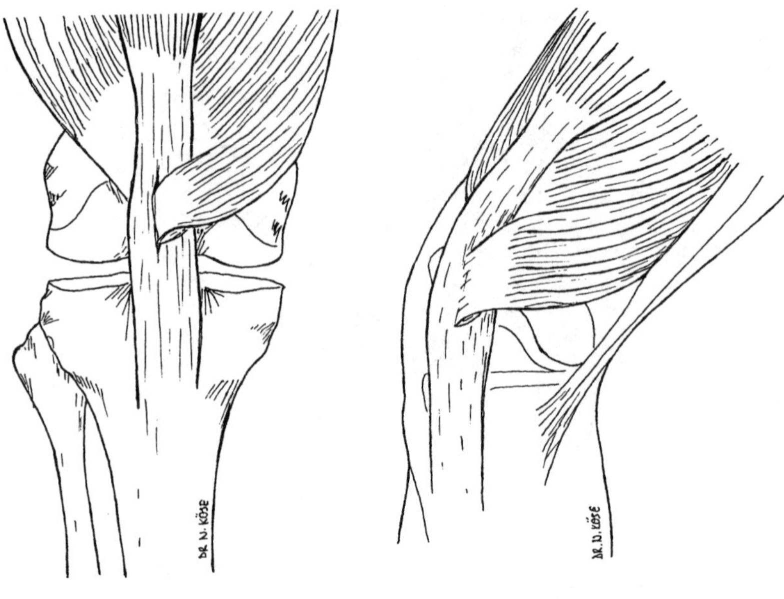

Fig. 1a   Fig. 1b

FIGURE 1.—Diagram to show vastus medialis obliquus advancement (**A**) anteroposterior and (**B**) lateral. (Courtesy of Günal I, Taymaz A, Köse N, et al: Patellectomy with vastus medialis obliquus advancement for comminuted patellar fractures: A prospective randomised trial. *J Bone Joint Surg Br* 78:13–16, 1996.)

have given dependably satisfactory results. A prospective, randomized trial evaluating the outcome of advancing the vastus medialis obliquus (VMO) in association with patellectomy at a minimum follow-up of 3 years was undertaken.

Methods.—A simple patellectomy (grade A, $n = 16$) or a patellectomy with VMO advancement (grade B, $n = 12$) was performed in skeletally mature patients with a comminuted fracture of the patella with at least 5 fragments observed radiographically (Fig 1). The male–female ratio was 9:7 in group A and 7:5 in group B, and the average age was 28 in both groups. Postoperative results were assessed using the criteria of Levack to evaluate pain, activity level, and quadriceps strength. Patients evaluated their function on a 3-point scale. Quadriceps strength was measured using a spring dynamometer and objective functional assessments, and range-of-motion measurements were made. Any development of heterotopic ossification was noted.

Results.—Thirteen patients in group A and 5 in group B had minimal pain, and 3 in group A and 7 in group B had no pain. The difference was almost significant. Significantly more group B than group A patients had unlimited activity (10 vs. 3). One patient in group A and all patients in group B had no loss of quadriceps strength. Three group A patients and all group B patients subjectively assessed their results as good. Objective functional assessments showed that significantly more group A than group B patients experienced discomfort during testing. All patients had a full range of motion, no heterotopic ossification was noted, and no patient experienced quadriceps rupture.

Conclusion.—When patellectomy is necessary, the procedure combined with VMO advancement gives superior functional results.

▶ The management of a comminuted fracture of the patella is difficult, and most methods leave quadriceps weakness. The authors of this paper compare simple patellectomy with patellectomy and advancement of the VMO; they report significant improvement in pain relief and functional activity after advancement.

C.B. Sledge, M.D.

Osteoarthritis

Association of Radiographically Evident Osteoarthritis With Higher Bone Mineral Density and Increased Bone Loss With Age: The Rotterdam Study
Burger H, van Daele PLA, Odding E, et al (Erasmus Univ, Rotterdam, The Netherlands)
Arthritis Rheum 39:81–86, 1996   5–52

Objective.—Although osteoarthritis (OA) and osteoporosis are common in elderly individuals, they rarely occur together. The relation between OA and femoral bone loss with age has not been studied. The relationship between radiographic OA of the knees and hips and the level of bone mineral density (BMD) and the rate of bone loss with age in a sample of the general population was investigated.

Methods.—Residents of Rotterdam, The Netherlands, 55 years or older, were interviewed and examined. Mobility measurements, anthropometric studies, BMD measurements, radiography, and hip and knee OA assessments were performed on 1,121 men and 1,624 women. Follow-up BMD measurements were performed in 714 men and 1,009 women.

Results.—Women with OA of the knee or hip or both had 3% to 8% higher BMD levels than women without OA. The differences were not significant in men. Levels of BMD increased significantly with increasing number of OA sites. The rate of bone loss was higher in men and significantly higher in women with OA. In women, the rate of bone loss was significantly related to the number of OA sites. Levels of BMD were significantly related to Kellgren scores for both men and women. Leg disability scores were related to Kellgren scores and the rate of bone loss for men and women. Disability and an increased rate of bone loss were significantly associated, although the higher rate of bone loss with increasing Kellgren score was independent of disability. Age and radiographically verified OA was significantly associated with increased bone loss and age in women for hips and knees and in men for hips only.

Conclusion.—Both BMD and the rate of bone loss are accelerated in men and women with OA of the hip or knee. Bone loss appears to increase with age in men and women 55 years or older. These results suggest an important difference in BMD earlier in life.

▶ One theory of the pathogenesis of OA is that increased pressure on articular cartilage leads to its degeneration. According to this theory, spongy, osteoporotic bone would absorb stress and protect the overlying articular cartilage. On the other hand, dense bone would transmit more force to the cartilage and lead to degeneration. The epidemiologic study reported by Burger and associates conforms to the theory by showing that radiographic evidence of OA is much more common in patients with high BMD than in those with normal or low density.

C.B. Sledge, M.D.

In Vitro Stimulation of Articular Chondrocyte mRNA and Extracellular Matrix Synthesis by Hydrostatic Pressure
Smith RL, Rusk SF, Ellison BE, et al (Stanford Univ, Calif; Veterans Affairs Med Ctr, Palo Alto, Calif; Univ of Washington, Seattle; et al)
J Orthop Res 14:53–60, 1996
5–53

Background.—Articular cartilage must tolerate the loading forces generated by normal physical activity. Both insufficient and excessive mechanical loading have been associated with cartilage degeneration. The effects of physiologic hydrostatic pressure were evaluated in high density articular chondrocyte monolayers.

Methods.—A servohydraulic testing machine was used to apply hydrostatic pressure (10 MPa) intermittently at 1 Hz or constantly for 4 hours to high-density monolayers of primary bovine chondrocytes in serum-free medium or medium containing fetal calf serum. Northern blots were used to quantitate mRNAs for aggrecan, type I and II collagen, and β-actin. Proteoglycan synthesis was quantified by $^{35}SO_4$ uptake into precipitable glycosaminoglycans. Immunohistochemistry was used to detect cell-associated aggrecan and type II collagen.

Results.—When intermittent hydrostatic pressure was applied to chondrocyte monolayers in serum-free medium, aggrecan mRNA increased 14%; when constant pressure was applied, type II collagen mRNA decreased 16%. When intermittent pressure was applied to chondrocyte monolayers in medium containing serum, aggrecan mRNA was increased 31% and type II collagen was increased 36%. Constant pressure did not affect either mRNA under these conditions. Both intermittent and constant pressure significantly stimulated glycosaminoglycan synthesis and increased cell-associated aggrecan and type II collagen.

Conclusions.—When bovine articular chondrocytes cultured in high density monolayers were treated with either intermittent or constant physiologic hydrostatic pressure, mRNAs for aggrecan and type II collagen, glycosaminoglycan synthesis, and cell-associated matrix proteins were increased. These results are in agreement with those of previous studies that suggested that cartilage responds to hydrostatic pressure and that physiologic hydrostatic pressure influences the extracellular matrix metabolism of articular chondrocytes.

▶ In keeping with the theory that pressure on articular cartilage is the stimulus for osteoarthritis, Smith and associates have shown that chondrocytes in culture are quite responsive to changes in hydrostatic pressure and synthesize more proteoglycan and type II collagen when stimulated by intermittent application of hydrostatic pressure. Their findings would also support the hypothesis that there is a normal threshold of force on articular cartilage that is necessary for its health; if the pressure is below that threshold, chondrocyte metabolic activity is depressed.

C.B. Sledge, M.D.

The Posteroanterior 45° Flexion Weight-bearing Radiograph of the Knee
Mason RB, Horne JG (Wellington Public Hosp, New Zealand; Wellington School of Medicine, New Zealand)
J Arthroplasty 10:790–792, 1995   5–54

Objective.—Biomechanical studies have demonstrated that radiographs of the osteoarthritic knee at 30–60 degrees of flexion provide a clearer picture of loss of articular cartilage than the knee in full extension. The posteroanterior (PA) radiograph of the knee at 45 degrees of flexion and the traditional anteroposterior (AP) weight-bearing radiograph in full extension were compared for assessing articular cartilage loss in the osteoarthritic knee.

Methods.—Anteroposterior and PA radiographs were taken of the knees of 35 patients (15 men), aged 42–81 years. Cephalocaudal joint dimensions of both medial and lateral compartments were measured on both radiographs and compared.

Results.—Of the 45 symptomatic knees (90 compartments), 27 knees (51 compartments) showed osteoarthritic changes. Ten other knees showed a normal or near normal joint space on the AP views but significant narrowing on the PA view in 45 degrees of flexion. These differences were significant.

Conclusion.—Posteroanterior radiographs of knees at 45 degrees of flexion detected significantly more osteoarthritic changes than AP radiographs.

▶ There is no entirely satisfactory way to obtain a radiograph that accurately demonstrates loss of articular cartilage in the knee in osteoarthritis. One-legged AP standing radiographs can be distorted by the patient shifting the center of gravity from 1 side to the other, either compressing or opening 1 of the compartments. In a bilateral stance, the patient will often shift the center of gravity over the less painful knee, thereby removing weight from the painful knee and leading to a false radiographic picture. As demonstrated in this paper, if the patient stands with both knees flexed it is very difficult to shift weight from 1 leg to the other, and a truer impression of the joint space is obtained. It is probably not important whether the angle of flexion is 30 degrees or 45 degrees, and this would simplify the technique considerably.

C.B. Sledge, M.D.

Articular Debridement Versus Washout for Degeneration of the Medial Femoral Condyle: A Five-Year Study

Hubbard MJS (Glan Clwyd Hosp, Rhyl, Wales; Robert Jones and Agnes Hunt Orthopaedic Hosp, Oswestry, England)
J Bone Joint Surg Br 78:217–219, 1996   5–55

Objective.—Although short-term trials of débridement vs. washout for treatment of degenerative arthritis of the knee have been reported, the extent of changes in the knee have not been completely described. In a prospective randomized study, arthroscopic débridement was compared with washout in patients with clearly defined levels of degeneration of articular cartilage of the medial femoral condyle.

Methods.—A total of 76 knees with an isolated degenerative lesion on the medial femoral condyle with an Outerbridge classification of grade 3 or 4 were selected for the study. There were 40 knees in the débridement group and 36 in the washout group. Patients were followed up for an average of 4.5 years in the débridement group and 4.3 years in the washout group. Debridement removed loose cartilage arthroscopically. In the washout group, 3 L of saline were run through the knee. Patients were reviewed, and knee stability and modified Lysholm score were determined at 3 months and annually for 5 years.

Results.—At year 1, significantly more patients in the débridement group ($n = 32$) than in the washout group ($n = 5$) were pain free. At year 5, 19 of 32 patients in the débridement group and 3 of 26 patients in the washout group were pain free. The modified Lysholm score at 1 year for the débridement group was 28, and for the washout group, it was 5. At 4 years, the score was 21 for the débridement group 21 and 4 for the washout group.

Conclusion.—Arthroscopic débridement of knee lesions of the femoral condyle with a grade 3 or 4 provides superior pain relief after 5 years.

▶ There have been isolated reports that arthroscopic lavage is a successful symptomatic treatment for osteoarthritis of the knee. Hubbard, in a carefully designed prospective, randomized trial of 76 knees, demonstrates quite conclusively that lavage gives inconsistent and transient results, whereas arthroscopic debridement produced improvement in 32 of 40 patients at 1 year. In 19 of 32 patients followed up for 5 years, there was still significant relief. Unfortunately, there is no mention of predisposing causes for osteoarthritis, such as varus angulation. The author states that there was "no deformity" in patients entered into the study, yet all had medial compartment degenerative changes. A clearer understanding of factors that predict or preclude a good result would be helpful.

C.B. Sledge, M.D.

Open-knee Magnuson Debridement as Conservative Treatment for Degenerative Osteoarthritis of the Knee

McEldowney AJ, Weiker GG (Cleveland Clinic Found, Ohio)
J Arthroplasty 10:805–809, 1995   5–56

Objective.—Although total knee arthroplasty (TKA) is a safe and effective treatment for osteoarthritis of the knee in older patients, the procedure may require subsequent revisions in patients younger than 65 years. The Magnuson open-knee débridement procedure has been reported to give satisfactory results in properly selected patients. The efficacy of the Magnuson procedure as an alternative treatment for degenerative osteoarthritis of the knee was investigated.

Methods.—Records of 11 patients (1 woman), average age 37 years, undergoing the Magnuson procedure at the Cleveland Clinic Foundation between July 1982 and December 1991 were reviewed. Patients were followed up clinically and radiographically for an average of 59 months. Patients completed the National Survey of Total Knee Replacement. Before surgery, 91% of patients had pain, 55% were unable to participate in recreational activities, 36% were unable to carry out activities of daily living, and 18% were unable to work or were unsteady on their feet.

Results.—Before surgery osteophytes were found in 3 compartments in 9 patients and in 2 compartments in 2 patients. At the most recent follow-up, osteophytes were found in 3 compartments in 6 patients and in 2 compartments in 5 patients. No change in alignment was detected in any patient. Nine patients were satisfied, 1 was dissatisfied, and 1 was neither satisfied nor dissatisfied. Three patients had a total of 4 additional surgeries to the affected knee. No patients required a TKA. There were no complications.

Conclusion.—In selected patients, the Magnuson open-knee débridement procedure provides satisfactory results in young individuals with osteoarthritis of the knee who do not wish to undergo TKA.

▶ Open débridement of degenerated cartilage and osteophytes as a treatment for osteoarthritis of the knee has been practiced for the last 50 years. McEldowney and Weiker report on 11 patients younger than 40 years who underwent open débridement of the knee; they report that 9 of the 11 were satisfied with the results in an average follow-up of nearly 5 years. Pain frequency and ambulation were both statistically significantly improved, and the authors recommend this as a conservative approach for the young patient with disabling osteoarthritis of the knee.

C.B. Sledge, M.D.

Arthroscopic Treatment of Osteoarthritis of the Knee: A Prospective, Randomized, Placebo-controlled Trial
Moseley JB Jr, Wray NP, Kuykendall D, et al (Baylor College of Medicine, Houston; Houston VA Med Ctr)
Am J Sports Med 24:28–34, 1996   5–57

Objective.—A number of studies indicate that arthroscopy is an effective approach to treating osteoarthritis of the knee, but a placebo effect has not been ruled out. A pilot study consequently was carried out before a planned randomized, controlled trial of arthroscopic treatment to ascertain whether the larger study should include a placebo control condition.

Study Design.—Ten patients less than 70 years of age with persistent symptoms of osteoarthritis of the knee despite at least 6 months of nonoperative measures were entered into the pilot study. All of them had moderate or severe knee pain. The patients, all men, had an average age of 46 years. Five patients were randomly assigned to undergo placebo arthroscopy that included local anesthesia and stab wounds but no instrumentation. Instruments were requested, however, in an attempt to simulate actual arthroscopic treatment, and the knee was manipulated. Three patients had arthroscopic lavage, and 2, standard débridement.

Results.—All groups had less pain when evaluated up to 6 months after surgery. There were no apparent physical changes, and the time for a 50-foot walk did not change in any group. Knee motion remained about the same 6 months postoperatively in all groups. All but 2 of 9 patients were satisfied with what was done 6 months postoperatively.

Conclusions.—There does appear to be a significant placebo effect associated with arthroscopic treatment for osteoarthritis of the knee, and this could be responsible for any benefit that accrues from this approach. Any large-scale study should include a placebo control group.

▶ This paper emphasizes the placebo effect seen with arthroscopy. This placebo effect may account for many of the good results reported from arthroscopic lavage in osteoarthritis of the knee. In this report, 10 patients were randomized into either arthroscopic débridement, arthroscopic lavage, or a placebo operation. Unfortunately, the numbers are extremely small with 5 patients randomized to the placebo group, 3 to the lavage group, and 2 to the débridement group. At follow-up at time intervals up to 6 months, all patients were improved and no significant differences were demonstrated. This was primarily a pilot study to demonstrate the feasibility of a larger study in terms of patient enrollment and retention in the study. Although this is a small and preliminary study, it serves to emphasize the degree of caution necessary in interpreting the results of treatment of osteoarthritis of the knee unless those studies are controlled for the placebo effect.

C.B. Sledge, M.D.

Proximal Tibial Osteotomy: A Subjective Outcome Study
Nagel A, Insall JN, Scuderi GR (Insall Scott Kelly Inst for Orthopaedics and Sports Medicine, New York City)
J Bone Joint Surg (Am) 78A:1353–1358, 1996   5–58

Objective.—Reports vary of long-term function and pain relief in patients younger than 60 years with unicompartmental osteoarthritis who undergo proximal tibial osteotomy. A retrospective study of the results of the highest level of activity achieved after proximal tibial osteotomy examined whether total knee arthroplasty would have been a better choice.

Methods.—After an average follow-up of 8 years, 34 male patients, aged 28–60 years, with 37 proximal tibial osteotomies were interviewed to determine their highest level of activity. Functional results were scored on a scale of 1–10 using the Tegner and Lysholm system. Patients answered a series of yes–no questions about manual labor and recreational activities, pain and swelling, and whether they would have the operation again. Based on their preoperative scores, patients were divided into groups 1 (scores of 4 or less) and 2 (scores of 5 or more). Results were compared using Fisher's Exact Test.

Results.—There were 12 group 1 patients (14 knees), aged 31–60 years, whose average preoperative score was 3.2 and whose average and postoperative score was 2.8. There were 22 group 2 patients (23 knees), aged 28–60 years, whose preoperative score was 6.5 and whose postoperative score was 5.9. Preoperative scores were the best predictors of postoperative scores. Activity caused mild pain in 9 patients and moderate pain in 2. Six patients had swelling after activity. Many of these patients engaged in activities postoperatively that would have been contraindicated after total knee arthroplasty. Patient satisfaction scores averaged 84 out of 100, and 9 group 1 patients and 19 group 2 patients said they would have the operation again. Six patients had had total knee replacement after an average of 7 years, 1 had anterior cruciate ligament reconstruction, and 1 had a fibular osteotomy.

Conclusion.—Proximal tibial osteotomy should be considered for younger, more active patients with osteoarthritis.

▶ Jackson and Waugh[1] popularized proximal tibial osteotomy in 1961 in England, and, later, Coventry[2] introduced the operation to a larger American audience. In this retrospective study, 82% of the patients were satisfied with the results, and most had returned to physical activities that would, as the authors point out, "lead to damage of the components of a total knee arthroplasty." Proximal tibial osteotomy carried out correctly and producing adequate correction of the varus deformity can produce highly satisfactory and lasting results. It should always be considered in medial compartment osteoarthritis in younger, more active patients.

C.B. Sledge, M.D.

References

1. Jackson JP, Waugh W: Tibial osteotomy for osteoarthritis of the knee. *J Bone Joint Surg Br* 43:746–751, 1961.
2. Coventry MB: Upper tibial osteotomy for gonarthrosis. The evolution of the operation in the last 18 years and long term results. *Orthop Clin North Am* 10:191–210, 1979.

Aneurysm Complicating High Tibial Osteotomy: A Case Report
Tandon SC, Kharbanda Y, Fraser AM (Keele Univ, Wolverhampton, West Midlands, England)
Acta Orthop Scand 67:73–74, 1996   5–59

Objective.—Reported is a case of a pseudoaneurysm of the lateral geniculate artery, a rare complication.

Case Report.—A man, 58, had increasing pain in his left knee for 18 months. He had quadriceps wasting, a stable joint with 5 degrees of varus misalignment, arthrosis of the medial component, and a closing wedge upper tibial osteotomy resulting in 10 degrees of valgus. The osteotomy was repaired with staples. On day 4 after surgery, knee pain and a foot drop developed. A blood blister on a wound hematoma was opened, but the hematoma developed a cavity with a bloody discharge. One month later, a venogram of the patient's swollen leg showed no filling of the calf veins. The patient was given anticoagulants, the discharge slowed, and the foot drop improved. After 2 months, the hematoma was still present and oozing. An angiogram revealed a pseudoaneurysm of the inferior lateral geniculate artery. A bleeding point was located along the subperiosteal sac and oversewn. The patient recovered slowly. At 1 year, his knee pain is greatly lessened, but the knee is still somewhat swollen.

Discussion.—Partial injury to the lateral vessel may occur as a result of surgery. The geniculate vessels are especially at risk during lateral knee surgery. The complication is rare after upper tibial osteotomy but may be difficult to avoid. The risk may be decreased by releasing the tourniquet before closing the wound and cauterizing any bleeding points.

▶ This case report of a pseudoaneurysm of the lateral geniculate artery raises a cautionary note regarding proximal tibial osteotomy, although it is a rare complication. Among the complications of the operation, injury to the popliteal vessels or peroneal nerve is more common. In the case reported, the patient had a persistent hematoma that raised suspicion. The foot drop resulted from pressure of the aneurysm sac on the peroneal nerve, which was reversed with correction of the aneurysm.

Although this is a rare complication, the authors emphasize the importance of releasing a tourniquet to identify bleeding vessels before closure of the incision after this operation.

C.B. Sledge, M.D.

6 Foot and Ankle

Introduction

The year 1997 continues to be an active one for foot and ankle research. The enclosed selections reflect the diversity of this ongoing research effort. Dr. Cracchiolo presents his latest work in first metatarsal phalangeal arthroplasty using a titanium grommet added to a traditional double-stem silicone implant. The current hallux valgus literature is expanded through the efforts of many researchers. Three current works present the treatment principles of advanced hallux valgus deformity, the results of Wilson osteotomy, and the complication of hallux varus. Pain and disability secondary to peripheral nerve injury or compression are very difficult and often unrewarding to treat. This area of disability is gaining more attention in the literature, and three articles selected here reflect this growing concern.

A wide variety of articles reflect research efforts in reconstruction of the hindfoot. Authors who previously researched core decompression techniques in the hip present their results in the talus. Other reconstruction articles include adult coalition resection, long-term total ankle arthroplasty follow up, and a tendon transfer for footdrop. Hindfoot trauma is heavily represented by quality articles this year. Midtarsal, subtalar, and ankle arthrodesis procedures are described, as well as a prospective ankle ligament treatment study. Two major prospective hindfoot trauma studies covering the pros and cons of internal fixation of calcaneus and pilon injuries are presented.

The literature reflecting foot and ankle research continues to grow in scope and quality. Particularly encouraging is the current emphasis on prospective clinical research and outcomes studies.

Michael G. Wilson, M.D.

Use of Titanium Grommets in Silicone Implant Arthroplasty of the Hallux Metatarsophalangeal Joint
Sebold EJ, Cracchiolo A III (Univ of California, Los Angeles)
Foot Ankle Int 17:145–151, 1996   6–1

Background.—Currently, a double-stem implant with a high performance silicone elastomer can be used in the treatment of arthritic hallux metatarsophalangeal joints with good overall results. However, silicone synovitis, destructive bone changes, and implant fractures have been re ported. Titanium grommets have been designed to protect the hinged portion of the implant to prevent such fractures. A group of patients who had received double-stem silicone implants protected by the titanium grommets were followed prospectively to determine outcomes.

Methods.—The hallux metatarsophalangeal joints in 47 feet of 32 patients were implanted with the double-stem devices with titanium grommets. The indication for surgery was painful joint destruction in all patients. The patients were mainly women, aged 34 to 76 years.

Findings.—Twenty patients with 30 affected feet were completely satisfied with their outcomes. Eight patients with 10 affected feet, all with rheumatoid arthritis, reported some minor problems postoperatively, mainly in the lateral toes. Two patients in this group reported too minimal hallux motion but no pain. In 1 patient with rheumatoid arthritis, deep sepsis developed in 1 foot, and the implant had to be removed. There was no radiographic evidence of implant fracture in any of these patients. The implant composite appeared to be tolerated well by surrounding bone. The implant used seemed much more stable when compared with another group of patients with no grommets. Implants protected by grommets showed significantly less evidence of radiolucency.

Conclusion.—Titanium grommets appear to effectively protect silicone implants, which may prolong the life of such implants. The most important criterion for achieving a good outcome is still appropriate patient selection.

▶ There continues to be a need for successful arthroplasty of the first metatarsophalangeal joint. Although fusion of this joint continues to be a serviceable operation for a majority of patients, the sacrificed motion prohibits certain types of shoe wear and athletic activities. In some patients with rheumatoid arthritis, arthrodesis of the hallux metatarsophalangeal joint can tend to increase stress at a deformed interphalangeal joint. Patients are often reluctant to accept the concept of arthrodesis at this joint, and the surgeon often believes that his informed consent borders on persuasion.

To his credit, Cracchiolo has contined to investigate the possibilities for arthroplasty of this joint, and this work reveals his experience with a third-generation device. The addition of titanium grommets appears to improve the radiographic condition of these implants at 3 to 6 years post surgery. However, Cracchiolo's method is flawed in certain aspects in that he uses an historical control group, the reading of the radiographs in terms of osteolysis is somewhat subjective and partially obscured by the titanium, and another 5 years of analysis will be required before firm conclusions can be drawn. No matter how encouraging these results appear to be, the clinician must remember that Silastic is a poor bearing surface, and the generation of micromolecules would seem to be inevitable. Indeed, there may be a threshhold effect in this group, with the titanium grommets contributing to precipitous failure, given slightly longer follow-up. The authors sensibly point out that arthrodesis remains the mainstay of treatment for the younger, active patient.

M.G. Wilson, M.D.

Advanced Hallux Valgus Deformity: Long-Term Results Utilizing the Distal Soft Tissue Procedure and Proximal Metatarsal Osteotomy

Dreeben S, Mann RA (La Mesa, Calif; Univ of California, San Francisco)
Foot Ankle Int 17:142–144, 1996   6–2

Background.—Many authors believe that metatarsocuneiform joint instability results in hallux valgus deformity and that if the joint is not stabilized, the instability will result in recurrence. The long-term results of the distal soft-tissue procedure and proximal metatarsal osteotomy in patients with advanced hallux valgus deformity were reported.

Methods and Findings.—Twenty patients with 28 feet with moderate-to-severe hallux valgus deformity and an intermetatarsal angle of 14 degrees or more were followed for a mean of 5.5 years. The mean correction of the intermetatarsal angle was 13.2 degrees. Average loss of correction was 1.4 degrees. The mean correction of the hallux valgus angle was 26.7 degrees. Average loss was 3.8 degrees. The deformity recurred in 3 feet. In another 3 feet, a hallux varus deformity occurred, being symptomatic in 2. Eighty-five percent of the patients were satisfied with their outcomes.

Conclusion.—In most patients with a hallux valgus deformity and an intermetastarsal angle of 14 degrees or more, the inherent stability of the first metatarsocuneiform joint is sufficient. Stabilization is not needed to obtain satisfactory long-term outcomes.

▶ This retrospective review of patients with hallux valgus deformity addresses the issue of first metatarsocuneiform instability and the role of proximal osteotomy vs. fusion of this joint. The senior author used an aggressive soft-tissue realignment with maximal displacement of the osteotomy as evidenced by the fact that in 3 cases, a postoperative hallux varus deformity developed. The described procedure of proximal osteotomy certainly prevented recurrent hallux valgus in this series.

The authors assume that these patients had instability of the first metatarsocuneiform joint if they displaced large preoperative intermetatarsal angles. This assumption is somewhat controversial, as Hansen's work would suggest that sagittal instability predisposes to recurrent hallux valgus deformity.[1] There is no way to know in this retrospective series how many of these patients truly had preoperative sagittal instability. Proximal osteotomy is also a demanding procedure in patients with a large intermetatarsal angle, although Dr. Mann has obviously mastered the technique. Perhaps there is room here for a good prospective, randomized study.

M.G. Wilson, M.D.

Reference

1. Klaue K, Hansen ST, Masquelet AC: Clinical quantitative assessment of first tarsometatarsal mobility in the saggital plane and its relation to hallux valgus deformity. *Foot Ankle Int* 15:9–3, 1994.

Clinical and Radiographic Evaluation of Wilson Osteotomy for Hallux Valgus

Pouliart N, Haentjens P, Opdecam P (Free Univ Brussels, Belgium)
Foot Ankle Int 17:388–394, 1996
6–3

Background.—The Wilson osteotomy is a treatment option for correcting hallux valgus. The preliminary results of this procedure in 1 group of patients were reported.

Methods and Findings.—Twenty-six patients underwent a total of 32 Wilson osteotomies. The mean follow-up was 20 months. Results were good or excellent in 90% of the feet according to the Bonney-MacNab classification. Patients' assessment of the outcomes was uncorrelated with the clinical results, based on objective, functional, and radiographic evidence. The occurrence of metatarsalgia or callosities was unassociated with shortening or angulation. Longer duration of follow-up was accompanied by a greater loss of correction. The tendency for recurrence was greater in patients older than 50 years than in younger patients.

Conclusion.—The Wilson osteotomy yields a high percentage of good and excellent results in patients with hallux valgus. Feet that show a tendency for recurrence may have a greater amount of loss of correction with a longer duration of follow-up. Although internal fixation with 2 K-wires appears to reduce the risk of shortening, its clinical implication could not be determined in this series.

▶ The authors conclude that the helal modification of the Wilson osteotomy for hallux valgus produces good and excellent results in 90% of patients. The Wilson osteotomy has been criticized before for producing excessive shortening of the metatarsal, with transfer of weight-bearing forces to the lateral metatarsals. The helal biplane osteotomy seeks to produce some plantar flexion of the distal fragment, thus minimizing this effect. It is concerning that in this study, 37% of the feet had shortening of the first ray, with an additional 37% having some elevation of the first ray. Twenty-one of the 32 feet had callosities under the second metatarsal, half of these having metatarsalgia under the lesser metatarsal heads. Given the fact that the main follow-up for this study was only 20 months, this clinically evident shortening of the first metatarsal could lead to a significant failure rate because of progressive pain under the second metatarsal head as further follow-up is achieved.

Successful correction of moderate-to-advanced hallux valgus deformity requires that the realignment of the first ray be achieved with a minimum of shortening. This report is important, and it represents a modern series concerning a procedure that is very popular in Europe. The authors' very careful review of their operative results reveals that the Wilson osteotomy, like the Mitchell osteotomy before it, can correct the inner metatarsal angle but at too high a cost of overall shortening.

M.G. Wilson, M.D.

Results of Hallux Varus Correction Using an Extensor Hallucis Brevis Tenodesis

Myerson MS, Komenda GA (Union Mem Hosp, Baltimore, Md)
Foot Ankle Int 17:21–27, 1996   6–4

Background.—Acquired hallux varus most commonly occurs after iatrogenic interruption of the lateral conjoined tendon with overpull of the abductor hallucis. Dynamic correction of the muscle imbalance with tendon transfers for hallux varus has been done using the extensor hallucis longus (EHL) tendon. The extensor hallucis brevis (EHB) as a static tenodesis was used as an alternative to the EHL in the correction of acquired hallux varus.

Methods and Outcomes.—Six patients aged 18 to 65 years were treated. Hallux varus developed after correction of hallux valgus deformity in 5 patients and after traumatic dislocation of the hallux in 1. All patients had flexible metatarsophalangeal and interphalangeal joints and no arthritis. The outcomes of surgery were excellent in all patients. These excellent results were maintained in all at a mean 28-month follow-up. Although there was a slight decrease in dorsiflexion (mean, 10 degrees) postoperatively, no other complications occurred. The mean American Orthopedic Foot and Ankle Society rating score improved from 61 to 85 postoperatively.

Conclusion.—An EHB tenodesis provides excellent correction of flexible, acquired hallux varus deformities. The complications associated with this procedure are minimal.

▶ Foot and ankle surgeons need a straightforward, reliable procedure to correct iatrogenic hallux varus deformities. If we use an aggressive surgical technique to treat hallux valgus—which is needed to prevent recurrences—a small percentage of patients will have a postoperative hallux varus deformity caused by overcorrection. The technique described by Myerson would appear to offer reliable correction of the deformity with minimal volarbidity because it is a relatively straightforward procedure. The small degree of lost dorsiflexion would appear to be acceptable. The interested reader can review the cadaver work by Myerson, which preceded this clinical investigation, in the same 1996 volume of *Foot and Ankle International.*

M.G. Wilson, M.D.

Surgical Treatment of Recalcitrant Plantar Fasciitis

Sammarco GJ, Helfrey RB (Ctr for Orthopaedic Care Inc, Cincinnati, Ohio)
Foot Ankle Int 17:520–526, 1996   6–5

Introduction.—Plantar fasciitis, a common condition affecting the hindfoot, has been referred to as heel spur syndrome, subcalcaneal pain syndrome, and calcaneal periostitis. Causes include chronic inflammation, heel spurs, microtrauma of the plantar fascia, increased calcaneal intraosseous pressure, fat pad degeneration, nerve entrapment, periosteal inflammation, and inflammation caused by seronegative arthritis. For those patients who do not respond to nonsurgical treatment—which can include heel cups, orthotic inserts, and stretching programs—surgical intervention may be necessary. Whether surgical treatment—including neurolysis of the nerve to the abductor digiti and partial plantar fasciectomy—achieves a good result was determined.

Methods.—Partial plantar fasciectomy with neurolysis of the nerve to the abductor digit quinti muscle was performed on 35 feet of 26 patients. The average patient age was 49 years. A subjective foot rating system was used to evaluate patients before and after surgery. These patients had been unsuccessfully treated with nonsurgical therapy. They filled out a complete questionnaire after surgery and were then followed for an average of 37.5 months.

Results.—A satisfactory functional outcome was assessed in 32 patients (92%). There was an unsatisfactory outcome in 3 patients (8%). The ratings were 21, excellent; 11, good; 3, fair; and 0, poor. The preoperative average of the foot rating system was 74.8/100 points; after surgery it was 90.6/100 points. Postoperative complications occurred in 4 patients who reported superficial wound infection, deep venous thrombosis, and superficial phlebitis. The conditions resolved with treatment. Some degree of heel pain was reported by 10 patients (28.6%) after surgery; however, their activity was not limited after surgery. It took an average of 5.6 weeks for patients to return to daily activity and restricted work duty. It took an average of 8.7 weeks to return to full work duty without restriction.

Conclusion.—In most patients who are treated for recalcitrant plantar fasciitis, a successful treatment outcome can be expected, although the length of time for partial or complete resolutions of symptoms is variable. Generally, surgery is recommended after 8 to 12 months of unsuccessful nonsurgical treatment.

► The care of recalcitrant plantar fasciitis has gone through an evolution in terms of theories of cause and treatment approaches. Because of the excellent work by Baxter and co-workers,[1] the role of compression neuropathy has assumed importance, and it may be that the majority of patients with heel pain who failed conservative treatment represent the small percentage of patients with a primary nerve compression. It also appears that most specimens of resected plantar fascia show signs of chronic inflammation and degeneration. These 2 causes, of course, may be interrelated, and it is perfectly reasonable to address both in every patient who undergoes surgery for heel pain. Sammarco's results of this approach are gratifying, with over 90% of the patients achieving a satisfactory outcome.

Several questions remain. What would be the natural history in those patients who undergo surgical treatment but derive no significant pain relief? If surgical treatment offers a 90% chance of pain relief, how long should we wait before offering this to patients who appear to have pain resistent to conservative measures, and will widening the indications diminish the percentage of satisfactory outcomes in future series? By exhausting traditional conservative measures, we may be selecting those patients whose underlying pathology is most amenable to the surgical treatment. This is, of course, what we should be doing, but we certainly need to find effective strategies to also hasten recovery for those treated with conservative modalities.

M.G. Wilson, M.D.

Reference

1. Baxter DE, Thigpen CM: Heel pain—operative results. *Foot Ankle* 5:16–25, 1984.

Recurrent Tarsal Tunnel Syndrome and the Radial Forearm Free Flap
Novotny DA, Kay DB, Parker MG (Akron Gen Med Ctr, Ohio)
Foot Ankle Int 17:641–649, 1996   6–6

Background.—Tarsal tunnel syndrome, characterized by pain, paresthesias, and vasomotor changes, results from posterior tibial nerve entrapment beneath the flexor retinaculum and deep fascia. The treatment of choice is surgical correction through flexor retinaculum release. The failure rate, however, is 10% to 20%. The treatment of 2 patients with recurrent tarsal tunnel syndrome by re-release of the retinaculum, followed by a radial forearm free flap for nerve coverage was described.

> *Case Reports.*—The 2 patients were a 48-year-old man and a 35-year-old woman with tarsal tunnel syndrome. In both patients, symptoms recurred after tarsal tunnel release. Re-release of the retinaculum and excision of scar tissue was followed by nerve coverage with a radial forearm free flap. No complications occurred. Postoperatively, both flaps were viable, and the patients' symptoms were improved dramatically. At 9 and 21 months, both were ambulatory, free of pain, and able to return to work. Both had a Takakaura score of 9.

Conclusion.—Recurrent tarsal tunnel syndrome does not respond well to conservative treatment. Re-release of the tunnel and scar tissue must be performed. The radial forearm free flap is recommended, especially in patients with hypertrophic scars and when multiple decompressions have failed. With this flap, adequate soft tissue over the posterior tibial nerve is provided, and scar formation that may predispose to symptom recurrence is limited.

▶ The treatment of patients with nerve pain in the foot and ankle is a daunting and frustrating challenge. Those patients that fail surgical release of the tarsal tunnel fall into this category and often require rigid ankle-foot orthoses; chronic medication; marked limitation of functional activities; and, occasionally, amputation. We do not know why some patients seem to readily reform the thick scar tissue released at the time of their primary tarsal tunnel release. For these patients, some additional strategy is clearly needed to alter the local biology so that the nerve and surrounding tissues remain pliable.

This report by Novotny et al., which covers only 2 cases, describes free tissue transfer to cover a surgically released nerve. To me, this approach makes good sense for several reasons. First, the addition of extra skin to the area will tend to decompress the dermal envelope. Second, the thick adipose layer from the radial forearm flap would cushion, protect, and possibly even improve the local vascularity. These results need to be verified on a larger scale, but the authors are justified in their aggressive approach to what could be a hopeless clinical scenario for patient and surgeon alike.

M.G. Wilson, M.D.

The Operative Treatment of Peroneal Nerve Palsy

Mont MA, Dellon AL, Chen F, et al (Johns Hopkins Univ, Baltimore, Md)
J Bone Joint Surg Am 78:863–869, 1996   6–7

Introduction.—Peroneal nerve palsy can occur after trauma or an elective procedure around the knee. Spontaneous resolution can occur, but if the palsy persists and is untreated, there may be severe functional disability. Operative treatment, however, is controversial. The results of operative decompression were reported for 31 patients treated between 1980 and 1990.

Patients and Methods.—The 20 women and 11 men had a mean age of 47 years. Peroneal nerve palsy had developed after a total knee arthroplasty in 6 patients, after a proximal tibial osteotomy in 4, after a distal femoral osteotomy in 1, and after a total hip arthroplasty in 1. The palsy appeared after fractures (tibia, knee, foot, or ankle) in 13 patients and as a result of a soft-tissue injury in 6. All had been initially managed nonoperatively for at least 2 months. The mean interval between development of the nerve palsy and operative decompression was 21 months. At the time of surgery, epineurial fibrosis and bands of fibrous tissue were found to be constricting the peroneal nerve at the level of the fibular head and at the proximal origin of the peroneus longus muscle.

Results.—The mean follow-up was 36 months. Sensory and motor function was scored preoperatively and postoperatively on a scale ranging from 0 to 5 points. Also assessed were need for an orthosis and function with regard to walking. Twenty-one patients (68%) had no remaining motor or sensory symptoms, 4 (13%) had complete or nearly complete relief, 5 (16%) had residual sensory or motor deficits, and 1 had little improvement. Overall, the mean palsy score improved from 4.5 points preoperatively to 1.5 points postoperatively. There was no relationship between patient age and recovery of neural function, but decompression was less successful with increasing delay of the procedure. No intraoperative or postoperative complications occurred. In a group of 9 patients treated nonoperatively during the same period, only 3 reported subjective and functional improvement.

Conclusion.—If peroneal nerve palsy does not resolve spontaneously, operative decompression is recommended to prevent lasting and severe functional disability. Electromyographic and nerve-conduction-velocity studies should be conducted at 3 weeks if the sensorimotor deficit continues, then repeated if the defect remains at 3 months; operative exploration should be performed within the fourth month of persistent dysfunction.

▶ These authors describe the results reviewed retrospectively of operative treatment of peroneal nerve palsy in 31 patients. Their results are remarkable and surprising. Remarkable in that 97% of their patients reported functional improvement and were able to discontinue the use of their ankle-foot brace and surprising in that good return of motor function was obtained despite time intervals to surgery of more than 24 months. According to the authors, 6 of 7 patients with moderate-to-severe motor loss regained useful function of their anterior compartment musculature, despite such a time lapse. Evidently, any muscular degeneration to prolonged denervation is not permanent. The authors' statement that early release correlated with better outcome is not supported by their data in that a high percentage of those with surgical relief of the nerve done later still enjoyed full or near-full functional recovery.

It appears that external paralysis of the peroneal nerve should be considered in treating postoperative palsies in the vast majority of cases, particularly because reconstructive options are suboptimal and dramatic recovery of nerve function can be expected. Corroboration of these results on a prospective basis is needed.

M.G. Wilson, M.D.

Centrocentral Anastomosis With Autologous Nerve Graft Treatment of Foot and Ankle Neuromas
Lidor C, Hall RL, Nunley JA (Duke Univ, Durham, NC)
Foot Ankle Int 17:85–88, 1996   6–8

Introduction.—Five patients with intractable nerve pain in the foot and ankle resulting from neuromas were treated by centrocentral anastomosis with an autologous nerve graft (CCA). Painful neuromas in these areas have been difficult to treat, and CCA was found to be effective in preventing and treating terminal or postamputation neuromas in hand surgery.

Methods.—The patients, 3 men and 2 women, ranged in age from 22 to 68 years. Three had undergone toe amputations with multiple operations, 1 had undergone 3 surgical attempts to excise a Morton's neuroma in the third web space, and another had neuroma in the superficial peroneal nerve as the result of a gunshot wound. End-to-end anastomosis of the nerve was performed in the 3 patients with stump neuromas that had developed after toe excision. The nerves were dissected proximally in the remaining cases, divided between the fascicular groups, and anastomosed end to end. An autograft of 5 to 10 mm in length was simultaneously performed in all cases. The outcome was evaluated by means of a 100-point scale, with 40 points allotted for measures of pain, 40 for function, and 20 for Tinel's sign.

Results.—The CCA procedures were performed at a mean of 12 months after the patient's last procedure; the mean follow-up was 22 months. Excised nerve tissue provided histologic confirmation for all neuromas. Four of the 5 patients had both subjective and objective improvement. The mean score on the assessment scale was 36 before CCA. With an average improvement of 52 points, the mean score rose to 81 points. The patient with the least improvement had recurrent Morton's neuroma.

Conclusion.—Centrocentral anastomosis with autologous transplantation is recommended for the prevention and treatment of symptomatic neuromas in the foot and around the ankle. Four of the 5 patients reported here experienced remarkable pain reduction. Histologic studies indicate that CCA is associated with cessation of axonal proliferation and reduction in the size of neuroma formation.

▶ Surgical treatment of neuromas has traditionally focused on removing the mechanical irritation of the nerve ending by either shortening the nerve or rerouting the nerve to deep muscle or bone tissue. A significant failure rate has been noted with these techniques, and the authors cite uncontrolled axonal regrowth as the source of continued pain. The significance of the study abstracted here is that this represents a biological approach to the problem of axonary growth. A CCA provides a control template for axonary growth after the surgical division of these nerves. The described surgical technique using an operative microscope would add significantly to the cost of treating primary Morton's neuroma, but the technique certainly would seem justified for any patient who has failed previous neuroma surgery.

M.G. Wilson, M.D.

Bridle Transfer for Paresis of the Anterior and Lateral Compartment Musculature

Prahinski JR, McHale KA Temple HT, et al (Walter Reed Army Med Ctr, Washington, DC)
Foot Ankle Int 17:615–619, 1996   6–9

Introduction.—The footdrop and steppage gait that results from paresis of the anterior and lateral compartments presents a considerable rehabilitative challenge. To obtain a brace-free balanced foot, orthopedic surgeons at the study institution have used the bridle tendon transfer procedure since 1985. The bridle (Riordan) transfer has been criticized, however, because its insertion is not into bone. Long-term outcome of the bridle transfer was reviewed for 10 patients, all with flaccid paresis involving musculature innervated by the peroneal nerve.

Methods.—The mean age of the patients at operation was 29.4 years; 8 of 10 were men and 7 were on active military duty at the time of the procedure. Eight patients had sustained traumatic peroneal nerve loss and 2 had a neuromuscular cause. In the bridle transfer, the posterior tibialis muscle as motor is routed through the interosseous membrane, then anastomosed into a "bridle" formed by the distal tibialis anterior and peroneus longus muscles. The ankle remains in neutral position with the foot in slight eversion; this position is maintained by a short leg cast for 6 weeks. A custom polypropylene ankle-foot orthosis is prescribed and worn for 6 months. At a mean follow-up of 61 months, patients were evaluated for functional status, ankle position and motion, findings on static electromyograms, and subjective satisfaction.

Results.—All patients were brace free after discontinuing the postoperative orthosis, but 4 later returned to bracing. Although all 10 could walk barefoot, 6 had a mild-to-moderate limp. Only 2 of 5 patients who had returned to running after the operation were still running at follow-up. Three of the 7 who were on active duty have returned to duty. Five patients agreed to have peroneal nerve exploration in conjunction with bridle transfer; transection was repaired in 2 and 3 underwent neurolysis. Static electromyograms revealed only insignificant nerve return in these 5 patients. All 10 patients expressed subjective satisfaction with bridle transfer.

Conclusion.—The Riordan bridle transfer works well for patients with low functional demands, but results are less satisfactory for high-demand patients such as active duty military personnel. Initially good results may deteriorate over time. Concurrent peroneal nerve exploration and repair offered no benefits in this small series of patients.

▶ The authors apply a pediatric reconstructive procedure to a new population—an active, useful population in the military with largely traumatic peroneal loss. Although initially encouraging, the results deteriorated significantly with time, with 40% of patients returning to bracing, 60% walking with a mild-to-moderate limp because of dragging the affected foot during swing phase, and only 60% of the patients having dorsiflexion to neutral. The results also must be viewed critically in that only 6 of the original 12 patients were able to be examined at the time of follow-up, four evaluated by questionnaire. One mode of failure in this small series appears to be soft-tissue failure at the point of a tendon weave, so direct transfer of the posterior tibial tendon to bone may improve long-term outcome. Interestingly, peroneal decompressions did not provide any anterior compartment recovery in this setting; results did vary from those of Mont et al. (Abstract 6–7).

M.G. Wilson, M.D.

Surgical Reconstruction of the Diabetic Foot: A Salvage Approach for Midfoot Collapse

Early JS, Hansen ST (Univ of Texas, Dallas; Univ of Washington, Seattle)
Foot Ankle Int 17:325–330, 1996   6–10

Objective.—When the diabetic neuropathic foot becomes grossly deformed, some have advocated surgical intervention. A retrospective review of surgical treatment of severe midfoot collapse was presented.

Methods.—Weight-bearing anteroposterior and lateral radiographs were taken of Charcot deformities of 21 feet in 18 patients, aged 35 to 72 years. Six patients had non–insulin-dependent diabetes mellitus. There were 12 Brodsky type I and 9 Brodsky type II deformities. Ten feet had a plantar midfoot ulcer, 1 grade I and 9 grade II, according to the Wagner classification. Five type I deformities underwent tarsometatarsal realignment and fusion. Seven type I deformities had fusion of part or all of the subtalar complex plus metatarsal stabilization. Type II deformities had subtalar complex stabilization and fusion of the midtarsal structures. There were no adverse reactions. Patients were fitted with a non–weight-bearing short cast and given IV cefazolin for 24 hours after surgery. Casts were changed at 2 and 6 weeks and then monthly thereafter. Patients were fitted with extra-depth, wide-toed shoes with soft custom inserts when there was radiographic evidence of body union.

Results.—Surgery was successful in 18 feet. Seven of 10 ulcers healed uneventfully in an average of 6 weeks and did not recur. Patients were followed for an average of 29 months. The average time to bony union was 5 months. One patient died in the hospital, and 2 patients with ulcers required below-knee amputations for postoperative osteomyelitis. Three patients with ulcers had wound dehiscence and 2 healed by 6 and 8 weeks. The third required oral antibiotics for a superficial wound infection. There were 2 long-term screw failures. Two patients with successul surgeries were unable or unwilling to walk unaided. A plantar midfoot ulcer developed in 2 patients.

Conclusion.—Surgery to reconstruct the diabetic foot was successful in 47% of patients. Midfoot ulcers healed uneventfully in 70% of patients. No midfoot ulcers recurred.

▶ The senior author's experience with late reconstruction of midfoot and hindfoot Charcot deformity is described. All patients had a history of midfoot ulceration, palpable peripheral pulses, and radiographic signs of consolidation. Key technical points included complete correction of the deformity by soft tissue release and/or osteotomy, rigid, ample internal fixation, and teno-Achilles lengthening. Two significant failures in patients who had ulceration at the time of surgery were caused by postoperative osteomyelitis. Although it was not used in this series, it would seem reasonable that patients with ulceration believed to be candidates for reconstruction should have screening examination for osteomyelitis. Magnetic resonance imaging appears to have excellent specificity for underlying bone involvement. Furthermore, in the absence of osteomyelitis, a healed skin envelope ought to be attainable before the time of surgical reconstruction.

Charcot arthropathy can occur bilaterally. Achieving a stable plantar weight-bearing surface in these patients would seem to provide tremendous long-term benefits.

M.G. Wilson, M.D.

Benchmark Analysis on Diabetics at High Risk for Lower Extremity Amputation
Pinzur MS, Stuck R, Sage R, et al (Loyola Univ, Maywood, Ill)
Foot Ankle Int 17:695–700, 1996   6–11

Background.—Diabetics with foot ulcers are at increased risk for multiple organ system disease and lower extremity amputation, yet most patients have not been scheduled for regular systematic foot examinations. Foot salvage clinics using a multidisciplinary approach are now recommended for addressing the complex nature of the diabetic foot. To provide benchmark data on whether such clinics have a positive effect, investigators followed a group of patients at high risk for lower limb amputation.

Methods.—The study population consisted of 1,346 patients with diabetes who were enrolled in a high-risk foot salvage clinic. All patients underwent an initial interview and a comprehensive foot examination by an orthopedic surgeon. Before establishment of the clinic, patients were referred only when a problem requiring treatment was identified. The new level of care included a self-care education program, therapeutic interventions and follow-up monitoring, and routine foot examinations every 2 to 4 months. Patient data were reviewed for clinical process factors related to successful outcome.

Results.—Of the 1,346 patients at high risk for foot ulceration and eventual amputation, 224 (16.6%) were admitted to the hospital. The hospitalized group comprised 104 men and 120 women with an average age of 65.5 years; the average length of hospitalization was 9.1 days. Seventy-four amputations of all or part of a lower limb were performed (5.5% of the patients). The patients who underwent amputations were younger and more severely ill than the group as a whole and required more frequent hospitalizations because of greater organ system involvement. The average length of hospital stay for amputation decreased from 22.3 days during the first year to 14.6 days during the final year of the study. Most amputees (73%) could be discharged to the home or to home care.

Discussion.—In this high-risk population, the rate of lower extremity amputations was 34.2 per 1,000, a rate lower than would be expected for diabetics with multiple risk criteria. In addition, the levels of amputation performed were significantly less debilitating than those reported in the literature. These preliminary benchmark data from a high-risk foot salvage clinic may provide a standard for the development and evaluation of further therapeutic interventions.

▶ This study following prospectively a group of diabetics at high risk for lower extremity amputation is unique in the literature. By describing the level of amputation, number of possible admissions, and length of stay, the authors create a standard for further comparison of treatment modalities and efficacy of hospital-based clinic screening practices. Such work aids in identifying risk factors for the diabetic population at large and also provides information for patient education. Conclusions are few in this study, but we will not know where we are going in this field unless we know where we started, and Pinzur's work provides an important starting point.

M.G. Wilson, M.D.

Gross, Histological, and Microvascular Anatomy and Biomechanical Testing of the Spring Ligament Complex
Davis WH, Sobel M, DiCarlo EF, et al (Miller Orthopaedic Clinic, Charlotte, NC; Beth Israel Hosp, New York; Hosp for Special Surgery, New York; et al)
Foot Ankle Int 17:95–102, 1996   6–12

Background.—Surgical treatment options for acquired pes planus resulting from posterior tibial insufficiency are based primarily on dynamic tendon transfers and/or static hindfoot fusions. Both methods have shortcomings, however, and a better understanding of the anatomy may be required before surgical outcome is improved. A cadaver study was conducted to gain additional information on the gross, histologic, and microvascular anatomy, as well as the biomechanics of the ligamentous structures surrounding the talonaviculocalcaneal (TCN) articulation, the site at which the breakdown of the medial longitudinal arch is most often seen in acquired pes planus.

Methods.—All investigations used adult, below-knee cadaver specimens with no gross evidence of disease or deformity. The gross anatomy was studied in a dissection of the medial aspect of 14 cadaver feet. Six feet were used to examine the normal histology of the calcaneonavicular (CN) ligament and 10 feet to determine its normal microvascular anatomy. The biomechanical properties of the CN ligament were measured in 8 feet. When 2 distinct failure regions were observed for each CN ligament, the biomechanical properties of the spring ligament complex were analyzed for each failure region.

Results.—In all specimens, there were 2 distinct structures that made up the ligamentous connection between the sustentaculum tali and the tarsal navicular: the superomedial CN (SMCN) ligament and the inferior CN (ICN) ligament. The SMCN ligament was the larger structure and had histologic properties that suggested significant load bearing. Its superomedial edge averaged 34.6 mm and its inferolateral edge averaged 17 mm. Each specimen was found to have an articular facet composed of fibrocartilage. The ICN ligament differed in both size (average length, 6 mm) and consistency from the SMCN ligament, and its histology indicated a pure tensile load function. In all specimens, the deltoid ligament and the posterior tibialis tendon had direct attachment to the SMCN ligament. Biomechanical testing showed the strength of both the SMCN and the ICN ligaments to be similar to that of ankle ligaments.

Discussion.—The term "spring ligament" is misleading because there is not a single structure at the medial and plantar TCN articulation. Instead, a complex of ligaments is created by the SMCN ligament, the ICN ligament, and the superficial deltoid ligament. Anatomical study suggests that the "spring ligament complex" functions more as an articular sling.

▶ The authors provide the definitive work to date on the anatomy and biomechanical characteristics of the 2 CN ligaments. More accurately characterized as the "sling" complex, elements not previously appreciated are presented here. For one, the complex nature of the SMCN ligament is described. It has meniscal characteristics to provide compressive support for the joint, but it is somewhat suboptimal in terms of tensile function. Also, the midportion is relatively avascular, which may preclude prompt healing after a stressful injury. The authors infer that a better understanding of the anatomy of this region will help in advancing the treatment of acquired flatfoot deformity. They will be proven correct in this assumption. This comprehensive work on the ligament complex is the result of a well-coordinated, multicenter effort.

M.G. Wilson, M.D.

Avascular Necrosis of the Talus Treated by Core Decompression
Mont MA, Schon LC, Hungerford MW, et al (Johns Hopkins Univ, Baltimore, Md)
J Bone Joint Surg Br 78:827–830, 1996   6–13

Introduction.—Avascular necrosis of the talus can occur as a complication of severe ankle injury and has also been reported in association with corticosteroid use, alcoholism, and various disease conditions. The results of treatment by core decompression are reported for 11 patients with nontraumatic avascular necrosis of the talus.

Patients and Methods.—Patients were 10 women and 1 man with a mean age of 47 years. Seven patients (11 ankles) were being treated with systemic corticosteroids for systemic lupus erythematosus and 2 (3 ankles) were receiving the drug for asthma or renal disease. In the remaining 2 patients (3 ankles), alcohol consumption was the suspected cause of the condition. Diagnosis was confirmed by biopsy in all cases. All patients had severe ankle pain on weight-bearing and either radiologic stage I or stage II avascular necrosis. None had responded to conservative treatment. After core decompression, performed as an outpatient procedure, patients were followed for a mean of 7 years.

Results.—Clinical evaluation was done by the Mazur ankle grading system in which pain, range of movement, and activity level are scored on a 100-point scale. Radiologic staging used the Ficat and Arlet classification. At final follow-up, results were judged excellent in 11 ankles and good in 3. The Mazur ankle score increased from a preoperative mean of 35 points to a mean of 92 points postoperatively. Three ankles required tibiotalar fusion at a mean of 13 months after core decompression but all united with excellent clinical outcome. There were no complications, and all patients were able to resume full weight-bearing after 6 weeks. Only 5 ankles progressed to radiologic stage III or IV (collapse).

Discussion.—The only options for symptomatic avascular necrosis of the talus that fails to respond to conservative treatment are various arthrodeses and core decompression. Hindfoot fusions are technically challenging and have a low success rate. For patients who have not progressed to end-stage tibiotalar arthritis, core decompression appears to be a satisfactory option.

▶ Having had previous experience with core decompression of hip and shoulder avascular necrosis, the authors extend the indications to early avascular change in the talus. This is important work because avascular necrosis in the talus appears to take 12 to 18 months to heal, and collapse of the articular surface can occur despite extended use of protected weight-bearing or an orthosis. Any procedure with minimal complication that could somehow affect this occurrance or speed revascularization would be useful, although the authors freely admit that the nature history of avascular necrosis of the talus is not defined to any degree.

Their results are encouraging, with the majority of patients achieving good pain relief and a stable radiographic picture. However, 5 of the 17 ankles did show progressive radiographic degeneration. Assuming all these, end stage arthritic change will develop in these ankles. The ultimate failure rate may not differ substantially from that of a given population treated with traditional conservative measures.

The early dramatic decrease in pain seen with decompression of the avascular area is a phenomenon recognized previously in a hip core decompression, as well as osteotomy for avascular necrosis. This early relief of pain did not always correlate with long-term successful outcome, however. The authors rightly state that this is an ideal area for a multicenter, prospective study.

M.G. Wilson, M.D.

Success of Calcaneonavicular Coalition Resection in the Adult Population

Cohen BE, Davis WH, Anderson RB (Carolinas Med Ctr, Charlotte, NC)
Foot Ankle Int 17:569–572, 1996   6–14

Background.—Arthrodesis is generally performed in adult patients with tarsal coalition or those with degenerative changes. Degenerative changes and the presence of a talar beak have been cited as contraindications to simple resection, which is generally performed in children or adolescents with tarsal coalitions. The results of resection for calcaneonavicular coalition in adults were reported.

Methods.—The experience included 13 feet of 12 adult patients with calcaneonavicular coalitions. The patients' average age was 33 years. Ten feet had documented degenerative changes and 7 had talar beaking. Eleven patients had less than 5 degrees of inversion/eversion. All patients had continued symptoms despite conservative therapy. Calcaneonavicular resection was performed on an outpatient basis using a modified Ollier approach. The surgeon took care to remove at least 1 cm of bone extending to the most medial aspect of the coalition. The patients were followed for an average of 36 months.

Results.—At follow-up, 10 of the 12 patients reported subjective relief from their preoperative symptoms. The average subtalar motion was 15 degrees. None of the patients required an orthosis, cast, or other device, and none had to alter their occupation or activity level. The 2 patients with persistent pain and restriction of motion were considered treatment failures. Both went on to have arthrodesis, which relieved their symptoms. The complication rate was 38%, including 3 cases of marginal wound dehiscence.

Conclusion.—Good results are reported with resection of calcaneonavicular coalition in adult patients. This may be a viable alternative to arthrodesis for patients in whom nonoperative treatment has failed. The long-term results remain to be determined, however.

▶ This is a nice sized study: 13 feet describing a fairly rare condition. By resecting the calcaneonavicular coalition in a young adult population (mean age, 33 years), the authors obtained good functional results with maintained hindfoot motion. Resecting the coalition is also an easier procedure than triple or double fusion, with a quicker recovery and fewer potential complications. These patients certainly may some day require subtalar or double fusion, but delaying the fusion may have benefits for the overall health and longevity of the ankle joint. Hopefully, these authors can continue to follow this cohort to 5- and 10-year follow-up.

M.G. Wilson, M.D.

Clinical Results of the Mayo Total Ankle Arthroplasty

Kitaoka HB, Patzer GL (Mayo Clinic and Mayo Found, Rochester, Minn)
J Bone Joint Surg Am 78:1658–1664, 1996   6–15

Introduction.—Total ankle arthroplasty has been proposed as an alternative to arthrodesis in patients with painful advanced osteoarthrosis of the ankle. This procedure does not appear to be as successful, however, as total hip and knee replacements. Long-term clinical and radiographic results were reported for 160 primary Mayo total ankle arthroplasties performed from 1974 through 1988.

Methods.—The patient group included 46 men and 97 women with a mean age of 54 years at the time of arthroplasty. Underlying conditions were rheumatoid arthritis (60%), posttraumatic osteoarthritis (35%), and osteoarthritis (5%). The mean duration of pain before arthroplasty was 8 years. All procedures were performed through an anterior incision. Patients were asked to return for physical and radiographic examinations at 1 and 2 years postoperatively and every 5 years thereafter. Adequate radiographs were obtained before arthroplasty and at follow-up for 63% of ankles. Overall results were rated as good, fair, poor, or failure.

Results.—In 31 ankles (19%), outcome was considered good; the patient believed the ankle to be much improved, had no pain, was able to walk more than 6 blocks, did not require a walking aid, and had no radiographic evidence of loosening. Results were fair in 35% of ankles; there was improvement, only mild pain, and no evidence of loosening, but walking was limited to 2–6 blocks and a cane was needed. Patients with poor outcome (11% of ankles) had no improvement; moderate or severe pain; required a cane, walker, or brace; and could not walk 2 blocks. The implant was removed in 35% of ankles; these procedures were classified as failures. Although there was radiographic evidence of loosening in 8% of tibial components and 57% of talar components, there was no association between clinical and radiographic results. Nearly half of the ankles (41%) had additional reoperations. Complications occurred after 19 arthroplasties; the most common were deep infection (6 ankles) and superficial infection (4 ankles).

Conclusion.—Primary total ankle arthroplasty with a Mayo implant yielded a good or fair result in 54% of ankles in this series, but 35% of procedures were considered failures and the rate of reoperation was high (41%). Thus, the procedure is not recommended for patients with painful rheumatoid arthritis or osteoarthritis of the ankle.

▶ This relatively constrained, cemented total ankle replacement performed poorly in this 9-year follow-up study. Two predominant modes of failure were noted: a high postoperative infection rate relative to other types of hip or knee arthroplasty and an even higher rate of mechanical failure with loosening or migration. A high postoperative infection rate points out the shortcomings of the anterior approach to the ankle which, because of a paucity of subcutaneous tissue, is unforgiving of any wound breakdown. Sometimes a deep capsular closure is not possible over the component, particularly in the rheumatoid population. Above all, however, the Mayo total ankle arthroplasty has a poor mechanical design, with predictable loosening at the bone-metal interface because of its constrained characteristics. Furthermore, the amount of bone lost because of the original cement technique makes arthrodesis of these failures quite challenging, as pointed out by Kitaoka and Romness in a previous work.[1]

Uncemented, less constrained designs for total ankle arthroplasty are now growing in popularity. We must bear in mind that the Mayo total ankle arthroplasty was promising at the 2-year mark, only displaying its failure at 5 years and longer. The orthopedic community must proceed slowly and with caution so that changes in total ankle design represent true incremental improvements. Current uncemented designs, for instance, may result in unacceptible degrees of osteomyelysis caused by particulate wear. Time will tell.

M.G. Wilson, M.D.

Reference

1. Kitaoka HB, Romness DW: Arthrodesis for failed ankle arthroplasty. *J Arthroplasty* 7:277–284, 1992.

Ankle Arthrodesis Using an Arthroscopic Method: Long-Term Follow-Up of 34 Cases
Glick JM, Morgan CD, Myerson MS, et al (Univ of California, San Francisco; Alfred I duPont Inst, Wilmington, Del; Union Mem Hosp, Baltimore, Md)
Arthroscopy 12:428–434, 1996   6–16

Introduction.—Arthroscopic ankle fusion was first reported in 1983. Compared with open fusion methods, the arthroscopic technique is associated with reduced morbidity and more rapid postoperative mobilization. The 34 ankle arthrodeses reported here indicate that arthroscopic methods also yield good long-term results.

Methods.—Thirty-four patients with an average age of 50 years underwent arthroscopic fusions between February 1983 and April 1989. Although 4 different surgeons performed the procedures, all used a similar technique. All patients had ankle joint arthrosis with significant pain and had failed to respond to at least 6 months of conservative treatment. None had active infection, a neuropathic joint, or severe joint deformity. The most frequent cause of ankle joint arthrosis was posttraumatic arthritis. Internal fixation was used in all cases, with crossed screws or pins to secure the fusion. (The operative technique is presented in detail.) Patients were followed for an average of 7.7 years.

Results.—Successful fusion was achieved in 33 of 34 ankles, and clinical results were rated excellent or good in 86% of cases. Subtalar pain resulted in a fair rating for 3 ankles; a nonunion and a malunion, both caused by surgical errors, accounted for the 2 poor results. One patient required a second procedure because of symptomatic hardware. No wound infections or neurologic injuries occurred. The average time to clinical and radiographic union was 63.5 days.

Discussion.—This largest reported series of arthroscopic ankle arthrodeses shows several advantages of the arthroscopic method over open methods of ankle fusion. Time to union is significantly reduced, thereby hastening recovery. The minimal soft-tissue stripping performed during the arthroscopic procedure appears to be the reason for shorter time to fusion. Most patients can be discharged on the day of surgery or after 1 night in the hospital. When patients have no contraindications for the procedure and the surgeon is well versed in both open and arthroscopic techniques, arthroscopic ankle arthrodesis can yield excellent long-term results.

▶ The results of this paper by surgeons in 4 different practice groups speak for themselves. Arthroscopic ankle arthrodesis can achieve a high union rate. Given the authors' straightforward operative technique and claim of early reliable healing, this article will no doubt inspire many orthopedists—hence, sports medicine specialists—to readily adopt arthroscopy as their primary technique for fusing ankles.

Several words of caution are in order. Arthroscopic ankle fusion is best performed by surgeons already well versed in open techniques. It is an unforgiving technique and, if not performed well, nonunions will result. Furthermore, although there may be some biological advantages to the minimal exposure required with this technique, the mechanical aspects of arthroscopic fusion are inferior if the cannulated screws can only be placed in cancellous bone of the talus, rather than the bicortical bites possible with open techniques. Finally, the authors claim that arthroscopic techniques provide earlier healing is, as yet, unproven.

This is not a prospective comparison of 2 techniques; the authors compare their series with older series in which time to fusion was more a casual observance of the studies than a subject of primary examination. Because x-ray studies are generally obtained on a monthly basis at most, time to fusion in these series is somewhat of an approximation. The greatest benefit of arthroscopic techniques for ankle arthrodesis is the resultant minimal postoperative pain. Often, these procedures can be performed on an outpatient basis.

M.G. Wilson, M.D.

Results of Arthrodesis of the Tarsometatarsal Joints After Traumatic Injury
Komenda GA, Myerson MS, Biddinger KR (Union Mem Hosp, Baltimore, Md)
J Bone Joint Surg Am 78:1665–1676, 1996   6–17

Introduction.—Operative treatment of fracture or dislocation of the tarsometatarsal joints yields better results than nonoperative management, yet many appropriately treated patients subsequently experience painful osteoarthrosis. In this retrospective review, investigators analyzed the results of arthrodesis of the tarsometatarsal joints for painful osteoarthrosis and deformity after traumatic injury of the midfoot.

Methods.—Forty-one patients were seen at the study institution between 1986 and 1992. All but 1 had been referred for evaluation after earlier management at another medical facility. Nine had undergone operative treatment of the initial injury and 23 had been treated nonoperatively. Various nonoperative modalities—including medications, an orthosis, and physical therapy—were tried after referral. If symptoms persisted for 3 to 6 months, an arthrodesis was recommended. Thirty-two patients underwent the procedure at a mean of 35 months after the injury. Rigid internal fixation was used in all cases; 24 patients with a defect created by débridement of the joints had an autogenous bone graft. Concomitant procedures were performed in 9 patients.

Results.—Eight patients with slight deformity had an in situ arthrodesis; the remaining 22 patients had arthrodesis with realignment. Fixation was removed once weight-bearing was started. Results of arthrodesis were evaluated by clinical and radiographic examination and scores on a clinical rating scale. Patients were evaluated at a mean of 50 months after the arthrodesis. Fusion occurred in from 8 to 12 weeks. The mean postoperative score on a midfoot rating scale (78 of a possible 100) was significantly better than the mean preoperative score (44 points). Complications included neuritis in 3 patients, metatarsalgia in 2, and malunion in 2; asymptomatic nonunion, wound slough, superficial infection, and reflex sympathetic dystrophy occurred in 1 patient each. Five patients had at least 1 subsequent procedure. Radiographic analysis, performed in the 24 patients who had realignment, showed satisfactory postoperative alignment.

Conclusion.—Patients who underwent arthrodesis of the tarsometatarsal joints after traumatic injury had marked improvement in function and relief of pain. It was not possible to show a relationship between functional outcome and extent of the arthrodesis, involvement of other joints in the hindfoot or forefoot, mechanism of injury, or whether the injury was work related.

▶ This is a wonderful article by the group in Baltimore describing their extensive experience with midfoot arthrodesis after trauma. I love this article because their clinical decision making is so sound, their operative technique so consistent, and their description of their technique is so detailed. I believe that the authors have addressed all the major clinical issues in this patient population. Their indications for reduction of deformity are sound, and their techniques of achieving reduction will be found useful by any orthopedist performing this procedure. Their high radiographic union rate is impressive and tests well to their technique and emphasis on autologous bone grafting.

Depite the authors' expertise in treating these injuries, it should be stressed that the main postoperative functional score was 78, which indicates that the majority of these patients still experienced functional limitation; this is a point that must be stressed clinically when educating patients before surgery. Although I think generalized functional scores are useful and allow some comparison of results between studies, some information is lost when authors present the total score without discussion of the makeup of the score. For example, many of these patients, although they will claim pain-free ambulation, still have significant limitations and often will require some type of supportive shoe or orthosis. The degree of this functional limitation should have been expanded in the text.

M.G. Wilson, M.D.

Primary Subtalar Arthrodesis for the Treatment of Comminuted Calcaneal Fractures

Buch BD, Myerson MS, Miller SD (Union Mem Hosp, Baltimore, Md)
Foot Ankle Int 17:61–70, 1996
6–18,

Introduction.—The choice of treatment for calcaneal fractures is controversial, but all authors agree that management of severely comminuted articular fractures is difficult. A retrospective review of patients treated between 1989 and 1992 examined the results of primary subtalar arthrodesis for severely comminuted articular fractures of the calcaneal.

Methods.—During the period of review, 112 calcaneal fractures in 108 patients were treated at the study institution: 9 with nonoperative methods; 83 with open reduction and internal fixation; and 20 with open reduction, internal fixation, and primary subtalar arthrodesis. Marked comminution with substantial displacement and/or severe cartilaginous damage of the posterior facet were indications for arthrodesis. Fourteen of 20 fractures treated with primary subtalar arthrodesis were available for review. The 14 patients (2 women and 12 men) had an average age of 40 years. Ten had been injured in falls and 4 in motor vehicle accidents. The time from injury to surgery averaged 14 days. An extensile lateral approach was used in the procedure. After calcaneal height and width were restored with standard fixation techniques, arthrodesis was performed with bone graft and fixation by 7.0-mm cannulated cancellous screws. Follow-up after surgery ranged from 12 to 54 months (mean, 26 months).

Results.—Patients remained non–weight-bearing on the affected extremity for an average of 8.6 weeks, but those with bilateral fractures began weight-bearing an average of 3 weeks later. Partial weight-bearing was started with a hinged range-of-motion walker boot or a firm surgical shoe. Full weight-bearing was accomplished by an average of 11.5 weeks. Radiographic union was present in all cases between 8 and 12 weeks after surgery. There were minor wound complications in 3 patients and a fourth required a split-thickness skin graft to cover the wound. Eleven of 12 patients who were employed before the injury returned to their original occupation at a mean of 8.8 months after injury. Pain at follow-up was absent in 3 patients, mild in 7, moderate in 3, and moderate-to-severe in 1. The patients' mean score on a rating scale of pain, function, and alignment was 72.4 points out of a possible 94 points. All reported limitations in their recreational activities and 9 of 14 reported some limitation in the activities of daily living.

Conclusion.—Primary subtalar arthrodesis yielded results comparable with those of other methods for treatment of comminuted calcaneal fractures. Although some discomfort and limitations were present in the affected extremity, the return-to-work rate was good.

▶ This retrospective review of 14 primary subtalar arthrodeses for comminuted calcaneal fractures describes 1 treatment option for this fracture pattern. The reader should be encouraged by the high radiographic union rate and absence of serious complications such as deep, persistent infection. Also, the majority of patients were able to return to work of some type, although clearly serious modification of activity level was a dominant feature. Also, many of the patients had persistent pain; only 3 were without pain or had moderate-to-severe pain postoperatively.

Primary subtalar arthrodesis is an appropriate surgical option for some patients, enabling restoration of extra-articular anatomy of the heel and avoidance of inevitable arthrodesis at a later date, given extensive loss of the cartilage integrity. This well-written article reports the results using modern techniques and CT scan indications. It is curious that the authors have not used the CT scan classification system of Sanders.[1] Coronal view classification of comminution of the posterior facet is straightforward and very useful in a clinical situation, although the authors correctly point out that, occasionally, intraoperative adjustment of the plan must be based upon an expected shear damage to the cartilage surface. I suspect that adequate coronal views to enable adequate classification were not obtained in all the patients preoperatively. This is a common problem, particularly in the multitrauma patient, as physician-supervised positioning is often required. Further results of series that compare results of fixation vs. fixation and arthrodesis in Sanders type II, III, and IV injuries as required.

M.G. Wilson, M.D.

Reference

1. Sanders R, Fortin P, DiPasquale T, et al: Operative treatment in 120 displaced intraarticular calcaneal fractures. Results using a prognostic computed tomography scan classification. *Clin Orthop* 290:87–95, 1993.

Operative vs. Nonoperative Treatment of Intra-Articular Fractures of the Calcaneus: A Prospective Randomized Trial
Thordarson DB, Krieger LE (Univ of Southern California, Los Angeles)
Foot Ankle Int 17:2–9, 1996   6–19

Introduction.—Studies comparing operative and nonoperative treatment of intra-articular fractures of the calcaneus have been limited in number and scope, and results have been quite mixed. This study is the first to use a prospective, randomized design in the comparison of operative and nonoperative treatment and the first in which current fixation methods and early mobilization were involved in operative treatment.

Methods.—Eligible patients were between the ages of 18 and 60 years and had no significant systemic illness. All underwent CT to define the anatomy of the fracture, especially involvement of the posterior facet, and the fracture was graded according to Sanders classification. Only Sanders type II (2 major articular fragments) or type III (3 major articular fragments) fractures were randomized into the study. Of 30 enrolled patients, 15 in the operative group and 11 in the nonoperative group were available for follow-up averaging 17 months and 14 months, respectively. All patients completed an outcome assessment questionnaire.

Results.—The 2 treatment groups were similar in demographic data. With 1 exception, the mechanism of injury was a fall from a height. Nonoperative treatment included ice, elevation, and a bulky Jones dressing. After edema subsided, patients were fitted with a removable posterior splint and started early range of motion exercises; weight-bearing was allowed at 8 weeks. Operative treatment involved open reduction and rigid internal fixation with a plate and screws through an extensile, L-shaped lateral approach. Range-of-motion exercises were started 3 days after surgery and full weight-bearing at 12 weeks. Results in the operative group were excellent in 7 cases, good in 5, fair in 2, and poor in 1; in the nonoperative group, results were excellent in 1 case, good in 3, fair in 1, and poor in 6. Although all fractures healed in both groups, differences in functional outcome between the 2 treatment methods were significant. The average functional score was 86.7 for the operative group but only 55.0 for the nonoperative group. All nonoperative patients, but only 25% of operative patients, experienced pain on extremes of motion.

Discussion.—This prospective, randomized trial confirms that current methods of operative treatment with early mobilization yield results that are clearly superior to those obtained with nonoperative treatment for patients with displaced, intra-articular calcaneus fractures. At short-term follow-up, pain was reduced and functional ability improved in the operative group.

▶ This is a remarkable study. Two important elements set it apart. One is that it is a prospective, randomized work with appropriate intra-articular fractures randomized to operative and nonoperative groups. Second, Thordarson has analyzed results in terms of outcome analysis, which is an approach that is becoming increasingly relevant in today's clinical setting. Much more than the extensive radiographic analysis or measurement of range of motion or alignment, the functional outcome data argue conclusively in favor of careful surgical fixation for these injuries. This is the kind of careful clinical work that should be adopted by major teaching institutions across the country. Hopefully, these 2 cohort groups will be available for further follow-up by the author at the 5-year mark.

M.G. Wilson, M.D.

Surgery Versus Functional Treatment in Ankle Ligament Tears
Kaikkonen A, Kannus P, Järvinen M (Univ of Tampere, Finland; UKK Inst, Tampere, Finland)
Clin Orthop 326:194–202, 1996
6–20

Background.—Nonoperative treatment is the accepted approach for grade I or II injuries of the ankle ligaments, almost always producing an excellent or good result. However, the best strategy for treating grade III sprains of the lateral ligament complex has not been established. Surgery was compared with functional treatment in patients with grade III lateral ligament injuries of the ankle in a prospective study.

Methods.—Thirty patients underwent primary repair plus early controlled mobilization, and 30 underwent early controlled mobilization alone. The 2 groups were matched by age, height, weight, gender, and sports activity.

Findings.—All but 1 patient in each treatment group had a stable ankle at 9 months. At 6 weeks, patients undergoing surgery had restricted range of motion of the ankle joint compared with those undergoing mobilization alone, but this normalized during follow-up. No restriction was observed in the latter group. According to a scoring scale developed for subjective and functional follow-up assessment of an injured ankle, 9-month outcomes were excellent or good in 87% of the functionally treated patients and in 60% of the surgically treated patients.

Conclusion.—In the short term, surgery plus early mobilization has no advantages over early mobilization alone in patients with grade III lateral ligament injuries of the ankle. Further research is needed to determine whether immobilization of any duration is required after lateral ligament ankle injuries.

▶ This randomized clinical trial compares anatomical repair and early mobilization with early mobilization alone for acute grade III ankle ligament tears. Postoperative stability was based solely on anterior drawer testing performed by the investigators, so some bias is possible. Also, anatomical repair and early mobilization is not commonly used in this country, as the popular Brostrom repair generally requires 4 to 6 weeks of mobilization. However, despite these potential drawbacks, this study clearly shows that grade III ligament sprains can do well with nonoperative functional treatment. Twenty-nine of 30 ankles in the functional group were stable by clinical examination at 9 months, none of the patients complained of the ankle giving way, and the functional group returned to work 5 weeks post injury compared with 7 weeks for the surgery group. These findings need to be coroborated by other authors, using a domestic population. Implications in the high performance athlete also need to be examined, as these patients are often treated with aggressive early surgical intervention.

M.G. Wilson, M.D.

Suggested Reading

VARUS MALALIGNMENT OF THE TALAR NECK

Daniels TR, Smith JW, Ross TI *J Bone Joint Surg Am* 78:1559–1567, 1996
> ▶ Fractures of the talar neck are some of the most difficult fractures in the foot to manage given their high frequency of nonunion, malunion, avascular necrosis, and subsequent osteoarthritis. Initial open reduction–internal fixation has become the treatment of choice for displaced talar neck fractures, and this article addresses 1 complication of these displaced fractures, that is, shortening with varus malalignment. This is a very common clinical entity inasmuch as these fractures of the medial column often involve compression and shortening, thus resulting in a varus deformity. The authors quantify the effect of shortening of the neck by measuring the decrease in hindfoot motion and degree of midfoot deformity after closing wedge osteotomy. Even relatively small amounts of shortening resulted in dramatic decreases in hindfoot motion, the implication being that such shortening cannot be accepted in the clinical situation. Often these fractures need to be bone-grafted to restore their length. It is also possible to overlengthen these fractures given too much bone grafting. It would be interesting to measure the effect of valgus malalignment as well.

MAJOR OPEN INJURIES OF THE TALUS

Marsh JL, Saltsman CL, Iverson M, et al *J Orthop Trauma* 9:371–376, 1995.
> ▶ This article reports a fairly large series of 18 open talus fracture-dislocations monitored for a reasonable amount of time. The majority of the patients were observed for more than 7 years. The authors confirm the impression that these are difficult injuries with a poor overall prognosis. The high rate of infection was caused by the multiple open joint cavities created by these injuries despite superficial soft tissue closure, as well as ischemia of the body of the talus. The series lacks the power to determine whether an extruded talar body should be excised or replanted; however, the study does suggest that a deep infection should be treated aggressively with consideration of radical débridement of infected bone. Reasonably good results were obtained after talar body excision and Blair-type fusion. Interestingly, a few of the patients were treated with talectomy and had a reasonably functional result, although the authors should have correlated the radiographic appearance of these feet with the requirement for braces to control instability.General treatment principles would seem to include replacement of the extruded talar body unless gross contamination is evident in which case talar body excision is recommended instead of reconstruction.

OPERATIVE TREATMENTS OF FRACTURES OF THE TIBIAL PLAFOND

Wyrsch B, McFerran MA, McAndrew M, et al *J Bone Joint Surg Am* 78:1646–1657, 1996
> ▶ This prospective study comparing primary internal fixation of plafond injuries with external fixation and limited internal fixation suggests that the primary consideration in treatment of these injuries should be care of the soft tissues. Of

the 3 common complications of these injuries, infection, shortening with varus deformity, and articular degeneration, only articular degeneration has a relatively straightforward solution, secondary arthrodesis. It follows that the primary treatment mode must focus primarily on protection of soft tissue to prevent infection and on restoration of length to the limb. Early application of an external fixator to span the medial column can maintain length of the tibia and thus fulfills both roles nicely. Furthermore, it appears that in these injuries degenerative changes will often eventually develop in even well reduced articular surfaces, so heroic attempts at anatomical articular reconstruction would not seem warranted if such an attempt in any way compromises wound healing and causes subsequent breakdown and skin necrosis. This important work stresses this important treatment principle. In fact, as long as the open injuries are adequately débrided and length and alignment are restored with external fixation, articular reconstruction can be delayed and carefully planned with CT scan imaging. A properly planned articular reconstruction can then often be carried out through small percutaneous techniques, and with extremely damaged joint surfaces, the patient and surgeon have the opportunity to consider early arthrodesis.

7 Trauma and Amputation

Introduction

This year's group of abstracts is representative of clinically relevant work using established techniques. Unfortunately, this year we have fewer examples of prospective clinical series that are controlled than we have had in the past 2 years. Nevertheless, there is a particularly valuable crop of abstracts within the amputation section and some very helpful manuscripts to assist clinicians in managing injuries in the lower extremity, in particular. In addition, several technological advances are presented in this year's group of abstracts. Potentially critical developments in terms of plate design and techniques for treating osteoporotic ankle fractures show great promise for the management of problem fractures.

Marc F. Swiontkowski, M.D.

Knee Injury

Arthroscopy for Acute Knee Haemarthrosis in Road Traffic Accident Victims

Lu KH, Hsiao YM, Lin ZI (Chung Shan Med & Dental College, Taiwan, Republic of China)
Injury 27:341–343, 1996

7–1

Background.—The need for early, complete diagnosis of acute knee injuries is accepted. Previous studies have described varying intra-articular lesions in patients with hemarthrosis of the knee. The characteristics of acute traumatic hemarthosis after road traffic accidents were investigated arthroscopically in a prospective study.

Methods.—Forty-six patients with 47 acute knee hemarthroses after road traffic accidents underwent arthroscopic examination of all suspicious structures with the use of anterolateral, anteromedial, superolateral, superomedial, posterolateral, and posteromedial entry portals.

Results.—Single damaged structures were found in 13 knees, and multiple damaged structures were found in 34 knees, for a total of 117 injuries in the 47 knees (Table 3). There were medial meniscus tears in 10.6% and

TABLE 3.—Arthroscopic Diagnoses in 47 Acute Knee Hemarthroses

Injury structure	Number
Anterior cruciate ligament	24
Posterior cruciate ligament	18
Medial collateral ligament	9
Posterior lateral complex	8
Medial meniscus	5
Lateral meniscus	19
Medial retinaculum	3
Fracture	
Femoral condyle	5
Tibial plateau and spine	21
Patella	2*
Synovial membrane	1
Medial patellar plica	2

*1 was lower pole patella fracture with patellar tendon rupture.
(Courtesy of Lu KH, Hsiao YM, Lin ZI: Arthroscopy for acute knee haemarthrosis in road traffic accident victims. *Injury* 27:341–343, copyright 1996, with kind permission from Elsevier Science Ltd., The Boulevard, Langford Lane, Kidlington OX5 1GB, U.K.)

lateral meniscus tears in 40.4%, with both menisci torn in 2 knees. One patient had a synovial tear and 3 patients had femoral osteochondral fractures. One patient had a patellar fracture, and 3 patellar dislocations were seen with medial retinaculum rupture. There were anterior cruciate ligament tears in 51.1%, with 4 distal avulsion fractures from the tibial spine, 4 complete tears, 15 partial tears, and 1 distal avulsion fracture from the tibial spine with a complete proximal tear. There were posterior cruciate ligament tears in 38.3%, with 9 avulsion fractures from the tibia, 6 complete tears, and 3 partial tears. Seven knees with posterior segment tears of the lateral meniscus also had 18 posterior cruciate ligament tears.

Conclusion.—Compared with the sports injury population, this road traffic accident population had a lower incidence of anterior cruciate ligament tearing and medial meniscal tearing and a greater incidence of posterior cruciate ligament and lateral meniscal tearing. The importance of arthroscopy in the diagnosis of acute knee hemarthrosis was confirmed.

Saline Load Test for Penetration of Periarticular Lacerations

Voit GA, Irvine G, Beals RK (Univ of New Mexico, Albuquerque; Oregon Health Sciences Univ, Portland)
J Bone Joint Surg Br 78:732–733, 1996

7–2

Background.—Intra-articular penetration and contamination can result from lacerations sustained next to joints. Local irrigation is usually done when a periarticular laceration does not penetrate the joint, but a more extensive operation is needed when penetration has occurred. Saline injections into joints can be performed to determine the best treatment. However, no data are available on the safety or efficacy of such a procedure.

TABLE 1.—Results of Clinical Prediction and the Saline Load Test
in 50 Patients

Saline Load Test	Clinical Prediction	% Error
Negative 36	Negative 22	*39*
	Positive 14	
Positive 14	Positive 8	*43*
	Negative 6	
Total 50	50	

(Courtesy of Voit GA, Irvine G, Beals RK: Saline load test for penetration of periarticular lacerations. *J Bone Joint Surg Br* 78:732–733, 1996.)

Methods.—A saline load test was performed on 50 consecutive patients with periarticular lacerations suggesting joint penetration. In addition, a surgeon had predicted whether the laceration penetrated the joint based on clinical findings.

Findings.—Joint penetration was demonstrated in 14 patients. In the remaining 36, no leakage was found. In a comparison of the surgeon's prediction and the test results, clinical findings were falsely positive in 39% of the patients and falsely negative in 43% (Table 1). No complications were associated with use of the test.

Conclusions.—Clinical assessment to determine whether a periarticular laceration has penetrated the joint is frequently incorrect. The saline load test is useful for evaluating periarticular lacerations.

▶ Knee injury is very common in motor vehicle accidents. Most clinicians believe that we are seeing an increasing incidence of this as vehicles have gotten smaller, particularly in North America. The first manuscript confirms our impression that arthroscopy for acute knee hemarthrosis in accident victims will have a very high yield. It would seem wise to make the diagnosis, perform meniscal repair or partial meniscectomy when indicated, and then discuss with the patient treatment options, surgical vs. nonsurgical for anterior cruciate and particularly posterior cruciate ligament injuries.

We have long suspected that in cases of penetrating knee injury, infiltration of the joint with sterile saline is a helpful adjunct in making the diagnosis. This nicely done study confirms that in 14 of 50 patients with periarticular lacerations, joint penetration does occur. With the high false positive and false negative results of clinical judgment, the saline load test should be used universally.

M.F. Swiontkowski, M.D.

Traumatic Skin Defects

Missed Closed Degloving Injuries: Late Presentation as a Contour Deformity

Hudson DA (Univ of Cape Town, South Africa)
Plast Reconstr Surg 98:334–337, 1996   7–3

Introduction.—Although open degloving injuries are common, usually obvious, and often associated with bony and neurovascular injuries, closed degloving injuries are uncommon, often missed or ignored while other more severe injuries are treated, and rarely associated with bony and neurovascular injuries. Even within the context of the rarity of closed degloving injury, those with an associated contour deformity are unusual. Seven patients treated over a 5-year period for a contour deformity after a missed degloving injury were reported.

Methods.—The records of 7 patients treated between 1990 and 1994 who had a closed degloving injury with associated contour deformity were reviewed. The mechanism and site of injury, associated injuries, reason for presentation, treatment, and outcome were noted.

Results.—All of the patients had been injured in motor vehicle accidents. Six were pedestrians and 1 was a passenger. They requested corrective cosmetic surgery for their contour defects between 14 months and 13 years after the original injury. The defect affected the lateral thigh in 5 patients and the calf in 2 patients. None had bone fractures under the contour defect, although 2 patients had bony injuries at other sites. The contour deformity had been diagnosed during the initial hospitalization in only 1 patient; the deformity was unsuccessfully treated with incision and drainage. No patients had functional deficits at the time they were seen for cosmetic surgery. Five patients were treated by liposuction; the patient with the largest contour deformity required 2 liposuction procedures. All of these patients had improved contour, although there was some persistent deformity in 2 patients. Two patients with irregular, gritty deformities underwent open incision with trimming and sculpting of areas of fat necrosis and/or heterotopic calcification after failed liposuction procedures. Both patients had improved contour but with some residual irregularity.

Conclusion.—Closed degloving injuries with associated contour deformity typically occur on the lower extremity, with the lateral thigh the most common site. Liposuction will improve the contour when the defect is soft and smooth. Irregular, firmer deformities may require open incision and sculpting.

Moving?

I'd like to receive my *Year Book of Orthopedics* without interruption.
Please note the following change of address, effective:

Name: ____

New Address: ____

City: _________________________ State: _________ Zip: _________

Old Address: ____

____

City: _________________________ State: _________ Zip: _________

Reservation Card

Yes, I would like my own copy of *Year Book of Orthopedics*. Please begin my subscription with the current edition according to the terms described below.* I understand that I will have 30 days to examine each annual edition. If satisfied, I will pay just $79.95 plus sales tax, postage and handling (price subject to change without notice).

Name: ____

Address: ____

City: _________________________ State: _________ Zip: _________

Method of Payment
O Visa   O Mastercard   O AmEx   O Bill me   O Check (in US dollars, payable to Mosby, Inc.)

Card number: _________________________ Exp date: _________________

Signature: ____

Your Year Book Service Guarantee:

When you subscribe to the *Year Book*, we'll send you an advance notice of future volumes about two months before they publish. This automatic notice system is designed to take up as little of your time as possible. If you do not want the *Year Book*, the advance notice makes it quick and easy for you to let us know your decision, and you will always have at least 20 days to decide. If we don't hear from you, we'll send you the new volume as soon as it's available. And, of course, the *Year Book* is yours to examine free of charge for 30 days (postage, handling and applicable sales tax are added to each shipment.).

BUSINESS REPLY MAIL

FIRST CLASS MAIL   PERMIT No. 762   CHICAGO, IL

POSTAGE WILL BE PAID BY ADDRESSEE

Chris Hughes
Mosby-Year Book, Inc.
161 N. Clark Street
Suite 1900
Chicago, IL 60601-9981

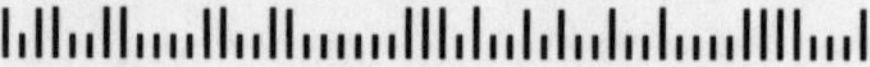

NO POSTAGE
NECESSARY
IF MAILED
IN THE
UNITED STATES

BUSINESS REPLY MAIL

FIRST CLASS MAIL   PERMIT No. 762   CHICAGO, IL

POSTAGE WILL BE PAID BY ADDRESSEE

Chris Hughes
Mosby-Year Book, Inc.
161 N. Clark Street
Suite 1900
Chicago, IL 60601-9981

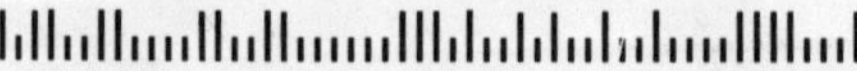

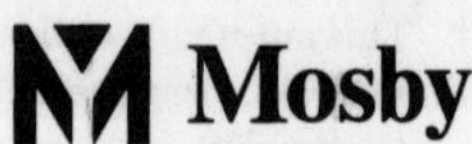

Dedicated to publishing excellence

External Tissue Stretching for Closing Skin Defects in 22 Patients
Bjarnesen JP, Wester JU, Siemssen SS, et al (Odense Univ, Denmark)
Acta Orthop Scand 67:182–184, 1996   7–4

Background.—A new device has been developed for rapidly stretching the skin. The device has 2 holding bars with a number of straps between them (Fig 1). There is a block on 1 end of each strap and a 1-way locking device on the other end. While the patient is under local anesthesia, the expander is placed under the skin, with the straps placed in the holding bars through a subcutaneous canal on each side of the defect. Tension is applied and increased twice daily with the 1-way locking device. The stretching is completed within 1–2 weeks. After the device is removed, the interjacent skin is excised and the wound is closed primarily. This skin stretching system was tested in the primary closure of a variety of defects.

Methods.—Twelve women and 10 men ranging in age from 15 to 67 years underwent skin stretching with the device for the closure of 9 fasciotomies and for preoperative skin extension before excision of 6 tattoos, 7 split–skin transplants, 4 giant nevi, and 3 cicatrices. The defects had widths ranging from 3 to 15 cm and lengths ranging from 6 to 31 cm. Pain intensity was recorded during expansion on a 10-point visual analogue scale. Skin biopsy specimens were obtained before expansion, during excision, and 3 months after excision.

Results.—Two to 11 days (mean, 4 days) were required for stretching. Fasciotomy defects required the least stretching time and the removal of split-skin transplants required the longest stretching time. The patients had a mean pain score of 2.2 during stretching. There were 2 complications: central rupture of the skin before excision of 2 split-skin transplants. These required earlier removal than planned but were nevertheless successful. All the patients were satisfied with their cosmetic results. The skin biopsy specimens showed no epidermal changes and slight dermal edema during excision; normal epidermis with mild reactive inflammation and perivascular mast cell infiltration in the dermis were seen at the 3-month evaluation.

Conclusion.—The external skin stretching device is highly efficient and effective and permits primary skin closure of large defects. Because a split-skin transplant may adhere to the subcutaneous tissue, excision of the split-skin before using the stretching device may be a better strategy.

▶ All experienced musculoskeletal trauma surgeons have seen patients with closed degloving injuries. It is a puzzling circumstance and treatment recommendations for patients are not uniform. This study is the first to pool a large group of these injuries and gives us useful information on what patients with these defects might expect. It is also helpful to note that few of these injuries were identified at initial hospitalization and seem to become more prominent as the hematoma liquefies. Liposuction seems to be a useful adjunct and can be offered to patients as a potential solution if the lesions prove bothersome.

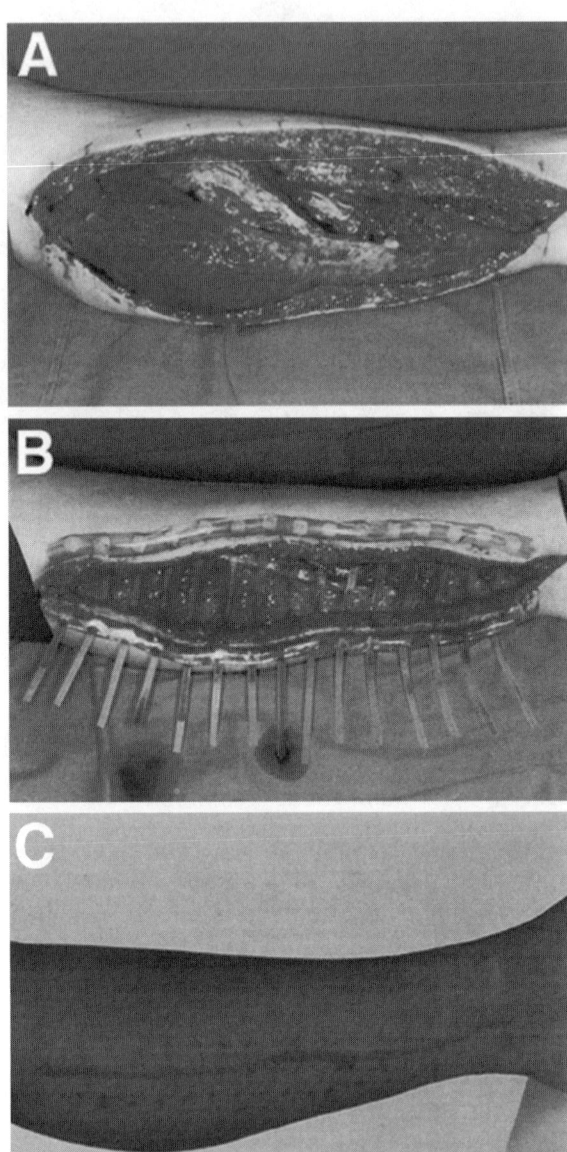

FIGURE 1.—**A,** medial fasciotomy of the lower leg, 30 × 15 cm. **B,** during expansion. **C,** 3 months postoperatively. (Courtesy of Bjarnesen JP, Wester JU, Siemssen SS, et al: External tissue stretching for closing skin defects in 22 patients. *Acta Orthop Scand* 67:182–184, 1996.)

Closure of traumatic skin defects is a difficult issue that involves judgment. The question is often whether to proceed with a skin graft or try to use suture techniques or skin hooks with multiple assistance to bring the skin edges together under tension. This new device seems to hold some promise in fasciotomy closure. It makes good sense for use with primary excision of skin lesions, as the authors have proved. The issue for the clinician then becomes the expense of this device vs. using multiple suture techniques and bringing them together with multiple clamps.

M.F. Swiontkowski, M.D.

Biomaterial Issues Related to Trauma

The Histologic Features of the Interfacial Membrane of Intramedullary Nails

Boss JH, Behar J, Misselevich I, et al (Bnai Zion Med Ctr, Haifa, Israel)
J Long Term Effects Med Implants 5:169–183, 1995   7–5

Background.—Because biomaterials are biocompatible in bulk form, interfacial membrane (IM) formation cannot simply be attributed to the effects of alloplastic material on the osseous environment. Interfacial membranes can develop at the bone-implant boundary, contingent on interfacial movements, deposition of implant breakdown products, and the inflammatory-granulomatous response. Adverse biomechanical conditions, a bioengineering predicament, or a design flaw may be related to or may exacerbate these events. The IMs of intramedullary nails used in the fixation of fractured long tubular bones were studied.

Methods and Findings.—Thirty-six IMs were obtained at the removal of intramedullary L316 stainless steel nails and assessed histologically. In a minority of cases, the membranes consisted of bland fibrous tissue. The nails were usually enclosed in a synovial-like membrane. The metallic surface of the nails showed abutment of palisading macrophages and fibroblasts. Foreign body giant-celled granulomas were scattered in the midzone of the membranes. Monokaryonic and polykaryonic macro-

TABLE 1.—Histologic Features of the Interfacial Membranes of Intramedullary Nails

Histological features of the IM	Number of patients	Percentage
Bland fibrous tissular membrane	3	8.3
Synovial-like interfacial membrane	33	91.7
Granulomatous response to metallic debris		
Finely dispersed metallic debris in some macrophages	25	69.4
Densely packed metallic debris in many macrophages	4	11.1
Granulomatous response to bony debris	16	44.4
Granulomatous response to lipidic compounds	7	19.4
Hemosiderin containing macrophages	7	19.4

Abbreviation: IM, interfacial membrane
(Courtesy of Boss JH, Behar J, Misselevich I, et al: The histologic features of the interfacial membrane of intramedullary nails. *J Long Term Effects Med Implants* 5:169–183, 1995.)

phages had phagocytized small metallic particles, necrotic bony debris, and occasionally lipid compounds. Some sites of previous bleeding were marked by aggregates of hemosiderin-containing macrophages. Remodeling was observed in bone underlying the membrane when present (Table 1).

Conclusion.—Intramedullary nails are enclosed in IMs. The nail apposes bone at few points on insertion, and osseous trabeculae at points of contact are removed later by osteoclastic activity. Consequently, the interfacial motion and accumulation of particulates recruit and activate macrophages, resulting in the formation of a synovial-like IM. The microscopic nuances of IMs are best viewed as an expression of the nearby foreign body and its breakdown products.

Titanium Plate Fixation: A Review of Implant Failures

Banovetz JM, Sharp R, Probe RA, et al (Univ of Missouri, Columbia; Texas A&M Univ, Temple)

J Orthop Trauma 10:389–394, 1996

7–6

Background.—The use of titanium plates and screws for fracture and osteotomy fixation is now widespread. Several early hardware failures in an institution's experience prompted a retrospective review of the occurrence of this complication.

Methods and Findings.—Hardware failure rates with titanium and stainless steel implants were compared in patients treated at 2 centers during a 2-year period. At 1 center, 51 fractures or osteotomies of the long bones were fixed using titanium implants and 101 were treated with stainless steel implants. Outcomes were known for 48 and 80 procedures, respectively. Postoperatively, failure occurred in 5 titanium implants and in 1 stainless steel implant. One set of broken implants obtained during

TABLE 1.—University of Missouri Hospitals and Clinics

	Stainless steel	Titanium
Platings	101	51
Patients	75	40
Location		
Humerus	13	5
Forearm	19	16
Femur	31	4
Tibia	14	10
Ankle	24	16
Nonunions	15	8
Lost to follow-up		
Platings	21	3
Patients	18	3
Nonunions	4	2
Hardware failure	1	5

(Courtesy of Banovetz JM, Sharp R, Probe RA, et al: Titanium plate fixation: A review of implant failures. *J Orthop Trauma* 10:389–394, 1996.)

revision surgery showed no manufacturing defects. At the second center, 21 titanium and 138 stainless steel platings were performed. Four titanium implant failures and 1 stainless steel implant failure occurred (Table 1).

Conclusions.—Titanium materials should be used cautiously in conditions of high load or when high tensile stresses will be applied to screws. Further research is needed to define when titanium implant use is appropriate.

Infection After Open Reduction and Internal Fixation With Dynamic Compression Plates—Clinical and Experimental Data

Arens S, Hansis M, Schlegel U, et al (AO/ASIF Research Inst, Davos, Switzerland; Universität Bonn, Germany; Chemisches Zentrallabor, Inselspital, Bern, Switzerland)

Injury 27:C27S–C33S, 1996

7–7

Introduction.—Infection rates associated with open reduction and internal fixation with dynamic compression plates (DCPs) have been reported to range from 0.8% to 29%. The higher infection rates were reported when DCPs were used in fractures with soft tissue trauma. The purpose of this study was to determine the rate of infection after open reduction and internal fixation using DCPs during a clinical and an experimental trial.

Methods.—A total of 281 open reduction and internal fixations were performed with stainless steel DCPs and titanium DCPs. Preoperative, intraoperative, and postoperative wound swabs were taken and drain tips and fluids were cultured. Initial bacterial contamination was classified as contaminated or noncontaminated. The rates of infection between the 2 groups were calculated. Patients were monitored for at least 6 months after surgery.

In a separate laboratory investigation, steel or titanium DCPs were implanted into the left tibia of white New Zealand rabbits. A range of doses of colony forming units (cfu) of *Staphylococcus aureus* were inoculated around the plate. After 4 weeks, bone and tissue surrounding the plate were examined for bacterial growth and clinical signs of infection.

Results.—A total of 281 cases of open reduction and internal fixation were performed. Based on initial bacterial findings, 41% of the steel and

TABLE 2.—Initial Bacterial Contamination for 281 Dynamic Compression Plates

%(m)	N	Non-Contaminated	Contaminated
Steel	154	41% (63)	59% (91)
Titanium	127	36% (46)	64% (81)
Total	281	39% (109)	61% (172)

(Reprinted from *Injury*, vol 27, suppl 3, Arens S, Hansis M, Schlegel U, et al: Infection after open reduction and internal fixation with dynamic compression plates—clinical and experimental data, pp C27–C33, copyright 1996, with kind permission from Elsevier Ltd, The Boulevard, Langford Lane, Kidlington OX5 1GB, UK.)

TABLE 3.—Infection Rates After Implantation of 281 Dynamic Compression Plates

%(n)	Infection Rate	Non-Contaminated	Contaminated
Steel	9.7% (15)	3.2% (2)	*14.3% (13)*
Titanium	6.3% (8)	2.2% (1)	*8.6% (7)*
Total	8.2% (23)	2.8% (3)	11.6% (20)

(Reprinted from *Injury*, vol 27, suppl 3, Arens S, Hansis M, Schlegel U, et al: Infection after open reduction and internal fixation with dynamic compression plates—clinical and experimental data, pp C27–C33, copyright 1996, with kind permission from Elsevier Ltd, The Boulevard, Langford Lane, Kidlington OX5 1GB, UK.)

36% of the titanium DCPs were classified as noncontaminated. (Table 2). Overall, after DCP implantation, the infection rates were 9.7% and 6.3% for steel and titanium DCPs, respectively (Table 3). Infection rates in the noncontaminated groups were lower than those in the contaminated groups and were similar for the titanium and steel DCPs. Infection rates in the contaminated groups were higher for steel DCPs than for titanium DCPs, but the differences were not significantly different.

In the animal study, a higher rate of infection was found with stainless steel DCPs than with titanium DCPs (75% vs. 35%, $P < 0.05$). An inoculum between 4×10^4 and 2×10^5 cfu resulted in the greatest differences in infection rates between the 2 materials.

Conclusion.—For noncontaminated titanium and steel DCPs, there was no difference in the rate of infection. Steel DCP implants had a higher rate of infection than did titanium DCP implants, but the differences were not significant. In the animal investigation, the rate of infection with titanium DCPs was significantly lower than that with steel DCPs.

▶ There has been an increasing move away from stainless steel for fracture implants toward titanium and titanium alloys. This group of articles (Abstracts 7–5–7–7) brings up several issues of relevance. The first one nicely identifies what the membrane is that we have all noted on removal of stainless steel intramedullary nails. This synovial-like membrane seems to have some element of foreign body reaction and lends some credence to the move toward titanium.

The article by Banovetz et al (See Abstract 7–6) cautions that particularly when we are speaking of plates and screws, the move toward titanium may not be so wise. They report a high rate of failure of titanium implants relative to their experience with stainless steel. It is likely that this series suffers from some selection bias but, nevertheless, seems a reasonable attempt at gathering a large number of cases over a 2-year period at 2 centers. The titanium failure rate seems to be well more than 2 times that of the stainless steel, which gives us pause.

The third article (See Abstract 7–7) combines a clinical and basic research study regarding the issue of infection as it relates to biomaterials. The difficulty with defining infection in the clinical scenario limits the utility of this aspect of the study. Judgment of redness and warmth is often difficult to quantify for an outcome of infection. Nevertheless, there does seem to be a higher rate of clinical infection for stainless steel implants in contaminated wounds. The authors confirm no difference in clean wounds between stainless steel and titanium implants. The animal investigation with highly contaminated wounds revealed a better outcome with titanium.

The ultimate decision of which material to use should be a combination of the cost, the perceived length of healing time, the level of contamination of the wound, and the experience of the surgeon. Titanium as a material for internal fixation warrants further prospective research in large, multicenter series.

M.F. Swiontkowski, M.D.

Bone Density and Fracture Risk

Dual-Energy X-Ray Absorptiometry Derived Structural Geometry for Stress Fracture Prediction in Male U.S. Marine Corps Recruits
Beck TJ, Ruff CB, Mourtada FA, et al (Johns Hopkins Univ, Baltimore, Md; Naval Health Research Ctr, San Diego, Calif; UCSD Med Ctr, San Diego, Calif)
J Bone Miner Res 11:645–653, 1996   7–8

Background.—Stress fractures, occurring mainly in the lower extremity, can cause significant morbidity among athletes and military recruits. These fractures are thought to result from bone structural failure caused by repetitive weight-bearing loads. Individual differences in bone strength are probably geometric. A technique for deriving cross-sectional geometric properties of long bones from bone mineral data acquired with absorptiometry scanners was used to prospectively study male Marine Corps recruits during a 12-week training program.

Methods.—Before their training period, 626 men underwent anthropometric measures and dual-energy x-ray absorptiometry (DEXA) scans of the femoral midshaft and distal third of the tibia. Data from conventional frontal plane DEXA were used to determine bone mineral density and to derive the cross-sectional area, moment of inertia, section modulus, and bone width of the femur, tibia, and fibula. Twenty-seven stress fractures in 23 recruits (3.7%) were confirmed radiologically during training. Sixteen patients with shin splints, periostitis, and other stress reactions not meeting criteria for fracture were excluded. Anthropometric and bone structural geometry measures in the remaining recruits with fractures and the 587 unaffected recruits were compared.

Findings.—The 2 groups did not differ significantly in age, femur length, pelvic width, and knee width at the femoral condyles. However, most anthropometric girth dimensions were significantly shorter, lighter, and smaller in the recruits with fractures. In addition, bone cross-sectional areas, moments of inertia, section moduli, and widths and bone mineral density in the tibia and femur were significantly smaller. After adjustment for body weight, the tibia cross-sectional area, section modulus, and width were still significantly smaller in recruits with fractures.

Conclusion.—Low body weight and small diaphyseal dimensions relative to body weight appear to predispose military recruits to stress fractures. Bone structural geometry measures derived from DEXA data may be useful in assessing the risk of stress fracture.

Risk Factors for Osteoporotic Fractures in Elderly Men

Nguyen TV, Eisman JA, Kelly PJ, et al (Garvan Inst of Med Research, Sydney, Australia; Vincent's Hosp, Sydney, Australia)
Am J Epidemiol 144:255–263, 1996

7–9

Introduction.—The problem of osteoporosis in aging women has received considerable attention, but few studies have included men. An epidemiologic study conducted in Dubbo, Australia, examined the pattern of age-related bone loss and the incidence and potential risk factors for osteoporotic fractures in men.

Methods.—Dubbo, a small city located 400 km northwest of Sydney, was chosen for an epidemiologic study of osteoporosis because the age and sex distribution of its population closely resembles that of the larger Australian population. Potential risk factors for osteoporotic fractures were assessed in 820 men aged 60 or older in 1989. A questionnaire administered at study entry gathered data on age, lifestyle factors, physical activity, and history of falls and fractures. Baseline bone mineral density (BMD) was measured in the lumbar spine and femoral neck of 752 (91%) men. Follow-up continued until 1994.

Results.—The men were divided into 4 age groups: 60–64, 65–69, 70–74, 75–79, and 80 years or older. Advancing age was associated with declines in weight, height, physical activity index, and quadriceps strength and an increase in body sway. Although lumbar spine BMD was stable or increased throughout the later decades, mean BMD decreased with age at the femoral neck, Ward's triangle, and the trochanteric areas. Femoral neck BMD was inversely correlated with age and smoking but positively related to weight, dietary calcium intake, and quadriceps strength. Similar trends were seen in a second BMD determination obtained in 442 men at an average of 2.5 years after the baseline studies. The rate of multiple falls increased from 3.9% in men aged 60–64 years to 9% in those aged 75 or more years. The incidence of atraumatic fractures and multiple fractures increased significantly with age. Independent risk factors for fracture in multivariate analysis were lower baseline femoral neck BMD, quadriceps strength, and body sway.

Conclusion.—The incidence of fractures increases with age in men as well as in women, but a more powerful predictor of fracture risk is bone mineral density, particularly at the femoral neck. Most fractures result from falls, and risk factors for falling include quadriceps weakness, impaired postural stability, shorter height, and a history of previous fractures and/or falls. A higher level of physical activity is protective against fracture risk in men.

▶ These 2 abstracts (Abstracts 7–8—7–9) prove the utility of DEXA as a technique for screening. In the first article, low body weight and small diaphyseal dimensions have proved a highly predictive measure for stress fractures in military recruits. In addition, DEXA showed promise as a technique for screening in the tibia and femur.

In elderly males, the issue of osteoporosis as it relates to low-energy trauma is not as widespread as the issue in women, but it is nevertheless important. This large, prospectively followed series showed that bone mineral density predicted by DEXA is a powerful predictor of fracture risk. Since the fractures are associated with trauma, the orthopedic community should continue with its major efforts in the prevention of falls. Exercise programs have shown to be efficacious in improving strength and balance and should be emphasized to all patients. Similarly, regular eye checkups and avoidance of shaggy carpets and poor footwear are issues we can all discuss with our elderly patients to prevent falls.

M.F. Swiontkowski, M.D.

Tibia Fractures

Effect of Loading and Fracture Motions on Diaphyseal Tibial Fractures
Sarmiento A, McKellop HA, Llinas A, et al (Univ of Southern California, Los Angeles; Los Angeles Orthopaedic Hosp)
J Orthop Res 14:80–84, 1996   7–10

Background.—Physiologically induced interfragmentary motions have been shown to be useful in the healing of diaphyseal fractures. Several investigators have introduced motion to stimulate consolidation when using otherwise rigid devices for stabilization. However, the amount and direction of the motions occurring in a fracture treated with a functional brace during healing have not been characterized fully. A computerized motion sensor was used to record the 3-dimensional components of interfragmentary motion during healing in 3 patients with closed, low-energy fractures of the tibial diaphysis treated with functional braces.

Methods and Findings.—Two weeks after fracture, the patients applied about 15 kg of load to the injured limb, producing 1–4 mm of translation of the fragments, which was recovered when the load was removed. The maximum rotational and angulatory displacements frequently occurred as the patients rose from a chair with no weight on the limb. These displacements were then often reduced as the 15 kg of load was applied. Maximum axial rotation and angular displacement were 3 degrees and 1 degree, respectively, under load. When the load was removed and the patient sat down again, the initial rotational and angulatory positions of the fragments were recovered, as with the translations. At 8 weeks full body weight was applied to the limb, resulting in a maximum interfragmentary translation of 0.5 mm and maximum axial rotation or angulation of 0.5 degrees. In all 3 fractures, abundant peripheral callus formed. These healed by 15 weeks through typical gradual consolidation and mineralization, accompanied by a corresponding reduction in interfragmentary motions.

Conclusions.—These findings are consistent with earlier findings showing recoverable elastic interfragmentary displacements of several millimeters or more in the absence of rigid fixation, indicating abundant callus formation and rapid consolidation to healing. The substantial elastic interfragmentary motions occurring in the early stages of treatment are consistent with and may promote favorable osteogenic effects.

Complications of Nailing in Closed Tibial Fractures

Williams J, Gibbons M, Trundle H, et al (Oxford Radcliffe Hosp, England)
J Orthop Trauma 9:476–481, 1995   7–11

Background.—Intramedullary nailing has become the treatment of choice for stabilization of closed tibial shaft fractures. The complications occurring with locked tibial intramedullary nailing were studied in patients with closed tibial shaft fractures over a 42-month period.

Methods.—A total of 102 patients with closed fractures of the tibial shaft treated with intramedullary nailing were studied, and complete follow-up was available for 94 patients. The patients were regularly followed until union was achieved or nonunion was established. All complications were reviewed.

Results.—Eighty-two patients underwent intramedullary nailing immediately, whereas the procedure was delayed in 3 patients with head injury and in 17 patients initially treated nonoperatively with a plaster cast. Of the 102 patients, reamed nails were used in 97 patients and unreamed nails were used in 5 patients. Of the 94 patients with complete follow-up, union was documented in 92 after a mean interval of 19 weeks. Malunion occurred in 37% of these patients: after the initial treatment in 33 patients and after excess shortening after dynamization in 2 patients. Common peroneal nerve (CPN) lesions were identified preoperatively in 10 patients; 2 of these patients had a persistent neurologic deficit. Another 19 patients had postoperative common peroneal nerve lesions; some degree of permanent neurologic loss remained in 4 of these patients. Seven patients had acute postoperative compartment syndrome requiring fasciotomy. There were superficial wound infections in 8 patients and deep infections in 3 patients.

Conclusion.—Intramedullary tibial nailing has many advantages but is technically demanding. Patients must be carefully monitored for complications and malunion (Table 3). The procedure is associated with a significant risk of transient or permanent nerve lesions. The risk of malunion is high without careful attention to technique in the reduction, reaming, and nail insertion.

TABLE 3.—Malunion Results Previously Published

Author	Method	Shortening	Sagittal	Coronal	Total (%)
Nicoll, 1964	POP	2.5% (>2 cm)	3% (>10°)	3% (>10°)	9
Sarmiento, 1974	Functional bracing	21% (>4.1 mm)	9% total (>5°)	9% total	30
Oni et al., 1988	POP	5.3% (>1 cm)	13% (>5°)	20% (>5°)	38.3
Hooper et al., 1991	POP	21%	33% total		54
Ruedi et al., 1976	AO plating	0%	0%	0%	0 (3 plate failures)
Batten et al., 1978	AO plating	0%	0%	0%	0 (2 plate failures)
Fisher et al., 1978	AO plating	0%	0%	0%	0 (4 plate failures)
Bilat et al., 1994	AO plating	0%	0%	2%	4
Bore and Johnson, 1986	IMN	5% (>1 cm)	3% total (>5°)	3% total	8
Alho et al., 1990	IMN	14% (>1 cm)	6% (5°)	11% (5°)	31
Court-Brown et al., 1990	IMN	3% (>1 cm)	0%	0%	2.5
Hooper et al., 1991	IMN	7%	0%	0%	7
Moed, et al., 1994	IMN	0%	0%	0%	0
O'Dwyer et al., 1994	IMN	0%	0%	2% Rotation	2
Sargeant et al., 1994	IMN	0%	0%	0%	0

Abbreviations: POP, plaster of Paris; *IMN*, intramedullary nailing.
(Courtesy of Williams J, Gibbons M, Trundle H, et al: Complications of nailing in closed tibial fractures. *J Orthop Trauma* 9:476–481, 1995.)

Tibial Diaphyseal Nonunions After External Fixation Treated With Nonreamed Solid Core Nails

Riemer BL, Sagiv S, Butterfield SL, et al (Med College of Pennsylvania, Pittsburgh)
Orthopedics 19:109–116, 1996

7–12

Introduction.—Although external fixation is frequently used to treat open tibial diaphysis fractures, complication rates are high, particularly when reamed intramedullary nails are subsequently used to correct nonunion. Plates have been used in fracture reconstruction with good long-term results. However, the exposure itself may make the reconstruction surgery difficult and bone may take longer to remodel. Previous reports of the use of nonreamed solid core nails suggest that they may be superior to reamed nails. The use of nonreamed nails for the treatment of tibial diaphysis nonunions is described.

Methods.—Twenty-nine patients with tibial diaphysis fractures who had nonunion after external fixation were treated with nonreamed solid core nails. The duration of nonunion ranged from 22 to 173 weeks, with an average of 51 weeks. An average of 32 weeks lapsed between external fixator removal and intramedullary nailing. Lottes, Alta, and Rush nails were used. Seventeen fractures were grade IIIB initially, 3 were grade IIIA, 7 were grade II, 1 was grade I, and 1 was a closed fracture.

Results.—Fractures were united in 27 patients within 14 weeks after 1 operation. Reamed exchange nailing was required in 1 patient whose fracture united 19 weeks after the procedure (58 weeks after nonreamed nailing). Reoperation was required in 1 patient who sustained a stress fracture 49 months after nonreamed nailing. Two patients had active wound infections at the time of nonreamed nailing. Débridement was necessary in 1 patient because of a mixed flora infection at the fracture site. In the second patient, the wound was débrided before nonreamed nailing and eventually closed with local care. Nonreamed nailing was successful in correcting prenail angular deformities of 10 degrees or more in 9 of 11 patients.

Conclusion.—Nonreamed solid core nails were effective in treating tibial diaphysis nonunion after external fixation. Fractures were united in 93% of the patients described within an average of 14 weeks. The rate of postnailing infections was low, and patients were able to be ambulatory during recovery.

Compartment Syndrome in Tibial Shaft Fracture Missed Because of a Local Nerve Block

Hyder N, Kessler S, Jennings AG, et al (York District Hosp, England)
J Bone Joint Surg Br 78:499–500, 1996

7–13

Background.—Fractures of the tibial shaft can be complicated by compartment syndrome, a serious condition requiring prompt diagnosis and treatment for a good prognosis. In the patient described, the diagnosis of compartment syndrome was delayed because of local nerve block given in the operating room after intramedullary nailing.

> *Case Report.*—Man, 28, sustained a closed fracture of the tibial shaft while playing football. No signs of neurovascular compromise or compartment syndrome were seen before surgery. After the fracture was treated, a triple nerve block using bupivacaine 0.5% was delivered for pain control. Postoperatively, the patient was pain-free but reported areas of altered sensation in his foot and leg. These regions varied and were thought to be caused by the nerve block. However, the symptoms persisted, and the patient was unable to actively extend his big toe. Pressure measures obtained 48 hours after surgery indicated a pressure of 108 mm Hg in the anterior compartment, and emergency fasciotomy was performed. Unfortunately, all the muscles in the anterior compartment were dead. Forty-hour hours later, with no sign of recovery, the whole anterior tibial compartment was débrided. This patient now needs an orthosis to walk.

Conclusions.—Nerve blocks should not be used when compartment syndrome is possible. When in doubt, clinicians should obtain intracompartmental pressure measures early. If the peak compartment pressure falls to within 20 mm Hg of the diastolic pressure, fasciotomy is indicated.

▶ Tibia fractures continue to be a common problem in general orthopedic practice. There has been a trend away from conservative care toward operative intervention, which sometimes does not seem logical. In the first article, Sarmiento et al. (See Abstract 7–10) has given a detailed picture of what happens during fracture healing with brace treatment in 3 patients with closed fractures of the tibial diaphysis. By 8 weeks after injury, the interfragmentary translation was minimal and the fractures all healed at 15 weeks. We should all consider closed treatment as the first line of management of patients with closed tibia fractures, particularly when their preference is to avoid surgical treatment with its inherent risks.

The second article (Abstract 7–11) attempts to quantify one aspect of the inherent risk. In 102 patients with closed fractures treated with intramedullary nailing, malunion occurred in 37% of the patients (94 with complete follow-up). Common peroneal nerve lesions were identified in 11%; 2 of these patients had persistent deficit. Superficial wound infection occurred in a significant number of the patients. This case series, without controls, gives us reason to pause in recommending the routine intramedullary interlocking nailing of closed tibial fractures, and these risks must be discussed with patients beforehand.

When nonunion does occur after external fixation management of open tibial fractures, a common method of treatment has been with reamed intramedullary nailing. This has been historically associated with a high rate of deep infection (24% in combined series). Riemer et al. (See Abstract 7–12) have shown us that these injuries can be managed with intramedullary chisels and unreamed tibial nails. It is highly possible that avoidance of reaming debris, which is potential culture material, could result in a lower rate of deep infection in fractures previously treated with external fixation. We need a comparative multicenter series contrasting fractures managed with reamed vs. unreamed nailing in this clinical scenario; the current series would lead us to believe that unreamed nailing has promise. An issue that would need to be addressed in a future series would be whether unreamed nailing is associated with a higher rate of mechanical failure than reamed nailing in this setting.

M.F. Swiontkowski, M.D.

Sequential Intramedullary Nailing of Open Tibial Shaft Fractures After External Fixation

Siebenrock KA, Gerich T, Jakob RP (Univ of Bern, Switzerland; Unfallchirurgische Klinik der Medizinischen Hochschule, Hannover, Germany)
Arch Orthop Trauma Surg 116:32–36, 1997   7–14

Background.—The introduction of unreamed interlocking intramedullary devices has intensified the debate on how to treat high-energy and open tibial shaft fractures. Authorities continue to disagree about the best treatment for severe open Gustilo type III fractures. One experience with sequential nailing of open tibial shaft fractures after primary treatment with an external fixation device was reviewed.

TABLE 1.—Average Treatment Data for Open Tibial Shaft Fractures Classified According to Gustilo et al.

	External fixation Treatment (median (days)	Time of Intramedullary nailing (median days)†	No interval‡ left	Interval >1 week	1–3 (4) weeks	Soft-tissue procedures per patient (n)
Type I* (n = 6)	32 (12–75)	39 (14–77)	2 (33%)	4 (66%)	0 (0%)	1.8
Type II (n = 10)	29 (5–150)	38 (5–150)	6 (60%)	3 (30%)	1 (10%)	2
Type III A (n = 7)	28 (7–105)	31 (7–120)	4 (57%)	1 (14%)	2 (29%)	2.6
Type III B (n = 9)	49 (16–94)	56 (16–108)	4 (44%)	2 (22%)	3 (33%)	3.2

*Type I group includes 2 patients with closed fractures.
†Time of intermedullary nailing after injury.
‡Interval is the time between removal of external fixation and intramedullary nailing. Soft-tissue procedures included débridement, secondary wound closure, skin grafts, and muscle flaps.
(Courtesy of Siebenrock KA, Gerich T, Jakob RP: Sequential intramedullary nailing of open tibial shaft fractures after external fixation. *Arch Orthop Trauma Surg* 116:32–36, 1997.)

TABLE 2.—Treatment Results for Open Tibial Shaft Fractures Classified According to Gustilo et al.

	Time to full weight-bearing (median weeks)	Malunion†	Non-union	Infection		Reduced joint mobility‡
				soft tissue	osteo-myelitis	
Type I* (*n* = 6)	15 (9–40)	0 (0%)	0 (0%)	0 (0%)	0 (0%)	0 (0%)
Type II (*n* = 10)	27 (18–42)	2 (20%)	0 (0%)	0 (0%)	0 (0%)	2 (20%)
Type III A (*n* = 7)	27 (10–33)	1 (14%)	0 (0%)	1 (14%)	0 (0%)	3 (43%)
Type III B (*n* = 9)	41 (18–128)	3 (33%)	1 (11%)	0 (0%)	1 (11%)	3 (33%)

*Type I group includes 2 patients with closed fractures.

†Malunion is defined as angulation greater than 5 degrees in frontal plane and greater than 10 degrees in sagittal plane, greater than 10 degrees of rotation, and greater than 1 cm of leg discrepancy.

‡Reduced joint mobility is defined as loss of motion in ankle joint greater than 10 degrees and knee joint greater than 20 degrees.

(Courtesy of Siebenrock KA, Gerich T, Jakob RP: Sequential intramedullary nailing of open tibial shaft fractures after external fixation. *Arch Orthop Trauma Surg* 116:32–36, 1997.)

Methods.—Thirty-two tibial shaft fractures were treated in 31 patients. Thirty fractures were open and 2 were closed, with severe blunt trauma requiring fasciotomy. Half of the fractures were Gustilo type III A and B. The mean time for external fixation treatment was 6.6 weeks. Secondary intramedullary nailing was done a mean of 7.4 weeks after injury. Secondary nailing was done at the time of external fixation removal in half of the patients.

Outcomes.—Overall, osteomyelitis occurred in 3.1% of the fractures, nonunion in 3.1%, and malunion in 19%. The mean time to weight-bearing was 31.2 weeks. Among the Gustilo type III B injuries, the incidence of osteomyelitis and nonunion was 11% and of malunion, 33%. The mean time to full weight-bearing in this group was 53 weeks (Tables 1 and 2).

Conclusions.—Sequential nailing after external fixation is effective in the treatment of severe tibial shaft fractures, including Gustilo type III A and B injuries. The risk of infection is not significantly greater when sequential intramedullary nailing is done at the same time as external fixation removal, provided there is no former pin tract infection. Aggressive soft-tissue management for early wound coverage and bone grafting is important in the treatment of severe open tibial shaft fractures.

▶ These authors have shown that conversion of open tibial fractures initially treated with external fixation to intramedullary nailing can take place at a mean of 7½ weeks after injury without a marked increase in the deep infection rate. This rate confirms that of Blachut et al.[1] The Vancouver group protocol relied on conversion in the first 2 weeks post injury. These authors have documented that with careful patient selection and excellent initial débridement technique, the risk of deep infection after conversion to intramedullary nailing is low.

M.F. Swiontkowski, M.D.

Reference

1. Blachut A, Meek RN, O'Brien PJ: External fixation and delayed intramedullary nailing of open fractures of the tibial shaft. *J Bone Joint Surg Am* 72:729–735, 1990.

Treatment of Tibial Pilon Fractures Using Ring Fixators and Arthroscopy
Kim S-K, Jahng J-S, Kim S-S, et al (Wonkwang Univ, Ik-San, Republic of Korea; Yonsei Univ, Seoul, Republic of Korea)
Clin Orthop 334:244–250, 1997   7–15

Objective.—The most common method for treating tibial pilon fractures is the AO technique. Some report a complication rate of more than 50% with internal fixation. Results of a new method of treatment using ring fixators and arthroscopy are reported.

Methods.—Ring fixators were used to repair 23 pilon fractures in 23 patients (6 women). Two patients were lost to follow-up. Of the 21 pilon fractures studied, 2 were Ruedi type I, 14 were type II, and 5 were type III fractures, including 1 grade I, 3 grade II, and 2 grade III open fractures. In Ruedi type I and II fractures, arthroscopy was used if the quality of the reduction was questionable and the reduction subsequently adjusted if necessary. Limited open reduction was performed instead of arthroscopy in all type III fractures and 4 type II fractures. Frames consisted of 2 or 3 full rings applied at the fracture site and 2 half rings joined by plates on a foot mounting. Wires were attached on the proximal ring and others were attached to the calcaneus and metatarsals. Reduction was accomplished by increasing the length of the external fixator. The ring fixator that connected the rods at the ankle was moved, and the rods were displaced.

Results.—Patients were evaluated an average of 37 months after surgery. The foot mounting was worn for 6–10 weeks. The ring fixators were removed in 20 of 21 patients between 16 and 28 weeks after bony union. One patient required a skin graft and another needed a second operation. Using the Bone clinical grading system, 15 results were good, 4 were fair, and 2 were poor. Satisfactory results were achieved in 2 type I fractures, 10 type II fractures, and 3 type III fractures. Complications included 8 pin tract problems, 1 loss of reduction, 1 patient with posttraumatic arthritis, and 3 with mild pain during vigorous exercise. No wound infections developed.

Conclusion.—Ring fixators for tibial pilon fractures yielded good results because soft tissue dissection, metal plates, and screws are not required. No deep wound infection resulted.

▶ There is widespread movement toward limited internal fixation with external fixation for articular fractures of the distal end of the tibia. These authors have demonstrated that arthroscopy has some potential as an aid for reduction with limited surgical exposure. Although this study is uncontrolled and is retrospective in design, it suggests to the reader that this technique is deserving of further study in prospective trials.

M.F. Swiontkowski, M.D.

Complications of Intramedullary Nailing

Fractures Below the End of Locking Humeral Nails: A Report of Three Cases
McKee MD, Pedlow FX, Cheney PJ, et al (Univ of Toronto; Harvard Univ, Boston; Emerson Hosp, Concord, Mass)
J Orthop Trauma 10:500–513, 1996   7–16

Background.—Locking humeral nails were introduced to address some of the shortcomings of previously available intramedullary implants for

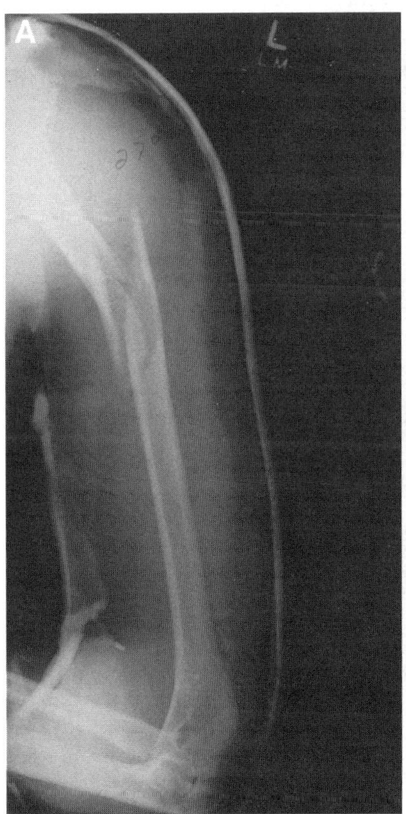
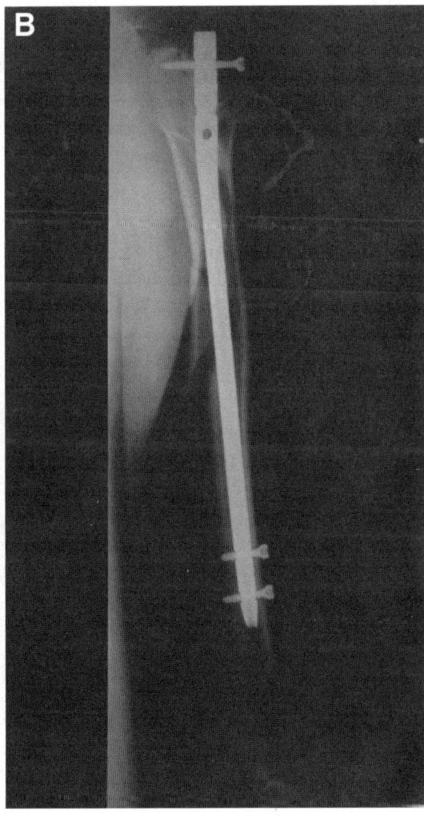

(Continued)

FIGURE 1 (cont.)

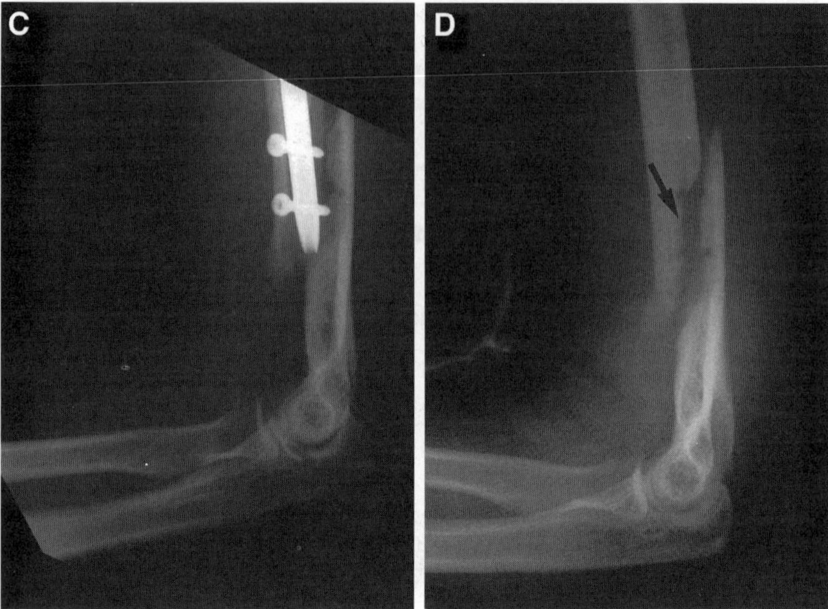

FIGURE 1.—**A,** humeral shaft fracture in patient 1 after a motor vehicle accident. A sugar-tong splint was applied, with angulation of the humerus into varus. **B,** a postoperative radiograph after reamed, locked humeral intramedullary nailing showed good reduction of the fracture and position of the nail. **C,** a lateral radiograph after fracture at the tip of the nail 10 weeks postoperatively revealed an oblique fracture line through both distal locking screw sites. **D,** a lateral radiograph after removal of the locking screws and humeral nail clearly showed propagation of the fracture line through both distal locking screw holes (*arrow*). (Courtesy of McKee MD, Pedlow FX, Cheney PJ, et al: Fractures below the end of locking humeral nails: A report of three cases. *J Orthop Trauma* 10:500–513, 1996.)

humeral shaft fractures. Because of the unique anatomy of the humerus, the tips of these nails end in diaphyseal bone. To date, there have been no reports of fracture at the tip of a locking humeral nail. Three patients were reported.

Case Reports.—The patients were 2 men aged 34 and 19 years and a woman aged 37. The first patient had been hit by a car, and the second and third patients had been in motor vehicle accidents. Interlocking humeral nails were secured with distal interlocking screws for humeral shaft fractures in each patient. At 8, 10, and 26 weeks after surgery, fractures occurred at the tip of the locking humeral nail, all through the distal interlocking screws after a rotational force on the arm (Fig 1). The distal interlocking screws were removed in all 3 patients to facilitate reduction, followed by open reduction and internal fixation in 1 patient and closed reduction and casting in the other 2. The fractures subsequently healed in 2 patients. The third is still in active treatment.

Conclusions.—This is the first report of fractures occurring below or at the tip of large-diameter locking humeral nails. Clinicians must consider this complication when deciding on locking humeral nails for the treatment of humeral fractures.

The Reconstruction Locked Nail for Complex Fractures of the Proximal Femur

Kang S, McAndrew MP, Johnson KD (Chung-Ang Univ, Seoul, Korea; Vanderbilt Univ, Nashville, Tenn)
J Orthop Trauma 9:453–463, 1995   7–17

Background.—Although many types of internal fixation have been described in the treatment of complex proximal femoral fracture, authorities do not agree on which is optimal. The outcomes of treatment with the reconstruction locked femoral nail in 1 series of patients with such fractures were reported.

Methods and Findings.—Thirty-seven patients were included in the analysis. Overall, union occurred in 92%. Thirty-five percent of the patients had complications. Complications included 3 nonunions, 1 delayed union, 2 leg-length discrepancies of more than 2.5 cm, and 2 cases of varus deformity exceeding 10 degrees and 2 of less than 10 degrees. There were also 4 revision surgeries, including 1 broken 13-mm nail; 4 proximal screws backing up and requiring removal; 2 cases of pudendal nerve palsy; and 1 case of heterotopic ossification. Complications occurred in 3 of the 4 patients with femoral neck and shaft fractures, in 6 of the 18 patients with intertrochanteric fractures with diaphyseal extension, and in 4 of the 5 patients with intertrochanteric fractures with diaphyseal extension in which anatomical reduction was not achieved. Six of the 9 proximal screws placed short in 9 fractures caused complications. More than 1 complication developed in 7 patients. Additional surgery was needed to treat complications in 11 of 13 patients (Table 4).

TABLE 4.—Femoral Neck and Shaft Fractures Treated With Reconstruction Nail

Authors	Aver. age	Year	No. of patients	Transcervical	Base of neck	Complications
Browner (7)	*	1991	11	10	1	Chondrolysis (1)
Wiss (23)	30	1992	14	4		Varus nonunion (1)
					10F	Varus nonunion (1)
						Implant removal (1)
Anderson (1)	42	1993	5	*	*	Delayed union (2)
						Varus deformity and shortening (1)
Young (13)	27	1993	4	3	1	*
Our series	57	1993	4	4	†	Varus nonunion (2)
						Revision (1)

*Information not available.
†Base of neck fracture was excluded.
(Courtesy of Kang S, McAndrew MP, Johnson KD: The reconstruction locked nail for complex fractures of the proximal femur *J Orthop Trauma* 9:453–463, 1995.)

Conclusion.—The reconstruction locked femoral nail is, apparently, not a good choice for ipsilateral intracapsular neck and shaft fractures. Anatomical reduction should be attained in all patients with the reconstruction femoral nail and is absolutely necessary in patients with intertrochanteric fracture with diaphyseal extension. The high rate of complications associated with reconstruction femoral nails is caused by the complex nature of the fracture as well as the device.

Femoral Nailing Without a Fracture Table

Sirkin MS, Behrens F, McCracken K, et al (New Jersey Med School, Newark; Roseland, NJ)

Clin Orthop 332:119–125, 1996

7–18

Introduction.—Fracture tables have been used during closed intramedullary nailing. Although these tables are widely used, the traction generated may cause complications and limit treatment of patients with multiple fractures. Use of a radiolucent table with manual traction during femoral fracture nailing is described in a retrospective study and compared with procedures using a fracture table.

Methods.—Patients who sustained a femoral shaft fracture during a 15-month period were included in the trial, which consisted 2 treatment groups. In group 1, fractures were treated with femoral nailing on a radiolucent table with manual traction. Patients in group 2 were treated by using a fracture table. Group 1 had 24 femoral fractures and group 2 had

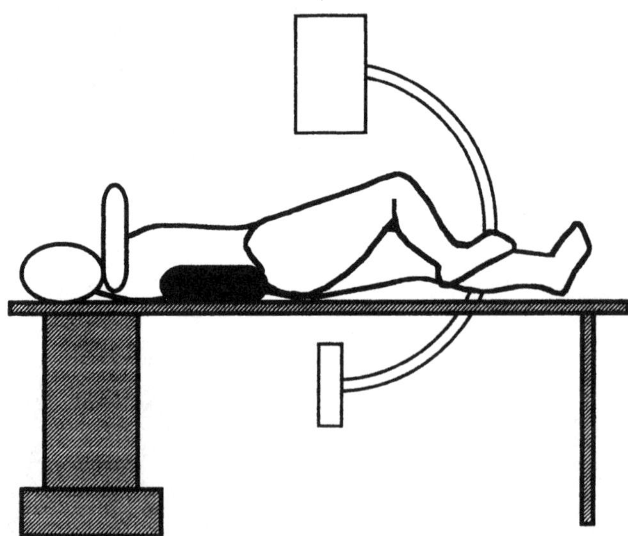

FIGURE 2.—Schematic representation of a patient viewed laterally. Rolled sheets are placed underneath the ipsilateral side of the trunk to elevate the hip 30 to 45 degrees. (Courtesy of Sirkin MS, Behrens F, McCracken K, et al: Femoral nailing without a fracture table. *Clin Orthop* 332:119–125, 1996.)

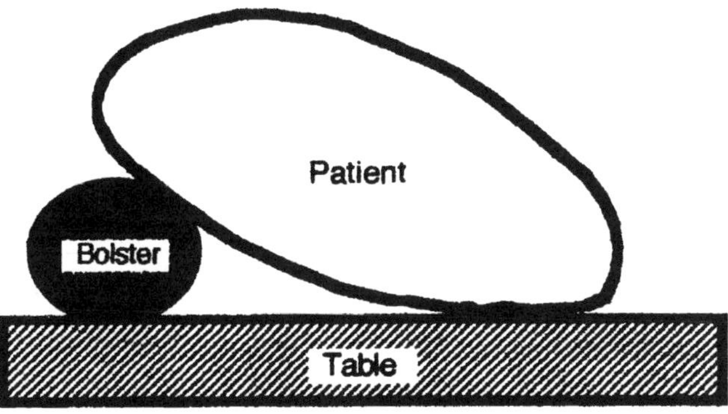

FIGURE 3.—Schematic representation of a patient viewed from the feet showing sloppy lateral position. (Courtesy of Sirkin MS, Behrens F, McCracken K, et al: Femoral nailing without a fracture table. *Clin Orthop* 332:119–125, 1996.)

59 fractures. Medical records and radiographs were reviewed and patient interviews conducted to obtain information. Data collected included the need for redraping or repositioning on a different table, complications, and postoperative alignment. During the procedure using the radiolucent table, a rolled sheet or similar support was placed under the patient to elevate the hip to a 30- to 45-degree angle (Figs 2 and 3). An image intensifier tube was positioned to obtain an anteroposterior and then a lateral view (Fig 4). Manual traction was used to bring the fracture fragments in line before nail insertion.

Results.—Multiple procedures were performed on 10 patients (43%) in group 1 without changing tables. Only a single preparation and draping were needed in 8 patients. In group 2, 12 of 19 patients who had multiple procedures required repositioning on a standard operating table. Significantly fewer patients in group 1 required redraping or table changes. Setup and operating times were similar between groups 1 and 2. One operative complication (radial nerve palsy) occurred in group 2. Malalignment of

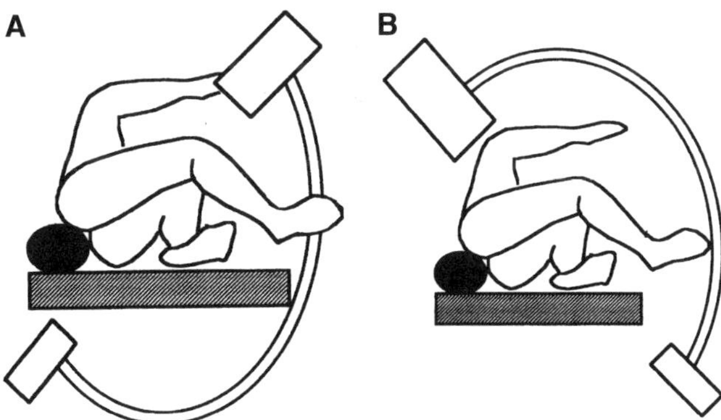

FIGURE 4.—Schematic representation of C arm position viewed from the feet to obtain anteroposterior (A) and lateral (B) images. (Courtesy of Sirkin MS, Behrens F, McCracken K, et al: Femoral nailing without a fracture table. *Clin Orthop* 332:119–125, 1996.)

fracture occurred in 2 of 24 fractures in group 1 and in 5 of 59 fractures in group 2.

Conclusion.—Use of a radiolucent table with manual traction during femoral shaft fracture nailing was not found to be associated with increased morbidity as compared with a fracture table. Multiple procedures were able to be performed without changing tables.

Unreamed Intramedullary Tibial Nailing: Fatigue of Locking Bolts

Boenisch UW, de Boer PG, Journeaux SF (York District Hosp, England)
Injury 27:265–270, 1996   7–19

Background.—Intramedullary nailing has proven to be an effective technique for the fixation of most nonarticular tibial fractures. Because unreamed nails damage less of the endosteal blood supply than reamed nails, these are attractive for use in open fractures. However, because unreamed nails have a looser fit in the bone than reamed nails, there are higher forces going through the interlocking bolts with these systems. The incidence of interlocking bolt failure was studied in patients undergoing insertion of interlocked intramedullary tibial nails over a 4-year period.

Methods.—Seventy-one patients with 72 diaphyseal tibial fractures underwent insertion of unreamed interlocked intramedullary nails and were followed for a mean of 15.2 months. The injuries were closed in 75% of cases and open in 25%, with fractures in the distal third of the tibia in 54%, in the middle third in 38%, and in the proximal third in 8%. Intramedullary nailing was performed primarily within an average of 20 hours after injury in 62 patients and as a secondary procedure in 11 patients. The patients were assessed clinically and radiologically for union. The occurrence of interlocking bolt failure was noted. Several of the failed

TABLE 3.—Comparison of Results With Those of Other Authors

	Whittle	Court Brown	Alho	Claudi	Whitelaw	Boneisch	Tscherne
Number	50	125	93	65	37	72	43
Types	G1–G3b	T0–G1	T0–G2	T0–G3b	G1–G3b	T0–G3b	T0–G3b
Nail	RT	GK	GK	AO/RT	Ender	AO/RT	AO prot.
Time to union	28 weeks	16.7 weeks	14.5 weeks	15 weeks	21 weeks	18.5 weeks	21.9 weeks
Nonunion	4%	1.6%	2.1%	3%	0%	1.4%	0%
Sup. inf.		2.4%	2.1%	1.5%	2%	2.7%	/
Deep inf.	8%	1.6%	3.2%	0%	/	0%	0%
Shortening >1 cm	/	0.8%	4.3%	7	/	1.4%	2.3%
Bolt failure	10%	0.8%	/	/	/	30%	16.3%
Varus			4.3%			1.4%	0%
Valgus	total	total	6.5%	total	total	4.1%	2.3%
Angulation	of 0%	of 2.4%	6.5%	of 7.2%	of 10%	1.4%	6.9%
rotation			0%			0%	16.3

Abbreviations: RT, Russel Taylor; *GK,* Grosse Kempf; *AO prot.,* AO prototype.

(Courtesy of Boenisch UW, de Boer PG, Journeaux SF: Unreamed intramedullary tibial nailing: Fatigue of locking bolts. *Injury* 27:265–270, copyright 1996, with kind permission from Elsevier Science Ltd., The Boulevard, Langford Lane, Kidlington OX5 1GB, U.K.)

interlocking bolts were evaluated after removal with scanning electron microscopy.

Results.—The nails were interlocked statically in 58% and dynamically in 42%. Union occurred after an average interval of 18.5 weeks overall—17.3 weeks in closed fractures and 22 weeks in open fractures. There was no restriction of knee movement, but ankle movement was restricted in 13 patients. Problems with union included shortening of 1 cm in 5.5%, valgus deformity in 4.1%, varus deformity in 4.1%, and anterior angulation in 1.4%. The most common complication was interlocking bolt breakage, which occurred in 30% of the patients. Bolt failure occurred both proximally and distally, in both statically and dynamically interlocked nails, an average of 8–10 weeks after partial weight-bearing began. Scanning electron microscopy revealed that, in all cases, failure was caused by fatigue.

Conclusion.—Fatigue failure is a major problem of intramedullary nailing with unreamed tibial nails. This occurrence was not related to clinical problems in this or other studies (Table 3). Therefore, efforts are needed to redesign the interlocking bolt.

A Comparison of One Versus Two Distal Locking Screws in Tibial Fractures Treated With Unreamed Tibial Nails: A Prospective Randomized Clinical Trial

Kneifel T, Buckley R (Univ of Calgary, Alberta, Canada)
Injury 27:271–273, 1996   7–20

Introduction.—Diaphyseal tibial fractures are most commonly treated with intramedullary nails. The use of interlocking screws increases bone stability by maintaining both length and alignment. However, failure of the interlocking screws has become an increasing concern. It is thought

TABLE 1.—Demographics

	One Screw	*Two Screws*	
Male	11	14	Pearson chi
Female	11	6	square = 0.19
			Prob. = 0.19
Age	38±10	34±12	ANOVA
			Prob. = 0.11
			f ratio = 2.36
Weight	78±15	77±12	ANOVA
			Prob. = 0.73
			f ratio = 0.31
	<u>Not failed</u>	<u>Failed</u>	T-test = 60.97
Prox. screw			P = 0.00
length	35 mm±4	38 mm±4	
Dist screws	36	38	
length			

TABLE 2.—Fracture Demographics

Compound Fractures	Number
Grade I	4
Grade II	5
Grade IIIA	3
Grade IIIB	1
Total	13

Fracture location	Percentage
Middle/distal third or distal third	78
Middle third	17
Proximal	5

Winquist comminution	Percentage
Type I	63
Type II	5
Type III	25
Type IV	7

(Reprinted from *Injury*, vol 27, Kneifel T, Buckley R: A comparison of one versus two distal locking screws in tibial fractures treated with unreamed tibial nails: A prospective randomized clinical trial, pp 271–273, copyright 1996, with kind permission from Elsevier Science Ltd, The Boulevard, Langford Lane, Kidlington OX5 1GB, UK.)

that the number of screws used may have an impact on the rate of failure. The purpose of this study was to determine whether the use of 2 interlocking screws in the treatment of diaphyseal tibial fractures would affect the rate of hardware failure as compared with the use of 1 screw.

Methods.—Forty-four patients with open or closed diaphyseal tibial fractures were randomly assigned to treatment using tibial unreamed nails with 1 or 2 distal interlocking screws. One proximal screw was used in all patients. Postoperative care was the same for both groups, with no weight-bearing activities allowed for 6 weeks followed by full weight-bearing. Clinical and radiologic evaluations were performed at 2, 6, and 12 weeks and continued until fracture healing.

Results.—No significant differences were found between the 2 treatment groups in regard to demographics, including wound grade, location, and comminution of the fracture (Tables 1 and 2). Seventy-eight percent of the fractures were located at the middle/distal third or distal third, and 63% were Winquist comminution type I. Significantly more failures were noted with 1 screw (59%) than with 2 screws (5%). Proximal screws failed in 17% of the patients, whereas distal screws failed in 33%. Significantly more failures occurred in women than in men, and patients who had failures had a higher mean body weight (79 kg). Proximal deep vein thrombosis developed in 1 patient 7 days postoperatively, and a common peroneal nerve neurapraxia occurred in another patient. Eight patients had delayed unions. Early dynamization was done in 6 patients; 3 patients had autogenous bone grafting. One of these 3 patients had sustained multiple trauma and eventually required a below-the-knee amputation because of intractable foot pain.

Conclusion.—Hardware failure occurred less often with the use of 2 distal locking screws to treat diaphyseal tibial fractures than with the use of 1 screw. However, proximal screws were found to fail more often in patients who received 2 distal screws. Consideration should be given to using 2 proximal and 2 distal locking screws.

▶ Intramedullary interlocking nailing is one of the most successful and reproducible techniques available to the orthopedic traumatologist. However, particularly with the advent of interlocking nailing, some additional complications have become apparent to the clinician. This nice group of 5 papers (Abstracts 7–16—7–20) helps delineate them. In the case of humeral nails, McKee et al (see Abstract 7–16) have demonstrated in an uncontrolled case report series that fracture distal to the end of a locking humeral nail is a real risk. Placement of distal interlocking screws through dense cortical bone can produce a stress riser that when associated with future torsional trauma, can result in a fracture. We should advise our patients that this could be a potential outcome and should caution them to limit activities that would place them at risk.

The reconstruction type of femoral nails has been a useful addition to the armament of the trauma surgeon for difficult proximal femoral fractures. These implants can be technically demanding. The uncontrolled series by Kang et al (see Abstract 7–17) demonstrated a high rate of complications, including diaphyseal extension and difficulties with proximal screw replacement, particularly with the use of this implant to manage displaced ipsilateral intracapsular neck and shaft fractures. This editor has long recommended against the use of this device for this fracture combination, and this series, although uncontrolled, would support such a recommendation. Femoral neck fractures should be given maximum priority with open reduction and screw fixation, and then the shaft can be managed with a retrograde femoral nail or plate.

One of the common difficulties in multiply injured patients with femoral fractures is the repositioning of patients on fracture tables. Sirkin et al. have provided us a nice, controlled series (although historical) supporting the original findings of Karpos et al.[1] that positioning of patients on radiolucent tables with manual traction has appeal. They showed a decrease in operative time and a relatively low rate of complications. The editor would caution readers that transverse fractures can be particularly difficult when using this technique and that an assistant and often multiple assistants are necessary to gain enough reduction to allow passage of the femoral nail. It is definitely a technique worthy of learning, particularly in patients with chest, abdominal, and/or head injuries.

With the advent of small-diameter, unreamed intramedullary nails for tibia fractures, we have seen an increasing incidence of fatigue fractures. The series by Boenisch et al. (see Abstract 7–19) confirms the 30% incidence of interlocking bolt breakage. Most prior series reported in the YEAR BOOK have shown the range to be 10% to 20% because with the smaller-diameter nail, the use of smaller-diameter screws is necessary. Patients should be cautioned that this could occur and might result in the need for a revision or could add difficulties when the implant is ultimately removed. Along these lines, Kneifel and Buckley (see Abstract 7–20) have examined the question of 1 vs. 2 distal bolts. It seems clear from their carefully followed series that

2 bolts at each end will result in a decrease in the ultimate rate of failure. This is probably the difference between the series previously reported in the YEAR BOOK and that of Boenisch et al. That is, in the other series 4 bolts were more commonly used, which would decrease the stress on an individual bolt. It seems prudent for most surgeons to use 4 bolts when using small-diameter nails in the tibia.

M.F. Swiontkowski, M.D.

References

1. Karpos AG, McFerran MA, Johnson KD: Intramedullary nailing of acute femoral shaft fractures using manual traction without a fracture table. *J Orthop Trauma* 9:57–62 1995.)

Amputation Surgery: Upper Extremity Issues

Long-term Follow-Up of 50 Duke Silicone Prosthetic Fingers
O'Farrell DA, Montella BJ, Bahor JL, et al (Duke Univ, Durham, NC)
J Hand Surg [Br] 21:696–700, 1996

7–21

Introduction.—Both emotional and physical trauma may result from the loss of a digit. Because of the high visibility of the hand, patients who undergo amputation of a finger may view themselves as deformed or different. Patient satisfaction and the functionality of custom-made digital protheses were assessed.

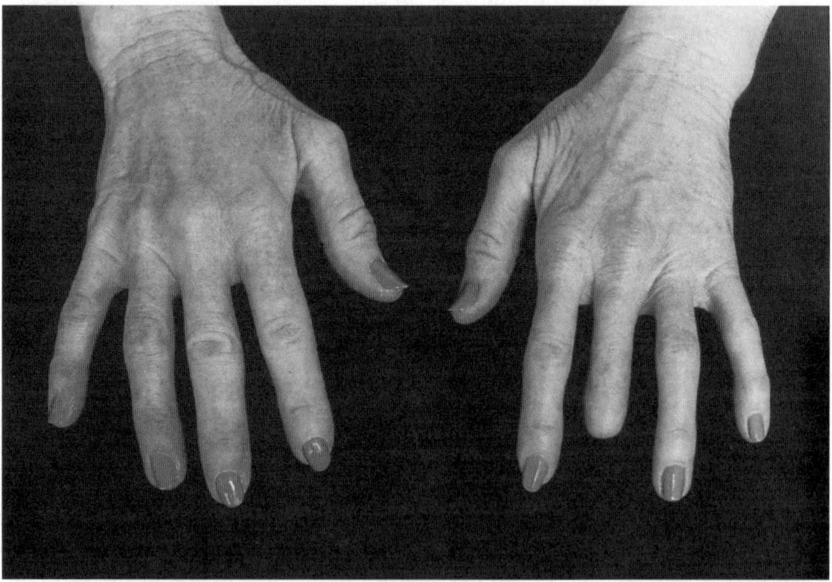

FIGURE 7.—Left middle finger amputation stump before fitting of the prosthesis. (Courtesy of O'Farrell DA, Montella BJ, Bahor JL, et al: Long-term follow-up of 50 Duke silicone prosthetic fingers. *J Hand Surg [Br]* 21:696–700, 1996.)

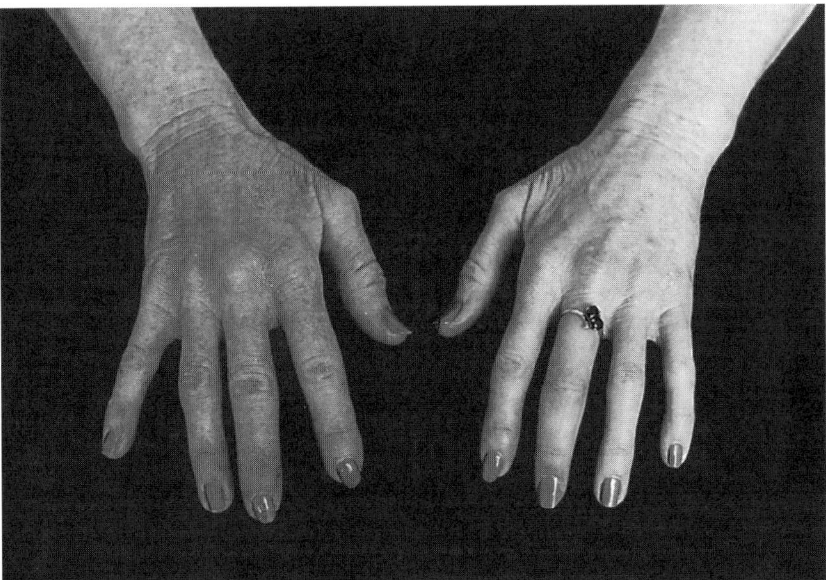

FIGURE 8.—Patient shown in Figure 7 after fitting of the prosthesis. (Courtesy of O'Farrell DA, Montella BJ, Bahor JL, et al: Long-term follow-up of 50 Duke silicone prosthetic fingers. *J Hand Surg [Br]* 21:696–700, 1996.)

Methods.—Digital prostheses were made for 33 patients who underwent a total of 50 digital amputations. Amputation was due to digital trauma for the majority of the patients, with tumor or congenital defects the cause in 3 patients. The prostheses were made from casts of the patients' hands taken with hard dental stone and dental base plate wax. After removal from the mold, the prosthesis was ground smooth and painted to match the patient's skin tone. Suction holds the prothesis to the affected finger (Figs 7 and 8).

Results.—Overall, 22 of 33 patients wore their prosthesis. Twenty-five patients returned to work, with 19 returning to their previous work and 12 wearing the prosthesis to work. Occupations of these 12 patients included typing or account keeping, machine operation, medical technician, teacher, social worker, factory worker, and housekeeper. The remaining 8 patients who did not return to work had multiple digit amputations. Most patients were satisfied with the appearance, fit, and/or color of the prosthesis. Twenty-six patients stated that the prosthesis was helpful psychologically, and 31 patients thought that the prosthesis improved their appearance. Activities such as writing, typing, and holding a cup were believed to be aided by the prosthesis.

Conclusion.—Overall, most patients were satisfied with the prosthesis, although one third of the patients did not wear the device. The prosthesis was helpful psychologically and functionally for most patients and improved activities such as writing, typing, or holding light objects.

▶ The 1 upper extremity amputation–related manuscript selected for this year reports on long-term follow-up of finger prostheses. It shows that prostheses that are molded according to the patient's uninjured hand are useful both functionally and cosmetically and should be offered to patients who have finger amputations. This is a helpful prosthesis and the technique should be more broadly disseminated in the orthopedic community.

M.F. Swiontkowski, M.D.

Amputation Surgery: Limb Salvage vs. Amputation

Amputation Versus Reconstruction in Traumatic Defects of the Leg: Outcome and Costs

Hertel R, Strebel N, Ganz R (Inselspital Univ of Berne, Switzerland)
J Orthop Trauma 10:223–229, 1996   7–22

Background.—The management of severely traumatized lower legs is controversial, with proponents of both primary amputation and reconstruction. However, there has been little comparison of the functional outcomes of these 2 treatment choices. Therefore, outcome and total costs associated with amputation and complex reconstruction of the leg were compared.

Methods.—Thirty-nine patients with grade 3B or 3C open fractures of the tibial shaft treated over a 10-year period were studied retrospectively. Of the 39 patients, 18 had undergone below-knee amputation, and 21 had undergone lower-leg reconstruction. All of the patients were interviewed regarding their pain, daily activities, function, treatment, work, social life, and psychological factors. Data were collected from medical and national insurance reports regarding hospitalization, costs, and compensation.

Results.—The patients underwent a median number of interventions of 3.5 in the amputation group and 8 in the reconstructed group. The median length of hospital stay was 101 days in the amputation group and 129 days in the reconstruction group. Rehabilitation required a median of 12 months in the amputation group and 30 months in the reconstruction group. Compared with the reconstruction group, the amputation group reported more pain, less walking ability, and similar standing ability. Patients in the amputation group were also more likely to abandon sports activities and to consider the trauma to have central importance in their daily lives. All of the amputation patients needed to be retrained for a physically less demanding job, whereas only 4 of the reconstructed patients had to change their occupations. The mean annual costs for the first 4 years were 15,112 Swiss francs in the amputation group and 17,365 Swiss francs in the reconstruction group. Patients in the reconstruction group also were paid loss-of-wages benefits for a period 2.5 times longer than those in the amputation group. However, 26% of the amputees and only 6% of the reconstructed patients were drawing a pension.

Conclusion.—In patients with potentially salvageable legs, reconstruction is superior to amputation because of its better functional outcome, relative avoidance of permanent social disintegration, and lower total costs (including pensions).

▶ In the only good article that revisits the topic of limb salvage vs. early amputation available for inclusion this year, Hertel et al. provided data that cast some doubt on the accepted belief that patients who undergo early amputation are better off functionally. With a careful economic analysis (admittedly subject to some bias), they show only a minor increase in the annual cost of limb salvage vs. amputation. They do report higher rates of return to work in the reconstructed patients, which may be selection bias, with the more severe injuries (some of which may have been multiple) having undergone early amputation. Nevertheless, this manuscript gives us food for thought and causes us to look forward to the upcoming published results from the lower extremity amputation trial currently under way in 8 centers under sponsorship of the National Institutes of Health.

M.F. Swiontkowski, M.D.

Amputation Surgery: Mobility After Amputation

Predicting Prosthetic Rehabilitation Outcome in Lower Amputee Patients With the Functional Independence Measure

Leung EC-C, Rush PJ, Devlin M (Univ of Toronto; Mount Sinai Hosp, Toronto)
Arch Phys Med Rehabil 77:605–608, 1996   7–23

Background.—The ability to predict the benefit to amputee patients of prosthetic fitting would be useful in their rehabilitation. The Functional Independent Measure (FIM) has been shown to have good reliability and

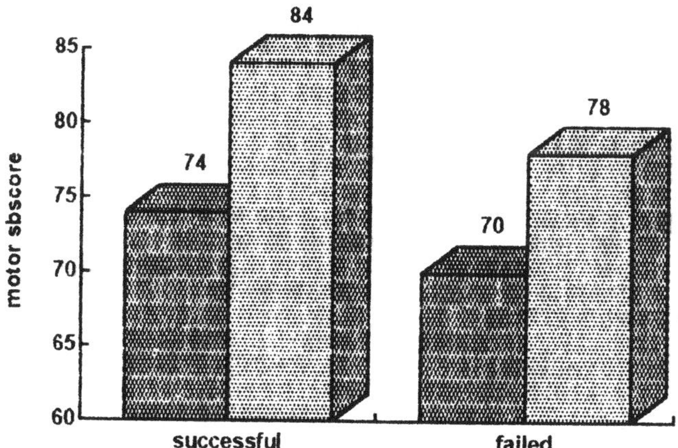

FIGURE 1.—Admission motor subscores (*solid bars*) and discharge motor subscores (*stippled bars*) of the successful and failed groups of prosthetic users. (Courtesy of Leung EC-C, Rush PJ, Devlin M: Predicting prosthetic rehabilitation outcome in lower amputee patients with the Functional Independence Measure. *Arch Phys Med Rehabil* 77:605–608, 1996.)

TABLE 3.—Studies on Success of Prosthetic Rehabilitation

Author	Criteria for Success of Prosthesis Rehabilitation	Significant Predictors
Weiss	Ambulation for 20 feet	Multiple disease and extensive atherosclerosis (negative predictor)
Moore	Ambulation on a daily basis with/without support	Level of amputation (proximal → worse)
Deluccia	Unclear, classified by interview into nonwearer, partial wearer, and full-time wearer	Level of amputation
Dove	Independent ambulation at least 100 feet with/without a cane	Age and level of amputation
Kerstein	Ambulation at least 100 yards	Age (older → worse)

(Courtesy of Leung EC-C, Rush PJ, Devlin M: Predicting prosthetic rehabilitation outcome in lower amputee patients with the Functional Independence Measure. *Arch Phys Med Rehabil* 77:605–608, 1996.)

validity, but its ability to measure the likelihood of prosthetic use in amputee patients has not been assessed. Therefore, the ability of the admission and discharge FIM data to predict prosthetic use was evaluated.

Methods.—Over a 15-month period, 41 consecutive amputee patients admitted to the rehabilitation unit were studied. The FIM was administered within 48 hours of admission and at discharge. Daily prosthetic use was assessed with the Houghton Scale, and a score of at least 9 defined successful prosthetic rehabilitation. Correlations between the Houghton Scale score and the admission FIM score, the admission motor subscore, the discharge motor subscore, and the difference between the 2 motor subscores were analyzed.

Results.—There were no significant differences between the patients with successful and those with failed prosthetic rehabilitation in admission FIM scores, admission motor subscore, or the difference between the 2 motor subscores. Only the discharge motor subscore correlated significantly with the Houghton Scale score (Fig 1).

Conclusion.—The discharge motor subscore did differentiate between the patients with and without a successful prosthetic rehabilitation. However, a discharge score is not useful in predicting before rehabilitation the success of prosthetic fitting, and neither admission FIM overall nor motor subscale score was useful. Other studies have identified age, the level of amputation, and the number of comorbidities as being significant predictors of prosthesis use (Table 3), and these patients confirmed the predictive importance of the level of amputation and comorbidity.

Pre- and Post-amputation Mobility of Trans-tibial Amputees: Correlation to Medical Problems, Age and Mortality

Johnson VJ, Kondziela S, Gottschalk F (UT Southwestern Med Ctr, Dallas)
Prosthet Orthot Int 19:159–164, 1995   7–24

Background.—Patient mobility, morbidity, and mortality after amputation can be influenced by medical problems, even those unrelated to the cause of amputation. Awareness of such problems is important in determining a patient's potential ability to use a prosthesis. Mobility before and after amputation and its association with medical problems were evaluated in a group of unilateral transtibial amputees.

Methods.—The charts of 120 men undergoing below-knee amputation at 1 veterans' hospital between 1983 and 1991 were reviewed. A 6-level scale, developed by Volpicelli, et al. was used to assess mobility.

Findings.—Changes in mobility after amputation were correlated with the presence of cardiac disease, chronic obstructive pulmonary disease (COPD), peripheral vascular disease (PVD), diabetes mellitus, degenerative joint disease, blindness, cerebral vascular accident, and age. Older men had more medical problems and lower mobility scores after amputation. However, regardless of age, patients with more medical problems had poor ambulation. Although individual medical problems did not affect mobility scores, the presence of COPD and PVD was associated with reduced mobility scores before amputation. Together or individually, cardiac disease and diabetes mellitus lowered postamputation mobility scores. Mobility scores were not affected by the cause of amputation per se (Tables 3, 4, and 5).

Conclusions.—Several medical problems are related to ambulation after amputation. Patients with more medical problems had poorer ambulation after surgery, regardless of their age.

TABLE 3.—Individual Correlation of Medical Problems, Age, and Mobility Scores

Variable	Spearman correlation coefficient (P value)
Age, number of medical problems	+0.28 (p=0.002)
Age, post-amputation score	−0.46 (p=0.0001)
Number medical problems, post-amputation score	−0.23 (p=0.01)*
Pre, post-amputation score	+0.52 (p=0.0001)
Age, pre-amputation	−0.25 (not significant)†
Number medical problems, pre-amputation score	−0.18 (not significant)

*N = 54.
†N = 120.
(Courtesy of Johnson VJ, Kondziela S, Gottschalk F: Pre- and Post-amputation mobility of trans-tibial amputees: Correlation to medical problems, age and mortality. *Prosthet Orthot Int* 19:159–164, 1995.)

TABLE 4.—Frequency of Number of Medical Problems and Means of Age, Post-amputation Mobility Scores

Number medical problems	Number of patients	Age	Post-amputation mobility scores
Zero	16	42.1	5.6
One	30	60.3	4.5
Two	44	60.1	4.5
Three	27	60.4	4.5
Four	3	66	3.0

(Courtesy of Johnson VJ, Kondziela S, Gottschalk F: Pre- and Post-amputation mobility of trans-tibial amputees: Correlation to medical problems, age and mortality. *Prosthet Orthot Int* 19:159–164, 1995.)

TABLE 5.—Medical Problem and Influence on Post-amputation Mobility Score

Medical problem	Influence on post-amputation score
CAD	−1.26
DM	−1.76
PVD + DM	−0.96
PVD + CVA	−4

Abbreviations: CAD, cardiac disease; *DM*, diabetes mellitus; *PVD*, peripheral vascular disease; *CVA*, cerebral vascular accident.

(Courtesy of Johnson VJ, Kondziela S, Gottschalk F: Pre- and Post-amputation mobility of trans-tibial amputees: Correlation to medical problems, age and mortality. *Prosthet Orthot Int* 19:159–164, 1995.)

Stump Length as Related to Atrophy and Strength of the Thigh Muscles in Trans-tibial Amputees
Isakov E, Burger H, Gregorič M, et al (Tel Aviv Univ, Ra'anana, Israel; Inst for Rehabilitation, Ljubljana, Slovenia)
Prosthet Orthot Int 20:96–100, 1996   7–25

Background.—The prosthetic rehabilitation outcomes of transtibial amputees are strongly influenced by stump length and thigh muscle strength of the amputated limb. An electrical dynamometer was used to measure and compare the strength of the quadriceps and hamstring muscles of both limbs in transtibial amputees.

Methods.—Twelve men and 6 women with transtibial amputations volunteered for the study. Their mean age was 45.7 years, and the mean time since amputation was 13.4 years.

Findings.—The thigh muscles of the sound limbs were significantly stronger than those of the amputated limbs. In the 9 subjects with a stump shorter than 15.1 cm, peak torque values and maximal mean torque were significantly weaker than in the 9 subjects with stumps longer than 15.1 cm. In subjects in whom muscle atrophy was accompanied by a thigh girth reduction of more than 5.9 cm, muscle strength was not significantly less than in subjects in whom thigh girth decline was less than 5.9 cm (Tables 2 and 3).

Conclusions.—Thigh muscle atrophy in subjects with transtibial amputations is accompanied by a significant reduction in strength. In amputees with short stumps, the short lever action interferes with the thigh muscles' ability to control the prosthesis efficiently during daily activities, such as standing and walking.

▶ Leung (Abstract 7–23) et al. looked at the functional independence measure as a predictor of the outcome of prosthetic rehabilitation. They did not find this measure to be useful as a predictor; instead, they found the often identified factors of medical co-morbidity and the level of amputation to be the most important predictors.

TABLE 2.—Means and Standard Deviations (Nm) of Muscles' Peak Torque (Isokinetic Contraction) and Maximal Average Torque (Isometric Contraction)

Muscle	Type of Muscle Contraction	Amputated Limb	Sound Limb	P
Quadriceps	Isokinetic concentric	40.4 ± 20.5	76.7 ± 31.0	0.001
	Isokinetic eccentric	112.0 ± 47.2	171.2 ± 45.4	0.002
	Isometric	46.0 ± 26.4	93.0 ± 34.0	0.001
Hamstrings	Isokinetic concentric	29.9 ± 20.0	74.6 ± 34.8	0.001
	Isokinetic eccentric	64.5 ± 37.3	128.2 ± 45.1	0.001
	Isometric	30.3 ± 20.4	52.6 ± 24.3	0.007

(Courtesy of Isakov E, Burger H, Gregorič M, et al: Stump length as related to atrophy and strength of the thigh muscles in trans-tibial amputees. *Prosthet Orthot Int* 20:96–100, 1996.)

TABLE 3.—Values of Muscles' Peak Torque (Isokinetic Contraction) and Maximal Average Torque (Isometric Contraction)*

Muscle	Type of Muscle Contraction	Stump length:		P
		<15.1 cm (N = 9)	<15.1 cm (N = 9)	
Quadriceps	Isokinetic concentric	32.6 ± 16.6	48.3 ± 21.9	0.113
	Isokinetic eccentric	87.0 ± 27.6	137.1 ± 50.6	0.016
	Isometric	35.4 ± 17.3	60.4 ± 31.7	0.112
Hamstrings	Isokinetic concentric	19.1 ± 6.0	40.6 ± 23.6	0.038
	Isokinetic eccentric	47.8 ± 10.5	81.3 ± 47	0.075
	Isometric	22.1 ± 12.6	38.3 ± 24.2	0.087

*Means and standard deviations (Nm) are related to stump length.

(Courtesy of Isakov E, Burger H, Gregorič M, et al: Stump length as related to atrophy and strength of the thigh muscles in trans-tibial amputees. *Prosthet Orthot Int* 20:96–100, 1996.)

Johnson et al. (Abstract 7–24) looked at these same issues of medical problems, age, and mortality and confirmed the same finding, that medical co-morbidity is a very strong predictor of ultimate function after an amputation.

In the third article Isakov et al. (Abstract 7–25) looked at the level of amputation and once again confirmed that short stumps in below-knee amputees are functionally a problem. They have identified thigh muscle atrophy as also being an important factor, and this problem is probably preventable with good physical therapy follow-up.

M.F. Swiontkowski, M.D.

Amputation Surgery: Amputation Technique

Syme's Amputation Revisited: A Review of 46 Cases
Gaine WJ, McCreath SW (Southern Gen Hosp, Glasgow, Scotland)
J Bone Joint Surg Br 78:461–467, 1996   7–26

Background.—Syme's amputation is indicated primarily for congenital deformity of the foot and trauma, and also possibly for vascular insufficiency with or without diabetes and forefoot infection. The important technical points in the classical procedure are preservation of the posterior tibial artery in the posterior flap, as this provides a blood supply to the heel flap; heel flap dissection from the calcaneum subperiosteally; and the division of the tibia at the level of the dome of the ankle, parallel to the floor. Although Syme's amputation continues to be popular in Canada and Scotland, it is less favored elsewhere. One experience with Syme's amputation was reviewed.

Patients and Outcomes.—Forty-six patients with Syme's amputation attending the Glasgow prosthetic clinics were included in the review. The clinical and radiologic condition of the stumps, level of function, and problems with prostheses were documented. Twenty-five of these patients were compared with a matched group of 25 patients who had had transtibial amputation (Table 2). Although function in the 2 groups was comparable, the incidence of prosthestic failure was greater in the

TABLE 2.—Comparison of the Mean Activity Level of Syme's Amputees and A Group of Transtibial Amputees

	Mean score*	
Activity	Syme's	Transtibial
Walking distance	2.4	2.0
Stair-climbing	2.5	2.0
Sports	1.3	1.3
Car-driving	2.0	1.4
Occupation	2.2	2.0

*3 = normal level of function; manual occupation; walking over 2 km without problems; able to drive manual car. 2 = reduced or limited level of activity; sedentary job; some restriction in walking and stair-climbing; able to drive automatic car. 1 = significantly disabled; not able to work; unable to drive or walk more than 200 m without stopping or needs cane.

(Courtesy of Gaine WJ, McCreath SW: Syme's amputation revisited: A review of 46 cases. *J Bone Joint Surg (Br)* 78B:461–467, 1996.)

patients who had had Syme's amputation. Overall, the Syme's amputees were satisfied with their prostheses and level of function. Patients undergoing Syme's amputation in childhood had fewer long-term stump and functional problems.

Conclusion.—Syme's amputation still has a place in the treatment of selected patients. It is undoubtedly useful for congenital foot deformities, fibular hemimelia, and severe foot injury, as long as the heel pad remains viable.

▶ Gaine and McCreath have revisited Syme's technique and, through their careful follow-up of 46 patients, bring the orthopedic trauma surgeon back to its use as a technique for severe foot injury, as long as the heel pad is intact. It does have some definite benefits for prosthetic fashioning and use, and it is often preferred by patients who have a below-knee amputation on the opposite side. We should continue to consider its use whenever the heel pad is intact.

M.F. Swiontkowski, M.D.

Amputation Surgery: Phantom Pain

Phantom Limb Pain and Etiology of Amputation in Unilateral Lower Extremity Amputees
Weiss SA, Lindell B (Connetquot Central School District, Islip, NY)
J Pain Symptom Manage 1:3–17, 1996   7–27

Background.—Broad etiologic categories, such as trauma, disease, and war wounds, may not account for the differences observed in phantom pain. The association of phantom limb pain with the etiology of amputation and occurrence of gangrene and/or infection was investigated.

Methods.—Ninety-two consecutive patients undergoing unilateral lower extremity (LE) amputation were studied. They were 61 men and 31 women, aged a mean 51.4 years. Fifty-five above-knee (AK) amputations and 37 below-knee (BK) amputations were performed. The indications for amputation included blood clots, nonclot diabetes, and other miscellaneous causes.

Findings.—Patients with blood clots had the highest levels of phantom pain before and after rehabilitation. These patients also had the longest interval between amputation and prosthetic fitting and the most medical conditions. A history of gangrene and/or infection was associated with greater phantom pain and a longer time to rehabilitation. Assessment by rehabilitation staff indicated that stump problems, including pain and sensitivity, before rehabilitation were variously associated with later stump pain and sensitivity.

Conclusions.—Compared to other amputation causes, blood clots are associated with greater levels of phantom limb pain before and after rehabilitation and a longer time between surgery and rehabilitation. This cause was followed by the nonclot diabetes and miscellaneous causes.

Evidence for a Change in Neural Processing in Phantom Limb Pain Patients

Larbig W, Montoya P, Flor H, et al (Univ of Tübingen, Germany; Humboldt-Univ, Berlin; Berufsgenossenschaftliche Unfallklinik, Tübingen, Germany; et al)
Pain 67:275–283, 1996   7–28

Introduction.—It has been suggested that phantom limb pain may be multifactorial, with involvement of both peripheral nerves and neural networks of the brain. The purpose of this study was to evaluate the response to pain-related word stimuli and to identify differences in neural processing and peripheral response in amputees who experience phantom limb pain (PLP) as compared with pain-free amputees and healthy controls.

Methods.—Eighteen amputees were assigned to 1 of 2 groups (PLP or pain-free group) based on information obtained during a prestudy interview. Thirteen healthy controls were also included in the trial. Word identification was used to assess differences in patients' perception of 40 pain-related, 40 neutral, and 40 body-related words. Physiologic testing (electroencephalography, bilateral electromyography [EMG]) electro-oculography, was performed to determine responses to word testing. Event-related potentials were determined for each word category and site.

Results.—Significantly more words produced responses in amputees than in controls. Amputees had a longer mean exposure time (15.9 and 17.2 msec for the PLP and pain-free groups, respectively) than did the control group (10.7 msec). N100 amplitude was reduced in the pain-free amputee group as compared with the PLP group (−1.14 vs. −4.99 µV, respectively). The N100 amplitude for the pain-free group was also reduced in comparison to controls (−1.14 vs. −5.42 µV, respectively). Patients in the PLP group showed a significantly greater late positive complex, which occurred at 500–800 msec after word stimulus, with mean amplitudes ranging from 19.60 to 20.35 µV. The corresponding values for controls and the pain-free group were 11.72–12.79 and 11.07–12.87 µV, respectively. Peripheral EMG responses also differed between the 3 groups. A greater EMG reaction was found on the contralateral side than on the stump side for patients in the pain-free group. Patients in the PLP group showed an opposite effect, with a greater response on the stump. For the control group, no differences in EMG response were found between the right and left sides.

Conclusion.—Processing of visual word stimuli was found to be significantly different in amputees who experience phantom limb pain as compared with pain-free amputees and healthy controls. Generalized neural changes may be involved in phantom limb pain, with involvement of peripheral factors as well.

▶ The troublesome aspect of "phantom limb pain" after amputation surgery is revisited in these 2 articles (Abstracts 7–27—7–28). Weiss and Lindell (Abstract 7–27) have identified deep venous thrombosis as an important, related cause. With our modern techniques of duplex scanning and prophylaxis with enoxaparin and/or heparin/warfarin (Coumadin), we may be able to have a favorable impact on this problem after amputation surgery.

Larbig et al (Abstract 7–28) looked at neural change processing in patients who have this phenomenon and identified a definitely different response in the processing of visual word stimuli, which may be indicative of generalized neural changes that may predispose patients to this clinical problem.

M.F. Swiontkowski, M.D.

Amputation Surgery: Postoperative Pain Management

Continuous Postoperative Infusion of a Regional Anesthetic After an Amputation of the Lower Extremity

Pinzur MS, Garla PGN, Pluth T, et al (Loyola Univ, Maywood, Ill)
J Bone Joint Surg (Am) 78A:1501–1505, 1996   7–29

Background.—The use of continuous perineural infusion of a long-acting local anesthetic to alleviate pain after lower extremity amputation is increasing in popularity. In a prospective, randomized clinical trial whether continuous bupivacaine infusion reduces the need for narcotics for pain relief after amputation was determined.

Methods.—Twenty-one patients scheduled for lower extremity amputation because of ischemic necrosis caused by peripheral vascular disease were assigned to a treatment or control group. After the amputation, a Teflon catheter was placed next to the transected end of the sciatic or posterior tibial nerve, and bupivacaine or normal saline solution was infused for 72 hours. Intravenous morphine delivered by a patient-controlled pump was allowed during infusion.

Findings.—Compared to patients in the control group, patients in the treatment group used less morphine on the first and second days after surgery. The groups did not differ in amount of morphine used on day 3.

Overall, 11 of 14 patients completing a questionnaire reported reduced pain between the third- and sixth-month assessment.

Conclusions.—Continuous perineural infusion of bupivacaine appears to be safe and effective for relieving pain after amputation. However, it did not prevent residual or phantom pain in this patient population.

▶ Pinzur et al. have done a nice job in examining continuous perineural infusion of a long-acting local anesthetic to alleviate pain after amputation. They identified positive benefits in terms of the overall use of narcotics and reduced pain at 3 and 6 months' assessment. This technique should be considered by surgeons who perform amputations. This study has a particularly sound clinical design as a randomized control trial, and although it suffers from low statistical power because small numbers, the study is very nicely done.

M.F. Swiontkowski, M.D.

Clinical Radiography

Value of Intraoperative Image Intensifier Prints in Trauma Surgery
Williams RL, Clarke AJ, Haddad FS (Univ College Hosp, London; Hosp for Sick Children, London)
Ann R Coll Surg Engl 78:512–514, 1996   7–30

Introduction.—Image intensifiers have the capability of printing thermal images with the use of digitized computer technology. The use of image intensifiers is increasing with the growing need for minimally invasive procedures during orthopedic surgery. The value of intraoperative image intensification during trauma surgery was evaluated over a 6-month period.

Methods.—Image intensification was used for intraoperative screening in 280 of 476 patients (58.8%) who underwent orthopedic surgery for trauma. Image intensification was used only when it was considered necessary and was never used solely for the purpose of obtaining prints. Each print was assessed for quality of the image and adequacy of coverage of the operative area, with particular attention paid to fixation devices.

Results.—Thermal prints were obtained in 278 of 280 surgical procedures using image intensification. No postoperative radiographs were required in 210 surgical procedures (75%). Both prints and radiographs were obtained in 68 procedures to ensure full coverage of the operative area.

Conclusion.—Thermal images can be considered a useful substitute for formal postoperative radiographs. Use of prints generated by image intensification can reduce patient discomfort, potentially decrease the cost and length of hospital stay, and save radiology and transporting manpower.

▶ In the era of increasing cost constraints, the routine use of postoperative radiographs has come under scrutiny in attempts to decrease costs. Most orthopedic trauma surgeons are using imaging intensifiers intraoperatively on an increasing basis. This group has confirmed that the permanent images obtained with these machines can be considered adequate and a substitute for formal postoperative radiographs, thereby decreasing costs.

M.F. Swiontkowski, M.D.

Clinical Value of Radiologists' Interpretations of Perioperative Radiographs of Orthopedic Patients
Clark R, Anderson MB, Johnson BH, et al (Southern Utah Ctr for Sports Medicine, Saint George)
Orthopedics 19:1003–1007, 1996   7–31

Objective.—Studies have shown that self-referrals result in increased utilization of services and increased cost to patients. That government agencies have restricted payments for self-referrals, including plain radiographs, has created a problem for orthopedic surgeons who provide radiographic services in their offices. Because no studies have examined the quality of radiologists' interpretation of plain radiographs, this study assessed the content and accuracy of such interpretations to determine whether radiology reports provide sufficient information to make clinical treatment decisions.

Methods.—A total of 371 preoperative radiographs from 211 orthopedic patients undergoing procedures at Dixie Regional Medical Center in Saint George, Utah, between August 1992 and March 1993 were retrospectively reviewed by 4 orthopedic surgeons after the initial report had been prepared by 3 staff radiologists to grade findings of fractures and implants and categorize their clinical usefulness.

Results.—Fracture locations were present in 92% (133 of 145) of the radiographs, absent in 2%, and incorrect in 6%. Fracture types were correctly described in 78%, absent in 22%, and incorrectly described in 0%. Fracture comminutions were correctly described in 88%, absent in 11%, and incorrect in 1%. Soft tissue findings were present in 83%, absent in 16%, and incorrect in 1%. Fracture alignment was generally described in 69%, precise in 21%, absent in 13%, and incorrect in 1%. Fracture displacement was generally described in 70%, precise in 24%, absent in 0%, and incorrect in 6%. Alignment and displacement were precisely described in 9%. Orthopedic implant–type descriptions were general in 72% (163 of 226) of the radiographs, precise in 12%, absent in 9%, and incorrect in 7%. Implant position was generally described in 54%, precise in 27%, absent in 16%, and incorrect in 3%. Implant effect was generally described in 55%, precise in 25%, absent in 17%, and incorrect in 3%. Implant stability was generally described in 21%, precisely described in 4%, absent in 75%, and incorrect in 0%. Radiologists' reports were not available until after the procedure in 61% of the surgeries. None of the reports changed the clinical course chosen by the surgeon. On average, descriptions were inaccurate 3% of the time.

Conclusion.—An accurate assessment of radiographic studies cannot be determined from the radiologists' report alone. The orthopedic surgeon should look at the radiographs.

▶ This very interesting article points out that radiologists are not routinely adding value to the radiographs themselves when orthopedists are primarily managing patients. This is particularly true for fractures. Orthopedic surgeons should be credentialed to read and interpret x-ray films, thus bringing about significant cost savings for the overall system of managing injured patients.

M.F. Swiontkowski, M.D.

Technical Advances

Strength Recovery in Fractured Sheep Tibia Treated With a Plate or an Internal Fixator: An Experimental Study With a Two-year Follow-up
Tepic S, Remiger AR, Morikawa K, et al (AO/ASIF Found, Davos, Switzerland)
J Orthop Trauma 11:14–23, 1997   7–32

Introduction.—The use of conventional compression plates for fractured bones usually requires a second operative procedure because of vascular damage leading to necrotic bone. The PC-Fix is a new internal fixation device that resembles a plate but functions as an internal fixator (Fig 3). It eradicates the need for direct contact with and compression of periosteum. The performance of the PC-Fix was compared to that of a conventional dynamic compression plate (DCP) in the treatment of experimental fractures in tibia of 56 adult Swiss mountain sheep.

Methods.—The right tibia of each animal underwent a standardized oblique fracture; sheep were then randomly assigned to the DCP or PC-Fix treatment group. The fractures were reduced and compressed by a lag screw before implants were applied. Animals were placed on restricted weight-bearing in individual stalls for the first 12 weeks and then were kept in groups. Callus size was measured using standard radiographs. The animals were killed, and the treated bone and contralateral bone were removed. Ultimate bending strength tests were performed with the plate side under tension at 12, 24, 48, and 96 weeks, with 6 sheep per group. Broken bones underwent histologic evaluation.

Results.—At 12-week testing, all 6 bones in the DCP group failed through the original fracture. At 24 weeks, 2 of 6 fractures failed through the fracture. At the 96-week time point, 1 of 6 bones in the DCP group failed through the original fracture and the rest through 1 of the screw holes (Fig 4). Histologic examination showed necrosis of the cortical bone underneath the plate in the DCP group. Intense remodeling activity surrounded the necrotic bone. There was only 1 failure through the original fracture at 96 weeks in the PC-Fix group. The strength values in the PC-Fix groups at 12 and 96 weeks were significantly higher than in corresponding DCP groups. Histologic evaluation indicated a filling of the gap between the PC-Fix plate and bone with periosteal bone formation. Small areas of

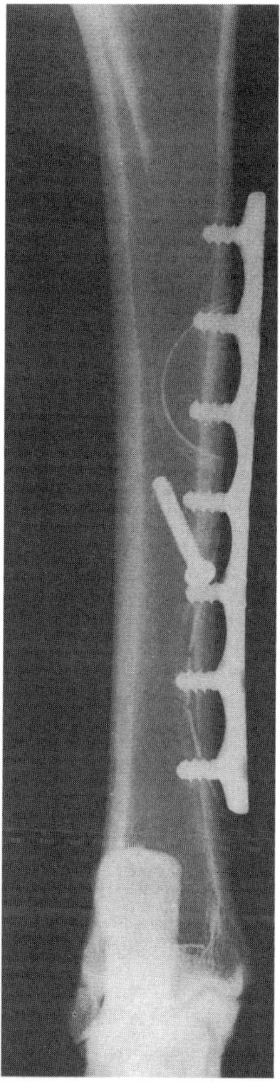

FIGURE 3.—Postoperative frontal radiograph of a fractured sheep tibia with a PC-Fix. (Courtesy of Tepic S, Remiger AR, Morikawa K: Strength recovery in fractured sheep tibia treated with a plate or an internal fixator: An experimental study with a two-year follow-up. *J Orthop Trauma* 11:14–23, 1997.)

remodeling activity were observed in the cortex at the very edge of periosteal bone apposition.

Conclusion.—The PC-Fix does not require an extensive amount of direct contact or compression between the implant and bone, thus minimizing the amount of necrotic tissue. The fracture callus in the PC-Fix group was significantly smaller, but the strength of the bone after implant removal was significantly higher at 12 and 96 weeks. The gap between the PC-Fix plate and bone caused new bone formation around the full circumference in continuation with the normal callus. The PC-Fix allowed

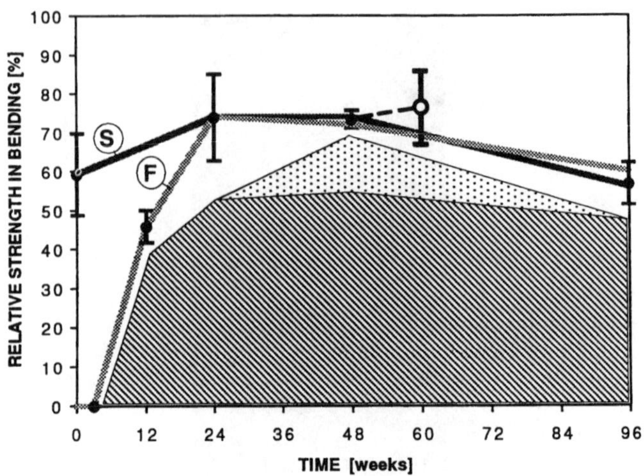

FIGURE 4.—Strength recovery of the fractured bones in the dynamic compression plate (*DCP*) group. Line F shows the average strength of bones that failed at the original fracture site; line S shows the average strength of bones that failed at a screw hole. The value of the S curve at time zero was established by testing fresh pairs of sheep tibias. The shaded area shows admissible bending loads after impact removal (average strength − 2 standard deviations). (Courtesy of Tepic S, Remiger AR, Morikawa K: Strength recovery in fractured sheep tibia treated with a plate or an internal fixator: An experimental study with a two-year follow-up. *J Orthop Trauma* 11:14–23, 1997.)

preservation of both the periosteal and endosteal blood supply. The PC-Fix offers advantages over conventional plates.

The Torsional Strength of Bones With Residual Screw Holes From Plates With Unicortical and Bicortical Purchase

Remiger AR, Miclau T, Lindsey RW (Kantonsspital, St Gallen, Switzerland; Univ of California, San Francisco; Baylor College of Medicine, Houston)
Clin Biomech 12:71–73, 1997   7–33

Background.—Dynamic compression plates compromise the cortical blood supply beneath the plate. The point-contact fixator (PC-Fix), recently introduced, contacts the cortical bone only at isolated points. Screws are used with unicortical purchase, which minimizes cortical vascular damage. The unicortical screw holes of the PC-Fix seem to heal faster than the bicortical screw holes of the dynamic compression plate (DCP), possibly reducing the time needed for postoperative protection. The effect of unicortical and bicortical screw holes on residual bone strength was assessed in cadaveric sheep tibiae.

Methods.—In 18 tibiae, screw holes were drilled and tapped through either a 7-hole bicortical DCP or a unicortical PC-Fix. Paired tibiae were grouped randomly and torsion tested. In group 1, unicortical screw holes were compared with intact bone; in group 2, bicortical screw holes were compared with intact bone; and in group 3, bicortical were compared with unicortical screw holes.

Findings.—The mean decrease in the torsional strength of unicortical screw holes in group 1 was 21.6%; that of bicortical screw holes in group 2 was 31.4% and in group 3, it was 26.7%. Within each group, mean torque values to failure were significant.

Conclusion.—Bones with unicortical screw holes are significantly weaker in torsion than intact bones but stronger than those containing bicortical holes. Thus, implants with unicortical purchase may be associated with less risk for early fracture on removal.

▶ These 2 articles (see Abstracts 7–32—7–33) provide information on the new development of the AO, the so-called PC-Fix plate. This plate has distinct advantages of not producing cortical bone necrosis directly underneath the plate because contact between the bone and the undersurface of the plate is limited. An additional, critical advance is the unicortical screw fixation. Avoidance of drilling across the endosteal surface and damaging the medullary sinus and/or nutrient artery is definitively shown in the first article (Abstract 7–32) to speed the rapidity and quality of bone healing. In the second article (see Abstract 7–33), the mechanical characteristics of unicortical fixation in terms of resistance to torsional stress is elucidated. Because of the rigid fit between the screwhead and the plate, plate contouring will be critical. We are waiting for clinical outcome studies on this technology to see whether it can be applied to common diaphyseal fractures such as adult both-bone forearm fractures. Clearly, this represents a technological advance. We need to wait for the effectiveness studies regarding clinical application.

M.F. Swiontkowski, M.D.

A New Technique for Complex Fibula Fracture Fixation in the Elderly: A Clinical and Biomechanical Evaluation

Koval KJ, Petraco DM, Kummer FJ, et al (Hosp for Joint Diseases Orthopaedic Inst, New York)
J Orthop Trauma 11:28–33, 1997   7–34

Background.—Open reduction and internal fixation is the treatment of choice for displaced ankle fractures. In older patients, however, this treatment may carry an unacceptably high risk. The use of augmented plate fixation of the fibula with intramedullary Kirschner wire to provide provisional fracture stabilization and enhance plate and screw fixation was reported in a series of older patients with comminuted and osteopenic fibula fractures.

Methods.—Twenty patients aged 50 years and older underwent treatment for 20 comminuted or osteopenic fibula fractures. Stabilization was achieved using plate fixation augmented with intramedullary Kirschner wires. Nineteen patients were followed for a mean of 15.4 months. In addition to retrospectively analyzing outcomes in these patients, a biomechanical evaluation was done to compare fixation of mildly osteopenic

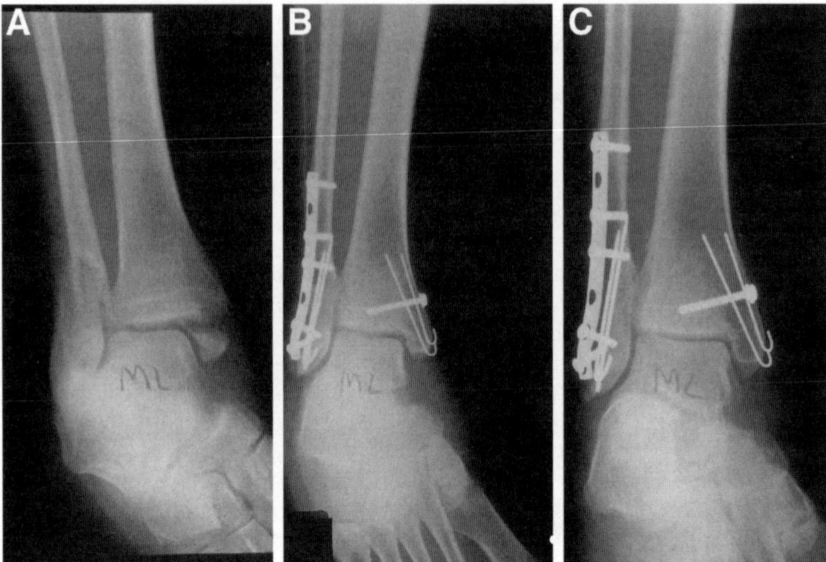

FIGURE 3.—Preoperative radiograph of comminuted bimalleolar ankle fracture in a 79-year-old woman (A). Initial postoperative radiograph (B) and radiograph at 1 year follow-up (C). The fracture united without loss of reduction. (Courtesy of Koval KJ, Petraco DM, Kummer FJ, et al: A new technique for complex fibula fracture fixation in the elderly: A clinical and biomechanical evaluation. *J Orthop Trauma* 11:28–33, 1997.)

fibulas using this method to the use of plate and screws alone. Nondestructive bending was done first, followed by destructive testing in torsion to determine stability and ultimate fixation strength.

Findings.—In all 19 patients available for follow-up, fractures united without loss of reduction. Eighty-nine percent of the patients had no, slight, or mild pain. Biomechanical assessment showed that the resistance to bending of the plated fibulas augmented with Kirschner wires was 81% greater than the fibulas stabilized with a plate alone. Torsional testing demonstrated that the augmented group had twice the resistance to motion of the plate group (Fig 3).

Conclusion.—Plate fixation augmented with intramedullary Kirschner wires appears to be an effective treatment of comminuted and osteopenic fibula fractures in elderly patients. This method results in better fixation than plate and screws alone in osteopenic bone. In addition, it may help prevent loss of fixation of these difficult fractures.

▶ This abstract presents an advance in terms of the management of spiral (Weber B) fracture of the distal end of the fibula in elderly, osteoporotic patients. The authors present critical biomechanical information coupled with a clinical series that shows definite value. The adjunctive use of Kirschner wires in this clinical situation of severe osteoporosis is one that can be recommended to orthopedists presented with this difficult clinical situation.

M.F. Swiontkowski, M.D.

Efficacy of Antibiotics Alone for Orthopaedic Device Related Infections
Isiklar ZU, Darouiche RO, Landon GC, et al (Baylor College of Medicine, Houston; Veterans Affairs Med Ctr, Houston; Univ of Texas, Houston)
Clin Orthop 332:184–189, 1996   7–35

Background.—Five percent to 20 percent of fracture fixation devices and 0.5% to 2% of joint prostheses become infected, despite compliance with infection control measures. Antibiotic treatment alone is thought to be inadequate for such infections. The efficacy of 4 antibiotic regimens in the treatment of orthopedic device-related infection caused by slime-producing *Staphylococcus epidermis* was tested in a rabbit model.

Methods.—A hole was drilled through the intercondylar notch and inoculated with bacteria, and a stainless steel screw was inserted into the femur. After 2 weeks, the rabbits were assigned randomly to 1 of 4 antibiotic regimens. For 2 weeks, 9 rabbits received vancomycin; 10, minocycline; 10, vancomycin plus rifampin; and 10, minocycline plus rifampin.

Findings.—Although levels of vancomycin were high in biofilm, vancomycin alone did not cure infection. Minocycline alone eradicated infection in only 20% of the rabbits. The highest cure rate—90%—was achieved with vancomycin and rifampin combined. Minocycline plus rifampin cured 70% of the infections (Table 1).

Conclusions.—Neither vancomycin nor minocycline alone appears to be effective in eradicating infection associated with orthopedic devices. The combination of vancomycin and rifampin merits further investigation in patients with infected orthopedic devices that cannot be removed.

▶ The clinical situation of posttraumatic deep infection remains one of infrequent occurrence but major significance. This article presents information on the efficacy of antibiotics alone for device-related infections in an animal model. The authors have shown that because of the nonviable surface presented, antibiotics alone provide limited ability to clear bacteria. This is not surprising, and herein lies the clinical value. Intravenous antibiotics in

TABLE 1.—Antibiotic Levels and Bone Cultures

| | Antibiotic Level | | | |
Antibiotic Regimen	Blood (μg/mL)	Bone (μg/g)	Biofim (μg/g)	Bone Culture (No. Positive/Total)
Vancomycin (Group A)	9.1 ± 3.3	5.0 ± 1.6	5.3 ± 37.5	9/9
Minocycline (Group B)	0.28 ± 0.01	0.22 + 0.06	ND	8/10
Vancomycin and	10.5 ± 4.0	3.9 ± 2.1	38.9 ± 38.0	1/10
rifampin (Group C)	1.56 ± 0.21	0.97 ± 0.36	ND	
Minocycline and	0.34 ± 0.04	0.25 ± 0.06	ND	3/10
rifampin (Group D)	0.55 ± 0.08	0.31 ± 0.2	ND	

Note: Antibiotic levels represents the mean ± standard deviation of the mean.
Abbreviation: ND, not detectable.
(Courtesy of Isiklar ZU, Darouiche RO, Landon GC, et al: Efficacy of antibiotics alone for orthopaedic device related infections. *Clin Orthop* 332:184–189, 1996.)

general do not completely eradicate infection when hardware remains in place. The orthopedist is foolish, however, to remove implants that offer stability before the fracture is completely healed. Based on these data, it seems as though vancomycin in combination with rifampin may have some promise in limiting the soft tissue extent of the infection associated with implants but will probably not eradicate it.

M.F. Swiontkowski, M.D.

Miscellaneous

Fracture and Dislocation Compendium
Orthopaedic Trauma Association Committee for Coding and Classification
J Orthop Trauma 10:5S–9S, 1996   7–36

Introduction.—There has long been a need for a systematic classification of skeletal fractures to enable simple, precise communication with unified terminology among orthopedic surgeons. In an attempt to meet this need, the Committee for Coding and Classification of the Orthopaedic Trauma Association has developed a classification system based on the AO Long Bone Classification System.

Definitions.—Glossary terms are derived from those established by the Long Bone Classification System: severity, location, segments, diaphyseal fracture type, impaction, center of fracture, specific terms for proximal and distal segments, partial articular fractures, complete articular fractures, and anatomical terms.

Fracture Characterization.—Classification of a fracture requires determining the following 5 characteristics: which bone, location in the bone, type (simple, multifragmentary wedge, or multifragmentary complex fractures), group (simple fractures: spiral, oblique, or transverse; wedge fractures: spiral, bending, or fragmented; complex fractures: spiral, segmental, or irregular), subgroup (unique from bone to bone).

Fractures of the Proximal and Distal Segments.—The same characteristics must be determined, but they may be defined differently. The bones may have 4 instead of 3 segments. The types of fractures are classified as extra-articular, partial articular, or complete disruptions of the articular surface from the diaphysis. The groups are defined as either avulsion fractures of ligamentous or tendinous insertions, simple metaphyseal fractures, or multifragmentary metaphyseal fractures.

Conclusion.—This classification system is proposed as the start of an evolving system, beginning with use and moving through problem identification and comment and criticism to acceptance.

▶ This 5-year work represents a major advance in musculoskeletal trauma research. It seems wise for all future authors to report injury severity with this coding system so that in the future, researchers who wish to collate series will have this universal yardstick as a reference point. This committee has taken pains to develop mechanisms for changing the classification on a

3-year cycle, which will make the evolving compendium relevant and useful in the future.

M.F. Swiontkowski, M.D.

Orthopedic Trauma Surgeons' Attitudes and Practices Towards Bloodborne Pathogens
McCarthy ML, Bosse MJ, Preas MA, et al (Johns Hopkins School of Hygiene and Public Health, Baltimore, Md; Carolinas Med Ctr, Charlotte, NC; Univ of Maryland at Baltimore; et al)
J Orthop Trauma 10:383–388, 1996   7–37

Background.—Because orthopedic trauma surgeons routinely perform invasive procedures with sharp instruments in emergency circumstances on a population at high risk for HIV, hepatitis B, and hepatitis C, they have a theoretically very high risk of occupational exposures to bloodborne pathogens. The individual attitudes and practices of orthopedic trauma surgeons regarding bloodborne pathogens were surveyed to determine their methods of minimizing this risk.

Methods.—A survey was distributed to practicing orthopedic trauma surgeons at 2 Orthopedic Trauma Association meetings. The survey addressed attitudes and practices toward HIV and hepatitis infections and their prevention, as well as the policies at their facilities.

Results.—Most respondents (93%) considered orthopedic trauma practice to carry a high risk of exposure to bloodborne pathogens, and 74% were moderately or very concerned about this potential. Mandatory HIV testing of patients was favored by 83% of respondents and of physicians by 56% of respondents. However, only 49% of the physicians were tested annually. Requiring disclosure of the patient's status to the physician was favored by 96%, whereas 78% reported that infected physicians should be required to disclose their status to their patients. However, less than half said that they would disclose their status to patients.

The respondents reported an average of 53.4 cutaneous exposures and 2 parenteral exposures annually, and half did not report any exposures to their facility. More than 40% did not routinely wear gloves when changing wound dressings. Although two thirds of the respondents had access to maximum protective equipment at their facilities, 83% of these physicians reported not routinely using such equipment to nail a femur fracture. Accessible maximum barrier equipment was routinely worn by only two thirds of physicians when operating on patients with HIV infection and by less than half when operating on patients with hepatitis infection. A large porportion of the respondents did not know all of their facility's specific policies, and 27% thought that their facility did not promote safe clinical practices. Many had not read guidelines, and more than half worked at facilities that trained orthopedic residents without requiring the residents to adhere to infection control standards.

Conclusion.—Many orthopedic trauma surgeons do not routinely comply with infection control practices. In addition, many institutions are not facilitating compliance and providing proper education regarding infection control. Strategies to reduce exposure to bloodborne pathogens should be implemented at the individual, institutional, and organizational levels. Senior orthopedic surgeons should be good role models for safe practices, motivating younger surgeons. Institutions should actively promote safe practice by periodically evaluating employee compliance and by encouraging employees to report all exposures, so that high-risk areas and procedures can be identified and studied to develop safer protocols. Professional organizations should provide education and motivation for maximally safe practice.

▶ McCarthy et al., through a survey methodology, evaluated the attitudes of orthopedic trauma surgeons toward infection control practices. Many surgeons do not seem to routinely comply. Since many of them work in teaching centers, their perception as role models is particularly concerning. Senior orthopedic surgeons should demonstrate universal precautions to minimize exposure of their trainees. We need to do a better job pressuring each other into not being reckless.

M.F. Swiontkowski, M.D.

Rehabilitation and Reintegration of Multiply Injured Patients: An Outcome Study With Special Reference to Multiple Lower Limb Fractures
Seekamp A, Regel G, Tscherne H (Medizinische Hochschule Hannover, Germany)
Injury 27:133–138, 1996   7–38

Objective.—Although multiply injured patients can be successfully treated, no studies have examined the quality of life after reintegration. The physical ability, rehabilitation, and social reintegration of patients with multiple limb fractures, torso, and head injuries were evaluated.

Methods.—Physical examinations were performed on 86 men and 18 women, aged 16–55 years, who had multiple injuries (Injury Severity Score > 20) for 2–4 years. Pattern and mechanism of injury, therapy, and back-to-work rate after 2 years were analyzed. Injuries were classified and scored.

Results.—Car and motorcycle accidents accounted for 88% of injuries, bicycle accidents for 4% and pedestrian accidents for 5%. The mean Injury Severity Score was 34.1. There were head injuries in 36 patients, thoracic injuries in 38, and abdominal injuries in 21. Most injuries were to the limbs. Group A patients had multiple ipsilateral leg fractures; group B patients did not. Most femur fractures were closed, and most tibia fractures were open. Neurologic disorders were present in 19 of 36 patients who had head injury. There was no significant range of motion reduction in 76 of 91 arm fractures (Fig 4). Of the 35 patients who had difficulty

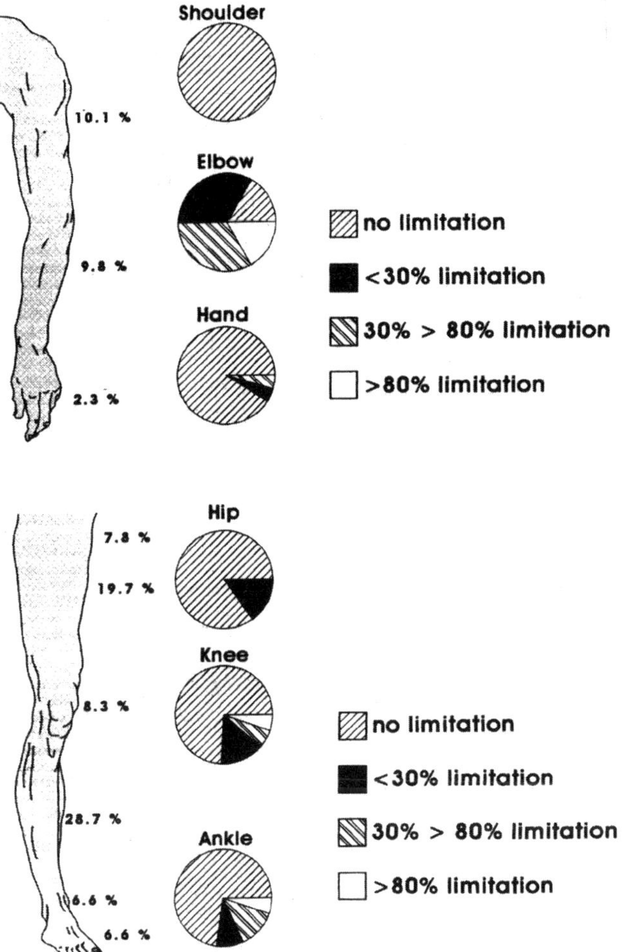

FIGURE 4.—Range of motion in upper (**above**) and lower (**below**) limbs. Numbers next to the illustration indicate the percentage of this location among all injuries in that limb. (Reprinted from Seekamp A, Regel G, Tscherne H: Rehabilitation and reintegration of multiply injured patients: An outcome study with special reference to multiple lower limb fractures. *Injury* 27:133–138, 1996, with kind permission from Elsevier Science Ltd, The Boulevard, Langford Lane, Kidington OX5 1GB, UK.)

walking, 24 had multiple leg injuries and 18 had open leg fractures. Rehabilitation lasted an average of 114 days. After 2 years, 7% of patients still could not work. Although 42% of group A and 46% of group B patients returned to their old jobs, 29% and 13.5%, respectively, had to change careers because of lower limb fractures in most cases (Fig 6). Reintegration was associated with age, the major prognostic factor of permanent disability was leg injury, and disability of more than 80% was associated with head or spinal injury. In group A and group B, 28% and 64%, respectively, were disabled by 20% or less (Fig 7). Seventy-three percent reported no change in social contacts, and 71% reported no

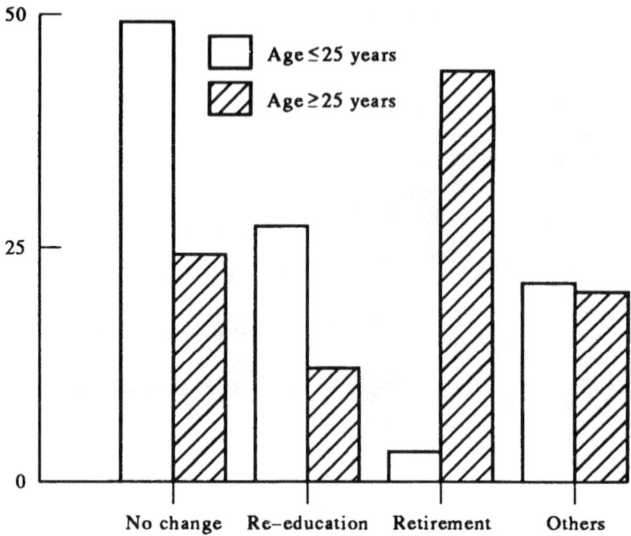

FIGURE 6.—Change in profession after injury with respect to patients' age. (Reprinted from Seekamp A, Regel G, Tscherne H: Rehabilitation and reintegration of multiply injured patients: An outcome study with special reference to multiple lower limb fractures. *Injury* 27:133–138, 1996, with kind permission from Elsevier Science Ltd, The Boulevard, Langford Lane, Kidington OX5 1GB, UK.)

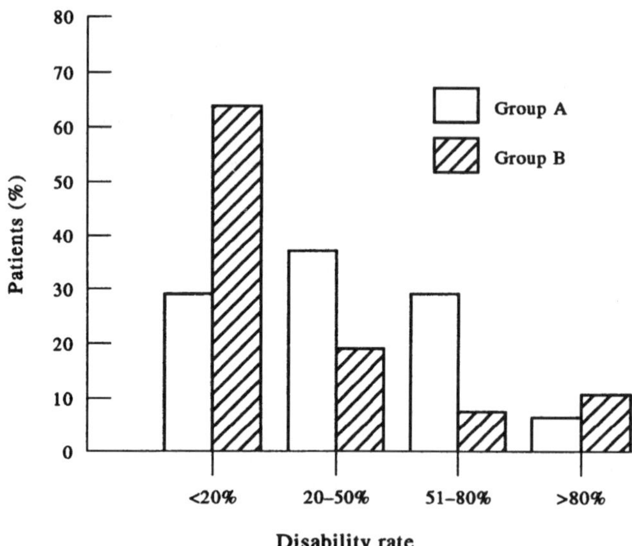

FIGURE 7.—Disability rate after injury according to the standards of insurance companies. (Reprinted from Seekamp A, Regel G, Tscherne H: Rehabilitation and reintegration of multiply injured patients: An outcome study with special reference to multiple lower limb fractures. *Injury* 27:133–138, 1996, with kind permission from Elsevier Science Ltd, The Boulevard, Langford Lane, Kidington OX5 1GB, UK.)

change in vacation plans. Forty-one percent remain active in sports. Daily activity mean total Functional Independence Measurement scores were 109.8 for group A and 113.4 for group B.

Conclusion.—Recovery and social integration after multiple injuries are generally good. Poor outcomes are the result of head and spinal injuries and multiple limb fractures. Younger patients appear to have a better prognosis. Rehabilitation is cost-effective but needs to be standardized.

▶ The functional outcome of patients with multiple lower extremity fractures has been studied in detail by McKenzie's group.[1] Seekamp et al. looked at a similar group with Functional Independence Measurement scores and found that particularly poor outcomes are associated with head and neurologic injuries. The rate of functional recovery goes down with multiple fractures in the lower extremity, a finding paralleling that of McKenzie et al., who used the Sickness Impact Profile to determine that functional outcomes in patients with more than 3 fractures in the ipsilateral lower extremity are definitely worse.

M.F. Swiontkowski, M.D.

References

1. McKenzie EJ, Siegel JH, Shapiro S, et al: Functional recovery and medical costs of trauma: An analysis by type and severity of injury. *J Trauma* 28:281, 1988.

Comparison of Intravenous and Oral Antibotic Therapy in the Treatment of Fractures Caused by Low-Velocity Gunshots: A Prospective Randomized Study of Infection Rates
Knapp TP, Patzakis MJ, Lee J, et al (Los Angeles County–Univ of Southern California Med Ctr, Los Angeles)
J Bone Joint Surg (Am) 78A:1167–1171, 1996   7–39

Background.—Although the optimal treatment of high-velocity gunshot wounds is established, the optimal treatment of low-velocity gunshot wounds is controversial, particularly regarding the role of antibiotics. The efficacy of oral and IV antibiotics in infection control was compared in patients with extra-articular fractures of long bones from low-velocity gunshots.

Methods.—A total of 190 patients with extra-articular fractures of long bones from a low-velocity gunshot were randomly assigned to receive either IV cephapirin sodium and gentamicin for 3 days (101 patients, 120 fractures) or oral ciprofloxacin for 3 days (89 patients, 102 fractures). The patients were followed until complete healing occurred, as evidenced by both clinical and radiographic union, and signs or symptoms of infection had been noted and treated.

Results.—The 2 groups were comparable in age, the time between injury and the institution of antibiotic therapy, and the anatomical location of fractures (Table 1). There was a 2% rate of infection overall and in each

TABLE 1.—Anatomical Distribution of Fractures

Location of Fracture	Group 1	Group 2	Total
Humerus	15	12	27
Ulna	12	9	21
Radius	6	4	10
Femur	13	10	23
Tibia	35	35	70
Fibula	26	21	47
Miscellaneous	11	9	20
Total	118	100	218

Note: The values represent the number of fractures. The fractures of the 4 patients who were lost to follow-up or who received additional antibiotic therapy during the period of the study were excluded.

(Courtesy of Knapp TP, Patzakis MJ, Lee J, et al: Comparison of intravenous and oral antibiotic therapy in the treatment of fractures caused by low-velocity gunshots: A prospective, randomized study of infection rates. *J Bone Joint Surg (Am)* 78A:1167–1171, 1996.)

group. All 4 infected fractures were located in the distal half of the tibia. There was an 11% rate of infection in the injuries to the distal half of the tibia. The 4 fracture sites were all infected with *Staphylococcus aureus*, and 1 was also infected with group-D gamma-hemolytic *Streptococcus*. All of these organisms were sensitive to both antibiotic protocols.

Conclusion.—Oral antibiotic treatment and IV antibiotic therapy are equally effective in controlling infections in extra-articular fractures of a long bone from a low-velocity gunshot. These findings are consistent with findings in previous studies (Table 2). However, injuries affecting the distal half of the tibia appear to have a higher risk of infection, regardless of the antibiotic protocol.

▶ The question of whether to use IV antibiotics after low-velocity gunshot wounds continues to be relevant and increasingly so in North American inner-city trauma centers. In this controlled trial (nonrandomized), the authors seem to confirm, within the limits of their study design, that oral antibiotic use is safe. Some clinical judgment will have to continue to be used for fractures associated with gunshot wounds in which there is a lot of contamination and surgical débridement is thought necessary. In this setting, IV antibiotics will probably still be indicated.

M.F. Swiontkowski, M.D.

TABLE 2.—Summary of Studies Comparing Rates of Infection Associated with Different Antibiotic Therapies in the Treatment of Fractures Caused by Low-Velocity Gunshots

| Study | Type of Study | Group Treated with Intravenous Administration of Antibiotics | | | Type of Therapy | Group Treated with Alternative Administration of Antibiotics | | | Comments |
		Total No. of Fractures	No. of Infections	Rate of Infection (Per cent)		Total No. of Fractures	No. of Infections	Rate of Infection (Percent)	
Freeark et al. (1961)	Retrospective	106	0	0	—	—	—	—	24 fractures lost to follow-up
Howland and Ritchey (1971)	Retrospective	19	2	11	None	53	0	0	No treatment protocol
Patzakis et al. (1974)	Prospective	51	3	6	None	27	1	4	Shotgun wounds included
Elstrom et al. (1978)	Retrospective	26	0	0	None	3	0	0	Fractures of forearm only
Brettler et al. (1979)	Retrospective	83	2	2	—	—	—	—	No control group
Marcus et al. (1980)	Retrospective	71	3	4	None	26	1	4	Also included soft-tissue wounds
Leffers and Chandler (1985)	Retrospective	32	2	6	—	—	—	—	30 of 41 fractures in total series lost to follow-up
Woloszyn et al. (1988)	Retrospective	63	0	0	Oral	52	2	4	32 fractures lost to follow-up
Dickey et al. (1989)	Prospective	36	1	3	None	37	1	3	22 fractures lost to follow-up
Geissler et al. (1990)	Prospective/ retrospective	25	1	4	Intra-muscular inject.	25	1	4	26 fractures involved hand or foot

(Courtesy of Knapp TP, Patzakis MJ, Lee J, et al: Comparison of intravenous and oral antibiotic therapy in the treatment of fractures caused by low-velocity gunshots: a prospective, randomized study of infection rates. *J Bone Joint Surg (Am)* 78A:1167–1171, 1996.)

Manual Assessment of Fracture Stiffness

Webb J, Herling G, Gardner T, et al (Nuffield Orthopaedic Centre, Oxford, England)
Injury 27:319–320, 1996

7–40

Background.—External fixation is often needed to facilitate fracture healing. The decision of when to safely remove the fixator is based on clinical and radiologic examination, but both have been shown to be unreliable. A previous study has shown that the external fixator can be safely removed when there is a bending fracture stiffness of 15 Nm/degree. The ability of orthopedic surgeons to accurately assess bending stiffness during clinical examination was assessed using a fracture model.

Methods.—Ten consultant orthopedic surgeons, 10 orthopedic trainees, 10 medical students, and 10 bioengineers were asked to manually estimate the bending stiffness of 7 models of midshaft diaphyseal fracture at different stages of healing, with and without a model soft-tissue envelope.

Results.—The consultants made significantly higher estimates of the bending stiffness than the true values, both with and without the soft-tissue envelope, with widely varying estimations in the group. There were no statistically significant differences in the accuracy of the 4 test groups. The surgeons considered 83% of the rods with a stiffness of less than 15 Nm/degree to be sufficiently united to safely remove the fixator and 13% of the rods with a stiffness greater than 15 Nm/degree to require prolonged fixation.

Conclusion.—The experienced orthopedic surgeons would have put 83% of patients at risk of refracture or malunion because of premature fixator removal and 13% of patients at risk of pin-track complications because of unnecessarily prolonged fixation. Clinical assessment of fracture stiffness is unreliable. Therefore, quantitative tests of fracture stiffness are needed.

▶ Bending stiffness as a measure of fracture healing is an attractive concept that has long been studied, particularly in the United Kingdom. This is a very clean study that evaluates surgeons' ability to predict bending stiffness and identify a safe time for fixator removal. Quantitative tests were shown to be highly accurate, and experienced surgeons could not adequately judge bending stiffness. In most of our practices, what this means is that we should leave the frames on longer rather than shorter to minimize the risk of malunion. Where available, quantification seems to be a useful adjunct.

M.F. Swiontkowski, M.D.

The Reinforcement of Cancellous Bone Screws With Calcium Phosphate Cement

Mermelstein LE, Chow LC, Friedman C, et al (Yale Univ, New Haven, Conn; American Dental Assoc Health Found, Gaithersburg, Md)
J Orthop Trauma 10:15–20, 1996   7–41

Background.—The use of polymethylmethacrylate (PMMA) in fracture surgery has been limited because of concerns about inhibition of the healing process and the possible formation of an inert barrier to bone in growth. The search for a more "biocompatible" cement has led to the development of a new calcium phosphate compound, which is the subject of the current study.

Methods.—The ability of calcium phosphate cement (CPC) to reinforce cancellous screws in previously stripped holes was assessed in canine femurs. Fifteen screws were placed in the distal end of 6 femurs. The pullout strength, failure displacement, stiffness, and energy absorbed were established for screws in intact bone. Then the stripped screw holes were packed with CPC, and the pullout test was repeated.

Findings.—The CPC reinforced the previously stripped holes and significantly increased the pullout strength and stiffness of the constructs.

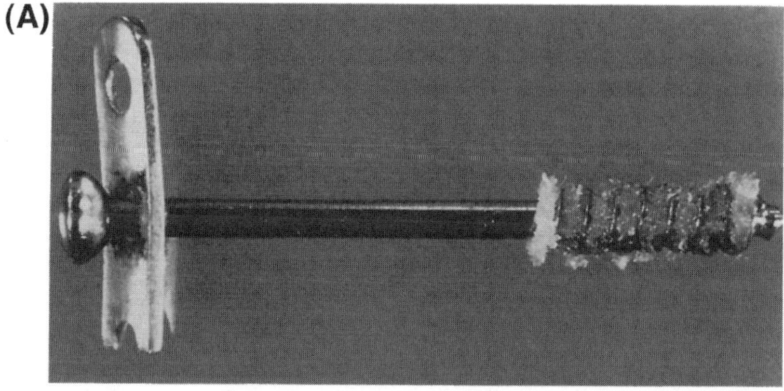

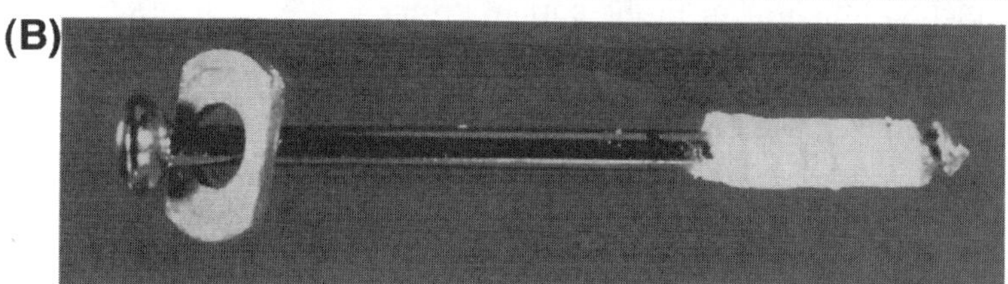

FIGURE 4.—**A** and **B**, photographs of screw specimens after pullout failure tests. The failure mechanism was the same in both the intact and the calcium phosphate cement–reinforced constructs. A core of cancellous bone (**A**) or cement (**B**) was extracted from the threads of the screws. There were no fractures of the lateral femoral cortex. The plate and washer in these photographs facilitated connection to the testing apparatus. (Courtesy of Mermelstein LE, Chow LC, Friedman C, et al: The reinforcement of cancellous bone screws with calcium phosphate cement. *J Orthop Trauma* 10:15–20, 1996.)

Energy absorbed by the constructs until failure was also increased. Failure displacement did not differ significantly (Fig 4).

Conclusions.—Filling a previously stripped screw hole in cancellous bone with CPC increases the average pullout strength by 189% of the original strength of the screw. In vivo data are now needed to further investigate the efficacy of CPC.

▶ Calcium phosphate cements are confirmed to be a useful adjunct in increasing bending, stiffness, and load to failure in proximal femoral fractures (both femoral neck and intertrochanteric fracture). This group has confirmed that calcium phosphate cement also improves screw pullout strength increases energy absorption, and is useful in cases in which screws had previously pulled out. These cements, once approved, will be an enhancement, particularly in the management in osteoporotic fractures.

M.F. Swiontkowski, M.D.

Outcome After Pelvic Ring Fractures: Evaluation Using the Medical Outcomes Short Form SF-36
Oliver CW, Twaddle B, Agel J, et al (Robert Jones & Agnes Hunt Orthopaedic Hosp, Oswestry, Shropshire, England)
Injury 27:635–641, 1996   7–42

Introduction.—Outcome measures after musculoskeletal injuries have historically been limited to measuring death or serious complications. Pelvic ring fractures are complex injuries that are often associated with considerable morbidity. The SF-36 medical outcome score measures 4 components related to physical health (physical function, physical role, bodily pain, and general health) and 4 components related to mental health (vitality, social functioning, emotional role, and mental health). Patient-oriented physical component scores (PCS) and mental component scores (MCS) from the SF-36 medical outcome score were assessed in patients with surgically stabilized unstable pelvic-ring disruptions and compared with a normative database to determine the degree of physical and mental impairment in the patient group.

Methods.—Fifty-five patients with unstable pelvic fractures treated by the same surgeon were followed as a consecutive, prospective cohort. Pertinent data on the patient, degree of injury, and treatment approach were recorded. Patients completed a SF-36 medical outcome questionnaire at a mean follow-up of 2 years.

Results.—Thirty-five of 55 patients were available to complete the SF-36 medical outcome questionnaire. Patient response indicated that physical activities were the most affected by injury and mental activities were affected least by the injury and surgery (Table 3). Compared with the normal population, the patient group had a 14% impairment in physical outcome score and a 5.5% impairment in mental outcome score. The incidence of open fractures, nerve injuries, and employment in the group

TABLE 3.—SF-36 Medical Outcome Scores for Pelvic Fracture and Normative Data from U.S. Population (Mean ± Standard Deviation)

	Pelvis fractures	*USA population*
Physical component score (PCS)	67.1 ± 26.3	78.3 ± 25.1
Physical functioning	64.3 ± 27.7	84.5 ± 22.9
Role physical	77.1 ± 26.5	81.2 ± 33.8
Bodily pain	62.9 ± 26.5	75.5 ± 23.6
General health	64.1 ± 24.6	72.2 ± 20.2
Mental component score (MCS)	71.1 ± 23.2	75.2 ± 23.6
Vitality	57.0 ± 22.4	61.1 ± 20.9
Social functioning	74.5 ± 26.2	83.6 ± 22.4
Role emotional	84.3 ± 23.3	81.3 ± 33.0
Mental health	68.6 ± 21.0	74.8 ± 18.0

(Reprinted from Injury 27: Oliver CW, Twaddle B, Agel J: Outcome after pelvic ring fractures: Evaluation using the medical outcomes Short Form SF-36. *Injury* 27: 635–641, Copyright 1996, with permission from Elsevier Science Ltd, The Boulevard, Langford Lane, Kidlington OX5 1GB, UK.)

of patients who responded was increased compared with nonresponders. In the nonresponder group, the incidence of urologic injury, lower- and upper-limb fractures, spine fractures, and tobacco and alcohol usage was increased compared with the responder group. Both groups were similar in Injury Severity Score, age, fracture classification, head injury, chest injury, abdominal injury, delay to pelvic fixation, transfer to a medical center for treatment, and pre-existing disease.

Conclusion.—Physical and mental health outcomes can be measured in patients with pelvic fractures and multiple injuries. At a mean period of 2 years after injury, patients indicated a 14% impairment in PCS and a 5.5% impairment in MCS compared with the general population.

▶ This study used a health status questionnaire to evaluate patient dysfunction after pelvic fracture. The authors used the Short Form SF-36, the most widely used health status instrument in the English-speaking world. Limitations of this study include passive follow-up (the questionnaires were not completed at the same time interval postinjury) and incomplete detail regarding associated injuries and medical co-morbidities. However, the information is useful to clinicians treating these injuries. Significant impact in the functional domains of physical and mental health are herein documented. With improved study design and further data collection, we will be able to learn a lot more about the effect of these injuries, as well as the treatments used to optimize anatomical results. The ultimate question may someday be addressed: "Does better reduction result in better patient function?"

M.F. Swiontkowski, M.D.

8 Pediatrics

Introduction

This year has produced an unusually large number of reports on fractures. Most of these are related to newer concepts for treatment, with the thrust being directed toward more aggressive use of open reduction and internal fixation. Dr. Pat Kelly has said that he did not want to be the first to try the new nor the last to discard the old. This is good advice as we carefully consider the treatment of fractures in children. Children's fractures heal rapidly, so open reduction–internal fixation is not needed for healing. Deformity will remodel to a large extent, and we must know within reason the extent of remodeling to be expected; therefore, anatomical alignment is not necessary. Hospital stay, the extent of temporary disability, and socioeconomic factors related to the family are legitimate factors to consider when choosing a method of treatment, but not at the cost of unnecessary risk. The inability of the orthopedic surgeon to reduce a fracture by closed technique and successfully immobilize the fracture with plaster may be a driving force for recommending open reduction–internal fixation. There is a question as to whether we are adequately teaching the art of reduction and plaster immobilization of fractures in children. The choice of treatment is usually one with which the physician has had previous success. Therefore, orthopedists will resort to open reduction of a particular fracture when their experience with the closed technique has been unsuccessful.

There continues to be a strong interest in hip problems. The unsolved problems presented by newer types of imaging bring new challenges to orthopedic surgeons. The section on hips includes the revival of some old surgical treatments, use of knowledge from new imaging, and long-term outcomes of some conditions.

In the section on bowlegs, the natural history, etiology, and treatment are covered in articles chosen for this section. Problems of early prediction of progression and prevention of recurrence after treatment are considered. More work on the prevention of recurrence in infantile Blount's disease is needed.

I included three excellent publications on infection. Musculoskeletal infection as a complication of varicella is not common, and the severity of bone and joint infections is not appreciated by most. Two papers address some controversial issues about the treatment of skeletal infection.

The miscellaneous section includes an outstanding paper by an experienced neurosurgeon on disk problems. The use of MRI may give an increased frequency of diagnosis of herniated disk, and it is important that we carefully consider the clinical fractures described by the author in the paper on pediatric disks in our decision making in children with back pain.

Other selections on scoliosis, torticollis, cerebral palsy, and talocalcaneal coalition are included in this issue. All of the articles selected either give a new approach to an old problem or have new information that needs to be considered in the diagnosis and treatment of musculoskeletal problems. Controversies are discussed in several papers. All of these articles are well worth careful study.

Paul P. Griffin, M.D.

Trauma

Open Reduction and Internal Fixation of Forearm Fractures in Children
Ortega R, Loder RT, Louis DS (Univ of Michigan, Ann Arbor)
J Pediatr Orthop 16:651–654, 1996   8–1

Background.—When closed reduction does not successfully treat both-bone forearm fractures, open reduction–internal fixation (ORIF) can be performed. However, ORIF is controversial in children before skeletal maturity. The indications for ORIF and outcomes were reviewed in a retrospective study of all children younger than 13 years of age who underwent ORIF of 1 or both forearm bones.

Methods.—The records of 16 children younger than 13 years of age with 17 fractures of the radius and/or ulna shaft treated with ORIF between 1988 and 1994 were reviewed. The reasons for ORIF were determined, and the final outcome was graded. The outcome was excellent if the patient had no complaints and/or a loss of less than 10 degrees of forearm rotation, good if the patient had mild complaints with strenuous physical activity and/or a loss of 11–30 degrees of forearm rotation, and fair if the patient had mild complaints during daily activities and/or a loss of 31–90 degrees of forearm rotation.

Results.—The patients had an average age of 9.4 years at surgery. Indications for ORIF were unacceptable fracture reduction after closed reduction of the radius in 14 children and unstable open injuries of the radius in 3 children. Interposed tissue complicated 7 fractures with unacceptable closed reduction. Open reduction–internal fixation was performed on the radius only in 12 forearms and on both bones in 5 forearms. Plates and screws were used for fixation in 8 fractures, percutaneous Steinmann pins in 7 fractures, and intramedullary Steinmann pins in 2 fractures. All patients had excellent results, with no delayed unions or nonunions and no infections or iatrogenic neurovascular injuries.

Conclusions.—Primary ORIF can have excellent results without an increased risk of complications in properly selected young patients. This approach may reduce the need for late osteotomy to correct malreduced fractures in these children.

Open Reduction and Internal Fixation of Pediatric Forearm Fractures

Wyrsch B, Mencio GA, Green NE (Vanderbilt Univ, Nashville, Tenn)
J Pediatr Orthop 16:644–650, 1996   8–2

Background.—Closed reduction is the standard of care for fractures of the forearm bones in children. However, residual deformity from malunion in children may result in loss of motion and dysfunction. Open reduction–internal fixation (ORIF) is controversial in children because of fears of potential complications. The results of ORIF of unstable forearm fractures in skeletally immature patients were studied retrospectively.

Methods.—The medical records and radiographs of 26 skeletally immature patients who underwent ORIF of forearm fractures between 1986 and 1993 were reviewed. The patients had a mean age of 11.5 years and were monitored for an average period of 39 months. Subjective evaluations of pain and function and objective measures of function were reviewed.

Results.—The 26 patients had 17 closed fractures and 10 open fractures. All of the patients with closed fractures initially underwent closed reduction with unacceptable results. The 10 patients with open fractures underwent primary treatment with ORIF. Stabilization was provided with plate fixation in 22 patients and with intramedullary fixation in 4 patients. All of the fractures healed, with an average time to union of 3.5 months. All but 3 patients had full range of motion. Of the 6 patients with preoperative nerve deficits, within 4 months the deficits completely resolved in 5. There were 3 complications: deep infection in 1 patient, initial nonunion in 1, and cross-union in 1.

Conclusions.—Although closed treatment is still the treatment of choice for pediatric forearm fractures, ORIF can be safe and effective treatment of unstable forearm fractures in children and may facilitate soft tissue management in children with open fractures. Either compression plating or intramedullary techniques provide reliable fixation in children. Open reduction–internal fixation is most likely to be needed for fractures of the proximal third of the radius and ulna and high-energy displaced and/or comminuted fractures.

Single-Bone Fixation of Both-Bone Forearm Fractures

Flynn JM, Waters PM (Children's Hosp, Boston)
J Pediatr Orthop 16:655–659, 1996   8–3

Background.—Recent studies have reported that internal fixation can be succcessful after failed closed reduction of forearm fractures in children. Another approach was developed that involved internal fixation of either the radius or ulna to treat pediatric diaphyseal both-bone forearm fractures. The outcome of children treated with this approach was studied retrospectively.

Methods.—Seventeen children aged 5–14 years have undergone single-bone fixation of a both-bone forearm fracture since 1989. Complete fracture of both bones was seen in 13 patients and a complete fracture of 1 bone with a greenstick fracture of the other bone in 4. Whenever possible, the ulna was fixed with an intramedullary pin; then the forearm was manipulated to reduce and stabilize the radius, and the arm was placed in a long-arm cast. When closed reduction of the radius was not possible, it was fixed with a tubular plate or intramedullary fixation; then the forearm was manipulated to reduce and stabilize the ulna. The patients were monitored up until the fracture was healed and function was either normalized or stable.

Results.—Complete follow-up was available for 16 of the 17 children. Healing was completed by 8 weeks for all fractures. Two children had a loss of 5 degrees of pronation; full motion of the elbow, wrist, and forearm was regained otherwise. No patients had infections, nonunions, malunions, synostoses, or refractures. Two patients had complications: 1 keloid and 1 transient superficial radial nerve neurapraxia.

Conclusions.—In children with failed closed treatment of both-bone diaphyseal forearm fractures, single-bone fixation is a safe and effective treatment involving the stabilization of 1 bone and rotation and reduction of the other bone. This approach avoids the need for repeated anesthetics and prevents malreduction without the need for plating of both bones. Intramedullary fixation is preferred because it is easier and safer to place and remove.

▶ These 3 articles describe the experience with open reduction with internal fixation of forearm fractures in children at 3 well-known institutions. Open reduction–internal fixation was successful in these reports. The reasons for open reduction were open fractures, inability of the surgeon to achieve an acceptable result, or inability to maintain the reduction with a plaster cast. The recommended management of an open fracture after reduction is internal fixation. This choice of immobilization is reasonable if wound care requires repeated débridement and/or dressings. The inability to obtain a satisfactory reduction is variable and in the gray zone. What is a satisfactory reduction? Is a distal angular deformity more acceptable than midshaft or a proximal angulation? Does age influence what is acceptable? A flaw in these articles is the age of the patients. In Abstract 8–1 they were all 5–12 years of age. In Abstract 8–2 only 4 were less than 11 years, and Abstract 8–3 reports a similar age group. A 12-year-old skeletally mature or nearly mature patient has problems with forearm fracture similar to adults and should be treated like an adult.

The institution reporting in Abstract 8–2 had an incidence of a requirement for open reduction and internal fixation of less than 2%, and around a third of these were open fractures. The institution in Abstract 8–3 had a 5% incidence of open reduction. There is a certain gratification we surgeons get from immediate restoration of anatomy deformed by a fracture, but this must not lead us to use open treatment of a fracture that can be treated by closed reduction. The most common reason for failure of closed reduction is inaccurate correction of rotation of the radius, and the 2 most common causes of loss of reduction are inaccurate correction of rotation and inadequate plaster application. We must remember that in open surgery, complications occur.

None of the articles addressed the inherent problems of plate removal. Plate and screw fixations look good on radiographs, but they interfere with appositional growth. The plate and screw can cause some ischemia in the cortex, which makes the bone more brittle for a period of time after the plate is removed.

Healing of forearm fractures occurs rapidly in children and does not require rigid fixation. Angulation can be controlled with an intramedullary pin in 1 bone in most cases. The intramedullary pin is easier to remove and does not affect the cortex. I think it is adequate and preferable to plate and screws.

We should use discretion in deciding to use open reduction, but I suggest you read an article by Evans[1] to better understand the mechanics of reduction, a report by Price et al.[2] to know what can be accepted and expect a good result, and a paper by Younger et al.[3] for an esoteric explanation of angulations that can be expected to correct.

P.P. Griffin, M.D.

References

1. Evans EM: Fractures of the Radius and Ulna. *J Bone Joint Surgery Br* 33:548–561, 1951.
2. Price CT, Scott DS, Kurzner ME, et al: Malunited forearm fractures in children. *J Pediatr Orthop* 10:705–712, 1990.
3. Younger ASE, Tredwell SD, Mackonjic W I, et al: Accurate prediction of outcome after pediatric forearm fracture. *J Pediatr Orthop* 14:200–206, 1994.

The Treatment of Supracondylar Fractures in Children With an Absent Radial Pulse

Garbuz DS, Leitch K, Wright JG (Hosp for Sick Children, Toronto)
J Pediatr Orthop 16:594–596, 1996   8–4

Background.—Volkmann's ischemic contracture related to vascular injury or compartment syndrome is the most serious complication of supracondylar fractures. The management of children with a supracondylar fracture and an absent radial pulse is controversial. Although children with an absent radial pulse and a cold and white hand after satisfactory closed reduction undergo exploration of the artery, the management of children with a satisfactory closed reduction and a well-perfused hand, but an absent radial pulse, has been debated. The outcome of children with a supracondylar fracture and an absent radial pulse was studied retrospectively.

Methods.—Between 1984 and 1992, 22 children had displaced extension-type supracondylar fractures of the humerus and an absent radial pulse on admission and were followed up. The children were divided into 2 groups defined by perfusion of the hand at admission. The final follow-up included evaluation of arm pain, claudication, functional limitation, range of motion, neurologic status, and radial pulse status.

Results.—Sixteen patients had an absent radial pulse and a well-perfused hand. Eleven underwent closed reduction, and 5 underwent open reduction and internal fixation. Exploration of the artery was performed in 4 of the 5 children who underwent open reduction, all of whom had a cold, white hand after reduction. Three of the 11 children had an absent radial pulse after closed reduction, but the hand was well perfused. These children were not given further treatment except for 48-hour inpatient observation. Final follow-up of the 16 children with a well-perfused hand revealed a normal radial pulse and no claudication in 15 children. One child who needed ligation experienced pain on the dorsal wrist with continuous writing. Of the 6 children with a cold, white hand at admission, all were without pain and claudication and had normal range of motion, carrying angle, neurovascular status, and function.

Conclusions.—Although a cold-white hand after a satisfactory closed reduction is an indication for open exploration of the artery, an absent pulse alone is not an indication for exploration of the artery, as long as the hand is well perfused and no compartment syndrome develops.

▶ This is a very important study that emphasizes the importance of immediate closed reduction for a supracondylar fracture with no radial pulse. After a satisfactory reduction, the pulse returns in most patients. For those patients in whom the radial pulse does not return but the hand is well perfused, observation is the only treatment required. The only patient who needs exploration of the artery is one with a white, poorly perfused hand after a satisfactory reduction. This paper should support observation rather than invasive arteriography for patients with no radial pulses after reduction of a supracondylar fracture when the hand is warm and well perfused.

P.P. Griffin, M.D.

Slipped Capital Femoral Epiphysis: Prediction of Contralateral Involvement
Stasikelis PJ, Sullivan CM, Phillips WA, et al (Texas Tech Univ, Lubbock; Univ of Chicago; Univ of Texas, Galveston)
J Bone Joint Surg Am 78:1149–1155, 1996   8–5

Objective.—Whether children with a unilateral slipped capital femoral epiphysis should undergo prophylactic fixation of the normal hip is controversial. Results of a retrospective review of the medical records and radiographs of children with unilateral slip to determine the risk of a later contralateral slip are presented.

Methods.—A review of records discovered 50 patients (21 girls), 38 black and 12 white, with unilateral slip treated between 1984 and 1991 with a single cannulated screw who had a complete set of radiographs taken at the time of injury and who had been monitored until evidence of partial physeal closure or a slip in the normal hip. Skeletal maturity was assessed by 4 different raters on a total of 442 observations of radiographs using a modification of the Oxford method. The relationship between scores and slips was determined.

Results.—Twenty children had slips in the contralateral hip. No significant difference between rater scores was noted. Modified Oxford scores varied between 16 and 24, with a score of 16 having an 85% risk of slip, and a score of 21 carrying a risk of 11%. Scores of 22 through 24 had a 0% risk of slip, and no slips occurred. For boys, younger age was predictive of slip, with slips developing in all 4 boys aged 11 years, 7 months and younger, in 9 of 22 boys older than 11 years, 7 months, and in no boys 15 years or older at the time of the initial slip. No age-associated risk for contralateral slip was noted in girls.

Conclusion.—Modified Oxford scores were associated with a risk of contralateral slip. Risk of contralateral slip was age related in boys but not in girls. No child with a score of 22 or higher had a slip.

▶ Should all patients with slipped capital femoral epiphysis have screw fixation of the normal hip? The maturity level determined by the Oxford method in this study defined the population that was not at risk for a slip on the contralateral side. It has been known that the more growth remaining at the time of an initial slip, the greater the chance of a slip on the contralateral side. I have found that the greater the loss of anteversion or the greater the degree of retroversion, the greater the risk of a slip of the contralateral hip. So immature patients with a score of 16 or less by the Oxford method who have retroversion are at such a high risk for slipping of the normal hip that bilateral screw fixation should be considered.

P.P. Griffin, M.D.

Flexible Intramedullary Nail Fixation of Pediatric Femoral Fractures
Carey TP, Galpin RD (Univ of Western Ontario, London, Ont)
Clin Orthop 332:110–118, 1996   8–6

Background.—Management of femoral shaft fractures in children has evolved toward a more operative approach in the past decade to speed recovery and avoid the negative effects of prolonged immobilization. Economic pressures have also prompted clinicians to adopt approaches that do not require prolonged hospitalization. Authorities have advocated external fixation, compression plating, and intramedullary nailing for the treatment of pediatric femoral shaft fractures. One experience with antegrade flexible intramedullary nailing in children was reviewed.

Methods and Findings.—Twenty-five children aged 5.7 to 10.9 years with a total of 27 femoral shaft fractures were treated. None had non-unions or significant malunions. Follow-up assessments of limb lengths and proximal femoral morphology demonstrated minor variations in articulotrochanteric distance and neck shaft angle. None of these variations were clinically significant. Minor limb length discrepancy measures showed no consistent pattern of overgrowth. Radiographic follow-up demonstrated no evidence of complete trochanteric growth arrest (Fig 1).

Conclusions.—This preliminary experience suggests that flexible intramedullary nailing is safe and effective in 6- to 12-year-old children with femoral fractures. This treatment reduces the risk of malunion, accelerates

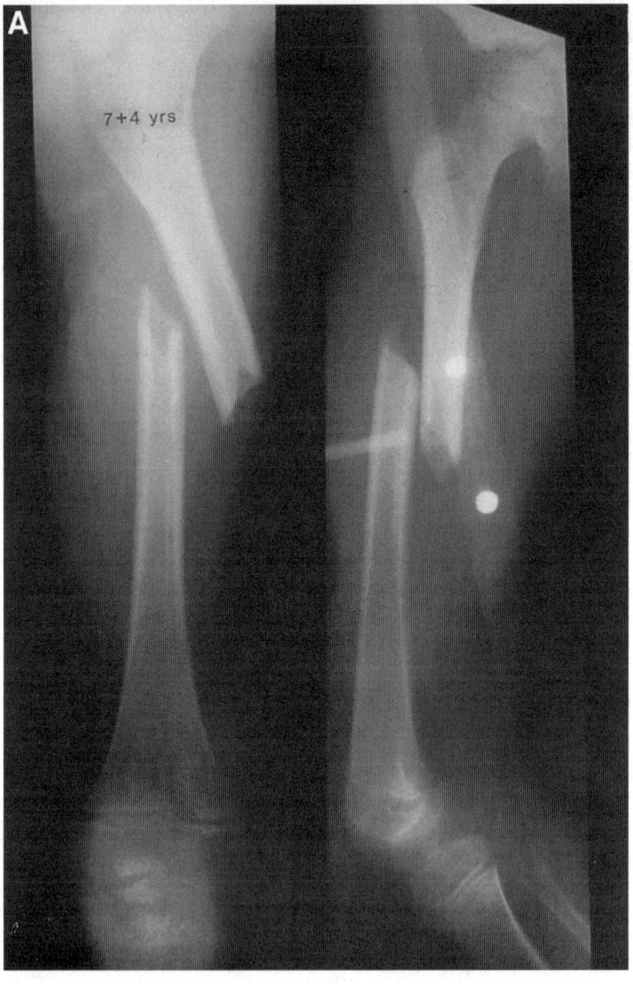

(Continued)

FIGURE 1 (cont.)

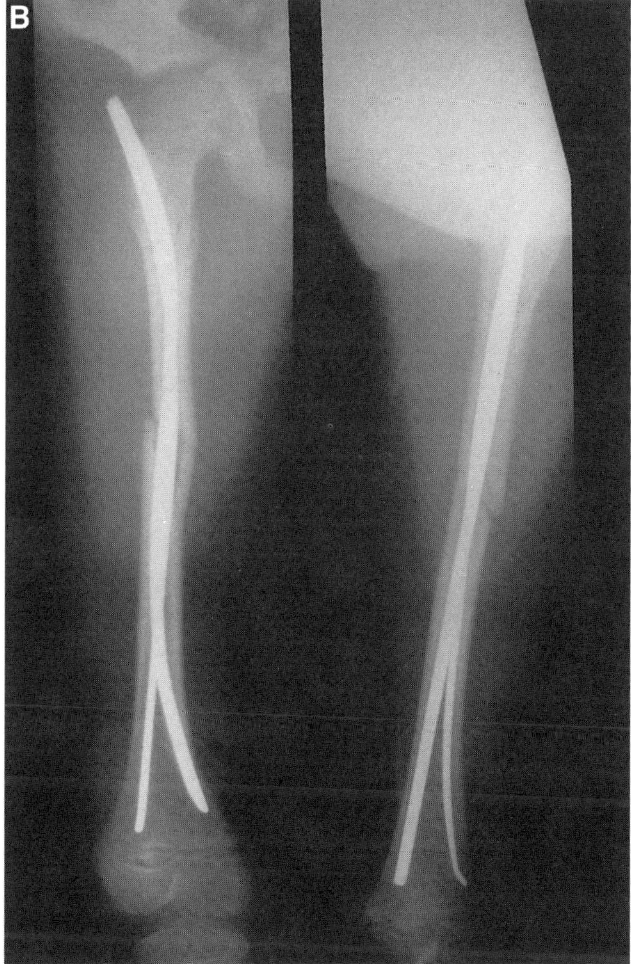

(*Continued*)

the rate of rehabilitation, and decreases the financial and emotional cost to the patients' families.

▶ Intramedullary (IM) fixation of fractures of long bones has become popular in Europe. Is IM fixation the treatment of choice for fractures in 4- to 10-year-olds? If well done, complications should be few. It may be that social conditions or family dynamics will drive this treatment. I know of few reasons to choose IM fixation in this population other than the necessity to accommodate the family.

P.P. Griffin, M.D.

FIGURE 1 (cont.)

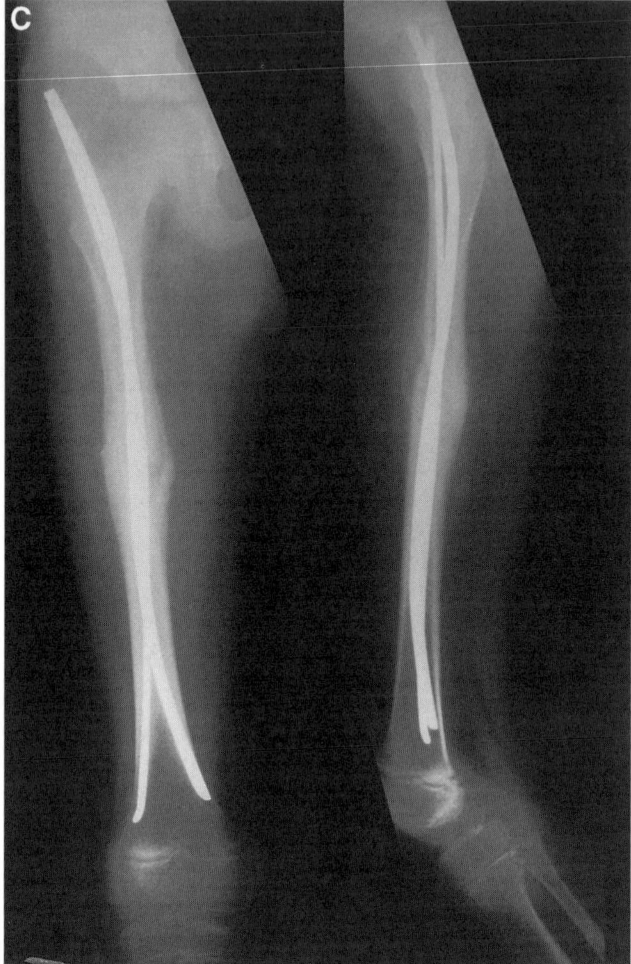

FIGURE 1.—A short oblique diaphyseal femoral fracture was sustained by a 7-year, 4-month-old boy in a motor vehicle accident. **A,** anteroposterior (AP, **left**) and lateral (**right**) radiographs before surgery. **B,** postoperative AP (**left**) and lateral (**right**) films showing fracture stabilization by 2 flexible intramedullary nails contoured into C and S shapes. **C,** 3-month follow-up AP (**left**) and lateral (**right**) films show healing with maintenance of alignment and abundant callus formation. (Courtesy of Carey TP, Galpin RD: Flexible intramedullary nail fixation of pediatric femoral fractures. *Clin Orthop* 332:110-118, 1996.)

Flexible Intramedullary Nailing as Fracture Treatment in Children
Huber RI, Keller HW, Huber PM, et al (Univ of Cologne, Germany; Univ of Utah, Salt Lake City)
J Pediatr Orthop 16:602–605, 1996   8–7

Introduction.—Intramedullary nailing with flexible titanium pins can be used as an alternative to plaster cast immobilization in children with fractures.

Methods.—Flexible intramedullary nailing is performed under general anesthesia and radiographic control. The 50-cm flexible titanium pins range from 2 to 4 mm in diameter to match different bone strengths. The principle involves transforming traction forces to compression forces on the fracture with 2 bent pins that cross each other and touch the bone at 3 points. Fractures of the femur, tibia, and humerus are stabilized with 2 crossing pins. Forearm fractures are splinted with a single pin. In radial head fractures, the displaced radial head is collected and anatomically reduced by a spin of the pin. Pins are removed after 10 weeks.

Results.—During 1991 and 1992, 28 children with fractures were treated by intramedullary stabilization with titanium pins. Wound healing was primary. A plaster cast was applied for 3 weeks to all fractures treated with 1 pin to avoid rotation. Children with lower extremity fractures were allowed partial weight-bearing the next day and full weight-bearing after 3 weeks. No intraoperative or postoperative complications were observed. The median hospital stay was 5 days. All fractures were successfully treated. The median follow-up was 6 months after pin removal.

Conclusions.—These authors recommend intramedullary stabilization with flexible prebent titanium pins for fractures in children aged 4–12 years. For children with multiple trauma, pin stabilization reduces operative time, exposure to x-rays, and postoperative immobilization.

▶ Internal fixation of femoral fractures in children may have socioeconomic value because of the shorter period of dependency. This report is on a technique for intramedullary (IM) fixation that avoids the problem of avascular necrosis associated with the standard IM fixation procedure. I think that in most femoral fractures, fixation with retrograde flexible nails is equally good and may be easier to do.

P.P. Griffin, M.D.

Severe (Type III) Open Fractures of the Tibia in Children
Buckley SL, Smith GR, Sponseller PD, et al (Emory Clinic, Atlanta, Ga; Children's Natl Med Ctr, Washington, DC; Johns Hopkins Hosp, Baltimore, Md; et al)
J Pediatr Orthop 16:627–634, 1996   8–8

Introduction.—In adults, type III open fractures of the tibia have been associated with an increased incidence of delayed union, nonunion, and infection. The delayed amputation rate is nearly 75% in adults with type IIIC open tibia fractures. The outcome of type III open fractures of the tibia in children is not known. Described are the complications and outcomes of severe type III open fractures of the tibia in children.

Methods.—The records of 20 children with acute type III open fractures of the tibial metaphyses or diaphysis were reviewed retrospectively. The average patient age was 9 years, 1 month. The fibula was fractured in all except 1 child. Fracture types were IIIA in 7, IIIB in 10, and IIIC in 3. Thirteen children had other injuries, including other fractures in 10, closed head injuries in 4, abdominal injury in 1, and 1 pulmonary contusion in 1. All fractures underwent irrigation and débridement in the operating room. Patients received prophylactic tetanus and parenteral antibiotics for at least 48 hours. Treatment approaches included external fixation in 15, above-knee casts in 3, internal fixation in 1 and a combination of external fixation and limited internal fixation in 1. Wound coverage included split-thickness skin grafts in 5, free muscle flaps in 6, delayed primary closure in 4, closure by secondary intention in 2, and a local muscle flap in 1. The remaining 2 wounds were clean and uncomplicated and were closed primarily.

Results.—The average time to fracture healing was 29 weeks in this patient series. Four and 2 patients, respectively, had delayed union and nonunion. The 2 patients with nonunion fractures were treated successfully with autologous bone grafting. A correlation was noted between the time to fracture union and the severity of soft tissue injury, fracture configuration, segmental bone loss, and infection. In 3 patients, osteomyelitis developed but was subsequently treated successfully. Two patients treated with external rotation had a leg length discrepancy of greater than 1 cm in the treated leg. No patients underwent late amputation.

Conclusion.—The incidence of osteomyelitis, delayed union, and nonunion occurs with similar frequency in adults and children with type III open fractures of the tibia. Children seem to respond to the treatment of these complications with a higher success rate than is observed in adults. With aggressive wound care and fracture management, children with type III open fractures of the tibia have a good prognosis for limb salvage.

▶ Children with severe open fractures will do well if soft tissue and bone are adequately débrided and the fracture is stabilized. However, complications such as nonunion, delayed union, and osteomyelitis do occur just as in adults, but children respond better to treatment of these problems than adults do. An external fixator has many merits, but this study shows that it can cause delayed union and leg length discrepancy.

P.P. Griffin, M.D.

Rib Fractures in 31 Abused Infants: Postmortem Radiologic-Histopathologic Study

Kleinman PK, Marks SC Jr, Nimkin K, et al (Univ of Massachusetts, Worcester; Commonwealth of Massachusetts, Boston)
Radiology 200:807–810, 1996

8–9

Introduction.—Most rib fractures in abused infants are the result of thoracic compression. Fractures near the costovertebral articulations are consistent with anteroposterior compression. Fractures involving the lateral and anterior rib arcs and the costochondral junction (CCJ) of the ribs in abused infants were examined to determine factors influencing radiographic visualization and gather information regarding the mechanism of injury of rib fractures in abused infants.

Methods.—Thirty-one infants who died of inflicted skeletal injuries underwent premortem or postmortem skeletal surveys taken with a single-emulsion, single-screen, high-detail imaging system. Anteroposterior radiography of the chest was performed. When rib fractures were suspected on the frontal radiograph, left and right posterior oblique views were taken. Histologic specimens were obtained and correlated with radiographic features.

Results.—The average infant age was 3 months. Eighty-four (51%) of 165 fractures in this series of abused infants were rib fractures. Thirty fractures (36%) were visible on the skeletal survey, and the rest required radiography of the specimen, pathologic analysis, or both. The distribution of the rib fractures was the rib head in 28, the costovertebral articulation in 27, the posterior arc in 8, the lateral arc in 5, the anterior arc in 6, and the CCJ region in 10. The lateral and anterior arc fractures had a tendency to impact along the inner cortex of the rib, and CCJ fractures were likely to involve the inner aspect of the osteochondral interface with an associated osseous fragment. The most common indicators of fractures were histopathologic features indicating healing: organizing hemorrhage with fibrosis, cartilaginous and bony callus, and subperiosteal new bone formation.

Conclusion.—Postmortem examination revealed that the rib cage was the most common site of fractures in abused infants. The fractures were not usually visible on standard radiographs. The most common indicators of fractures were histopathologic features of healing. Imaging protocols with high-detail, screen-film systems may be used in living and dead infants to maximize detection of indicators of infant abuse. Oblique views of the thorax should be included.

▶ It seems that child abuse is recognized more frequently than in the past. The diagnosis is not always obvious, but the consequences of missing the diagnosis can be devastating. This study shows that rib fractures are common in child abuse. The presence of a posterior rib fracture is, in my opinion, diagnostic of abuse. When abuse is suggested, oblique as well as anteroposterior and lateral views of the chest should always be taken.

P.P. Griffin, M.D.

Musculoskeletal Complications of Varicella

Schreck P, Schreck P, Bradley J, et al (Children's Hosp, San Diego, Calif)
J Bone Joint Surg Am 78:1713–1719, 1996   8–10

Introduction.—Varicella has some uncommon, but serious complications in children that can be life and limb threatening: osteomyelitis, necrotizing fasciitis, septic arthritis, and abscess. The association between varicella and serious secondary musculoskeletal infections requiring operative treatment was evaluated in a large series of children. The etiology of these infections was analyzed.

Methods.—The records of all children hospitalized with a diagnosis of varicella and its complications over an 11-year period (1984–1994) were retrospectively reviewed. Pertinent demographic, laboratory, imaging, surgical, pathologic, and patient data were collected. There were 417 admissions.

Results.—The average patient age was 4.1 years. Twenty-six patients had 27 admissions for musculoskeletal complications of varicella that required surgery. All 26 children were immunocompetent. Complications included osteomyelitis in 7, septic arthritis in 4, necrotizing fasciitis in 5, deep tissue abscess in 10, and toxic shock syndrome requiring multiple limb amputations in 1. A significant increase was noted in the ratio of admissions for varicella-related complications to total hospital admissions in 1994 as compared with previous years. Eleven (41%) of the 27 admissions for musculoskeletal complications requiring surgery occurred in 1994. The causative bacterial pathogen was identified in 25 of the 27 infectious complications. Twenty-one (78%) of 25 were caused by group A β-hemolytic streptococci: 5 of 7 patients with osteomyelitis, 2 of 4 patients with septic arthritis, 3 of 5 patients with necrotizing fasciitis, and all 10 patients with deep tissue abscess. Osteomyelitis was caused by *Staphylococcus aureus* in 1 patient. In 1994, group A β-hemolytic streptococcus was the causative organism in 9 of the 11 musculoskeletal complications requiring surgery.

Conclusion.—Group A β-hemolytic streptococcus was the predominant cause of musculoskeletal complications of varicella in an 11-year period in a series of patients hospitalized in San Diego, California. Physicians must have a high level of suspicion for musculoskeletal infection when examining children with varicella who have localized warmth and erythema, swelling, and pain and refuse to bear weight. Prompt and effective medical and surgical treatment is required to prevent the spread of infection and loss of life or limb.

▶ The increased frequency of musculoskeletal infections complicating varicella may be peculiar only to the San Diego area. When a child with varicella complains of pain in an extremity, a musculoskeletal infection must be ruled out as the cause. We should teach our medical friends to be alert to this complication because prompt treatment is necessary for success.

P.P. Griffin, M.D.

Hip Problems

Magnetic Resonance Imaging of Knee Injuries in Children
King SJ, Carty HML, Brady O (Royal Liverpool Children's NHS Trust, England)
Pediatr Radiol 26:287–290, 1996   8–11

Background.—Magnetic resonance imaging is superior to other imaging techniques in revealing internal derangement of the knee, and it is useful in diagnosing tears of the meniscus. Meniscal appearance in children undergoing MRI has not been previously described. The significance of meniscal appearance and the frequency of abnormalities detected via MRI were evaluated in a large series of children with knee injuries.

Methods.—Magnetic resonance imaging was performed on 74 children aged 5–16 years with unfused epiphyses (78 consecutive imaging studies). Conventional grading techniques were used to evaluate the menisci, and the chi-squared method was used to compare the frequencies of medial and lateral meniscus and anterior cruciate ligament tears. The results were compared with published data for children.

Results.—The sensitivity (100%) and specificity (89%) of MRI for meniscal tears were calculated by using arthroscopic data from 26 children. Most studies (82%) revealed grade I or II signal intensity in 1 or both menisci. In the 33% of this group evaluated arthroscopically, all had normal menisci. Injuries of the anterior cruciate ligament were less frequent than previously reported and were significantly less frequent than tears of the medial and lateral menisci.

Conclusions.—These data indicate that grade I and II intrameniscal signal intensities are a normal finding in children. Medial and lateral meniscal tears are significantly more common in this population than are tears of the anterior cruciate ligament. Meniscal MRI appears to be reliable in children.

▶ This study defines MRI criteria for the diagnosis of a meniscal tear in children. Arthroscopic evaluation was done in a third of the patients and the accuracy of MRI confirmed. Treatment of meniscal and anterior cruciate ligament (ACL) tears in children has not yet been defined. We need to know the outcome of known meniscal and ACL tears treated conservatively.

P.P. Griffin, M.D.

Hip Abnormalities Detected by Ultrasound in Clinically Normal Newborn Infants
Terjesen T, Holen KJ, Tegnander A (Trondheim Univ, Norway)
J Bone Joint Surg Br 78:636–640, 1996   8–12

Background.—Ultrasound evaluation of the hips of newborn infants can detect abnormalities that are not evident clinically. However, whether such abnormalities require treatment from birth has not been established.

To further elucidate the clinical course of ultrasonically detected hip abnormalities in newborns, a series of children with US but without clinical hip lesions were studied.

Methods.—Ultrasonographic evaluation of the hips was performed on 9,952 newborn infants. Clinical examination was also conducted by both a pediatrician and an orthopedic surgeon; hips were considered potentially abnormal if the femoral head coverage was less than 50% or the joint seemed unstable during manipulation. The examinations were repeated after 2 to 3 months for infants with normal clinical examination results and abnormal US results. Infants with continued US abnormalities underwent a third evaluation, including a standard anteroposterior radiograph at 4 to 5 months of age. Treatment with an abduction splint was instituted for infants with abnormal findings on both US and radiologic examination.

Results.—Of the 9,952 newborns undergoing US evaluation of the hips over a period of 6 years, 306 had abnormal findings (31 per 1,000 live births). At the 2 to 3-month follow-up, 245 infants had normal hips. At the 4- to 5-month follow-up, 291 infants had normal hips. The 15 infants with abnormal hips showed no pronounced deterioration or frank dislocation and all became normal after treatment.

Conclusions.—Treatment from birth does not appear necessary in newborn infants who have hip abnormalities evident via US but normal clinical findings. Delay in beginning treatment did not affect outcome in these patients, but if US evidence of dislocation or clinical instability is detected, immediate treatment is reasonable. Otherwise, treatment may be postponed until the age of 4 or 5 months because most hip abnormalities resolve spontaneously. Treatment should be based on the results of both radiography and US.

▶ Many studies have been published about US and developmental dysplasia of the hip (DDH). This study found US findings that are considered by current standards to be abnormal in children who had normal physical findings. Without treatment, only 15 of 306 such hips had abnormal US measurements at 4 or 5 months of age. This study confirms that static US measurements alone are not sufficient evidence to treat an infant for DDH. The important aspect of management in this group of infants who have a normal physical examination with abnormal US findings is careful repeated evaluations. When there is progressive improvement in acetabular development, continued observation is appropriate.

P.P. Griffin, M.D.

Organism Isolation and Serum Bactericidal Titers in Oral Antibiotic Therapy for Pediatric Osteomyelitis

Marshall GS, Mudido P, Rabalais GP, et al (Univ of Louisville, Ky)
South Med J 89:68–70, 1996   8–13

Background.—Oral antibiotic therapy for pediatric ostcomyelitis is considered acceptable provided that, among other caveats, the etiologic organism is identified and serum bactericidal titers (SBTs) are monitored. However, no causative organism is isolated in many cases of osteomyelitis, and no evidence definitively links SBT monitoring with clinical outcome. The validity of these conventional prerequisites for oral treatment of skeletal infection was examined.

Findings.—Records were reviewed for 36 patients in a children's hospital (median age, 4 years) in whom acute hematogenous osteomyelitis was diagnosed over a 5-year period. Ten patients underwent treatment with IV antibiotics for a median of 45 days. Causative organisms were isolated in 5 of these children and 5 had SBTs determined; all outcomes were excellent. Sequential parenteral-oral antibiotic therapy was received by 26 children (median durations of therapy: IV, 17 days; oral, 27 days). Causative organisms were identified in 17 of these children; SBTs were determined for only 7. All these children also did well, with no incidence of residua or relapse after a median follow-up of 1 year.

Conclusions.—For pediatric patients with acute hematogenous osteomyelitis, isolation of an etiologic organism may not be an absolute prerequisite for changing from IV to oral therapy. Oral therapy may be an acceptable alternative, especially for older children who respond favorably to initial empirical IV antistaphylococcal antibiotic treatment. Furthermore, if compliance is rigorously assessed and clinical improvement is documented via interval histories and serial examinations, SBT monitoring of patients receiving oral therapy may not always be necessary.

▶ It has been taught that to use oral antibiotics in the treatment of acute hematogenous osteomyelitis, certain prerequisites are necessary, namely, good response to the initial IV antibiotic, isolation of the etiologic organism, an effective oral agent, assurance of compliance, and the ability to monitor serum bactericidal levels. This study showed that oral antibiotics after an initial period of IV treatment can effectively treat osteomyelitis without monitoring the serum level of the antibiotics. The response to treatment— decreased swelling, pain, and temperature—gives the most reliable information as to whether the treatment is effective. The authors support their conclusion that oral therapy is effective without the need for isolation of an etiologic agent or the necessity of having SBT available. The clinical response to treatment is the most important guide to the effectiveness of treatment, but the aforementioned prerequisites, where available, should be considered.

P.P. Griffin, M.D.

Effect of Early Hip Decompression on the Frequency of Avascular Necrosis in Children With Fractures of the Neck of the Femur
Ng GPK, Cole WG (Hosp for Sick Children, Toronto)
Injury 27:419–421, 1996   8–14

Objective.—Recent studies have suggested that the incidence of avascular necrosis in fractures of the neck of the femur in children is reduced by early decompression of the hip with reduction and internal fixation of the fracture. The effect of early hip decompression with reduction and internal fixation of displaced high-risk fractures was prospectively evaluated in 32 children treated between January 1967 and January 1993.

Methods.—Reviews were performed on 32 children (14 girls) with an average age of 9 at least 18 months after injury. Four type I, 11 type II, 12 type III, and 5 type IV fractures were treated within 36 hours of injury. Internal fixation with supplementary hip-spica immobilization was used for 26 fractures. Decompression by aspiration or capsulotomy was performed in 2 and 11 children, respectively.

Results.—Nine children had type I (7), type II (1), and type III (1) avascular necrosis within a year after fracture in 3 type I, 5 type II, 1 type III, and no type IV fractures. Seven patients with avascular necrosis had displaced fractures. Avascular necrosis occurred in 3 of 6 patients with displaced type II and type III fractures without decompression and in 1 of 10 patients with decompression. When data from these patients were combined with data from similar patients, avascular necrosis was found in significantly more patients without decompression (22 of 54, 41%) than in patients with decompression (3 of 39, 8%).

Conclusion.—Early decompression reduces the likelihood of avascular necrosis in children with type II and III fractures of the neck of the femur. Avascular necrosis was more likely to develop in displaced fractures. Reduction and internal fixation minimize nonunion, malunion, and premature closure.

▶ The effect of tamponade from intracapsular pressure has been discussed for years as a factor in the frequency of avascular necrosis (AVN) after fractures of the femoral neck. In this study, hips with type II and III fractures that had early hip aspiration had a significantly lower incidence of AVN than did those hips not aspirated. For now it appears from this study that type II and III fractures of the hip in children should have early aspiration of the hip as routine management.

P.P. Griffin, M.D.

Conventional Radiography and Bone Scintigraphy in the Prognostic Evaluation of Legg-Calvé-Perthes Disease

Kaniklides C, Sahlstedt B, Lönnerholm T, et al (Univ Hosp, Uppsala, Sweden)
Acta Radiol 37:561–566, 1996   8–15

Background.—In Legg-Calvé-Perthes disease (LCPD), avascular necrosis results in growth disturbance in the femoral head. The involved segment may collapse and cause various femoral head deformities. Because incongruity between the articular surfaces may result in early degenerative changes, early identification of hips with an unfavorable prognosis is important. The prognostic value of radiography and bone scintigraphy on LCPD was investigated.

Methods.—Seventy-five children with 86 affected hips were monitored until primary healing. Conventional radiography was performed at the initial assessment, at the time of maximum capital head involvement, and at the end of the healing process. Findings on conventional radiography were compared with early bone scintigraphy features.

Findings.—When compared with initial radiographs, bone scintigraphy provided more accurate information on the extent of the necrotic process. It also determined revascularization and, consequently, disease stage. However, bone scintigraphy did not predict the outcome of disease in some patients, especially if it was performed late after symptom onset. Conventional radiography contributed important information about other parameters such as head-at-risk signs, which facilitated treatment decision making. Metaphyseal changes as well as lateral subluxation strongly predisposed to severe deformity of the hip joint.

Conclusions.—Bone scintigraphy performed early in the course of disease can provide information about disease stage and detect the extent of necrosis in most patients. Conventional radiography provides information about the shape of the hip joint and demonstrates changes important in prognostication. Combining these 2 modalities is of greater prognostic value than using either alone. Clinicians should assess bone scans and radiographs at the same time.

▶ I believe that surgical treatment of Legg-Calvé-Perthes disease improves results over the natural history of the disease. Poor results are related to the extent of deformity at healing. Selection of patients for surgical treatment (those with over half of the head involved and minimal or no deformity) can best be done by the use of well-performed scintigraphy and conventional radiographs. Scintigraphy done early will show the extent of involvement and, if done later, will show whether revascularization has taken place, in which case further collapse is not likely to occur, particularly if the lateral column is revascularized.

P.P. Griffin, M.D.

Vascularity of the Neonatal Femoral Head: In Vivo Demonstration With Power Doppler US
Bearcroft PW, Berman LH, Robinson AHN, et al (Univ of Cambridge, England; Addenbrooke's Hosp, Cambridge, England)
Radiology 200:209–211, 1996   8–16

Background.—Avascular necrosis resulting from compromise of the blood supply to the developing femoral head is an iatrogenic complication of treatment of hip dysplasia in infants with positional abduction restraints. Power Doppler US was used to study the intrinsic blood supply of the unossified neonatal femoral head in vivo, and whether blood flow was reduced with hip abduction was determined.

Methods.—Power Doppler US was performed in 1 hip of 13 neonates. Vessels in the femoral head were identified, and the thigh was slowly abducted. The angle at which flow became undetectable was recorded. Spectral Doppler tracings were recorded in all neonates.

Findings.—In all babies, intrinsic blood flow of the femoral head was demonstrated. In 11 of the 13, flow became undetectable during hip abduction but reappeared during adduction. Flow became undetectable at angles ranging between 60 and 85 degrees. A mixed arterial and venous trace was seen on spectral Doppler.

Conclusions.—Power Doppler US may be useful in identifying neonates at risk of avascular necrosis. This imaging modality allows a simple, real-time assessment of the femoral head blood supply.

▶ The demonstration that the epiphyseal vessels of the femoral head can be identified by power Doppler US contributes another valuable evaluation to the treatment of developmental dysplasia of the hip. If vascular flow is compromised with less than 60% of abduction, the Pavlik harness may not be a good choice for management of the dysplastic hip. It would be interesting to detect the point in abduction at which the flow is stopped before and after treatment to see whether it is the degree of abduction or the pressure against the femoral head that impedes vascular flow.

P.P. Griffin, M.D.

Use of the Milwaukee Brace for Progressive Idiopathic Scoliosis
Noonan KJ, Weinstein SL, Jacobson WC, et al (Orlando Regional Med Ctr, Fla; Univ of Iowa, Iowa City)
J Bone Joint Surg Am 78:557–567, 1996   8–17

Objective.—For many years, the Milwaukee brace and other braces have been used for the nonoperative treatment of idiopathic scoliosis. However, it is still uncertain whether bracing is effective in halting the progression of scoliotic curves. The results of Milwaukee bracing in a large group of patients with idiopathic scoliosis at high risk of progression are reported.

Methods.—The study included 102 patients who began using the Milwaukee brace for idiopathic scoliosis when they were at least 8 years old. For patients managed nonoperatively, it had been an average of 6 years from the cessation of bracing until the latest radiographs were made. The brace's effects in preventing progression of the curve were analyzed. Certain variables were examined for their possible effects on treatment, including sex, skeletal immaturity, curve pattern and magnitude, rotation of the apical vertebra, spinal balance, the response of the curve, and patient compliance. Statistical analyses were performed in 88 patients.

Results.—In the statistical analysis, the curve progressed by an average of 4 degrees from the start to the finish of bracing. For patients who did not undergo arthrodesis, the amount of additional progression after cessation of bracing was 5 degrees. Progression at the time that brace use stopped exceeded 5 degrees in 48% of the patients, and 42% underwent surgery or had a curve sufficient to warrant an operation. The average correction of the Cobb angle in patients whose curve did not progress or who did not require surgery was 20% as compared with 8% in patients in whom bracing failed. Patients meeting the criteria for arthrodesis averaged 1 year younger and had curves of greater magnitude than did those who did not require arthrodesis.

Conclusions.—In contrast to previous studies, this study questions whether the Milwaukee brace truly alters the natural history of progressive idiopathic scoliosis in immature patients. Bracing will maintain the scoliotic curve in some patients, but it may progress after bracing stops. Bracing has no effect on curve progression in other patients who are candidates for arthrodesis. A controlled, prospective study with long-term follow-up of patients at similar risk is needed to determine the true efficacy of bracing.

▶ The effectiveness of a spinal orthosis in changing the natural history of idiopathic scoliosis continues to be controversial. This study is as thorough as a retrospective study can be, but yet cannot prove or disapprove that bracing scoliosis prevents progression. The excellent analysis of the multiple variables in the small number of patients available for study in this paper gave results that raised the authors' doubts that brace treatment of scoliosis is effective. More prospective long-term studies are needed.

P.P. Griffin, M.D.

Torticollis Secondary to Ocular Pathology

Williams CRP, O'Flynn E, Clarke NMP, et al (Southampton Univ, England)
J Bone Joint Surg Br 78:620–624, 1996   8–18

Introduction.—Torticollis is one of the most frequent causes of abnormal head posture in children. A review was prompted after seeing a child with torticollis but no structural muscle contracture. The child was referred for ophthalmic evaluation after no response to physical therapy or manipulation under anesthesia. The abnormal head posture resolved after treatment of a palsy of the superior oblique muscle. From that time on, all children with torticollis of unknown etiology were referred for ophthalmic assessment.

Methods.—Over a 12-month period, all children referred with torticollis but no obvious orthopedic cause underwent ophthalmic evaluation. The age range of 9 girls and 5 boys was 3 months to 4 years. One patient was a girl 15 years of age. The children underwent plain radiographs of the cervical spine. The teenager had MRI of the neck and posterior fossa of the skull. All patients underwent history and full ophthalmic assessment, including extraocular muscle balance and binocular status. Before referral, no patients had any apparent ocular abnormalities.

Results.—Eight children with normal ocular examinations had plagiocephaly. Of 7 children with abnormal ocular examinations, 3 had plagiocephaly. Five of 7 children with abnormal ocular examinations had ocular causes of torticollis. In the nonocular group, 3 had congenital dislocation of the hip. Of these 3, 1 child had congenital vertical talus and renal insufficiency and 1 had partial deletion of chromosome 10. There were no other diagnoses in the group of children with ocular causes of torticollis. Two and 3 children in the ocular group had an abnormal head posture at birth and 3 months of age, respectively. In the nonocular group, torticollis was diagnosed at birth in 7 children and at 3 months, 3 years, and 13 years in 1 each. In the nonocular group, 8 children had no family history of any ocular mobility disorder and 2 had a history of a second-degree relative with strabismus. In the ocular group, 2 children had no family history of ocular disorder, 2 had a first-degree relative with a squint, and the father of 1 child with nystagmus was similarly affected. All children had full symmetric range of cervical movement. One and 5 patients in the ocular and nonocular groups, respectively, had a palpably tight sternomastoid muscle at maximum tension.

All 3 patients with underaction of the superior oblique muscle required extraocular muscle surgery to weaken the inferior oblique muscle of the affected eye. In 2 patients, this reduced the head tilt. In the remaining patient, restoration of binocular single vision eliminated the abnormal head posture. The child with nystagmus has a cosmetically acceptable variation of head posture that has not required surgery. One patient with paresis of the sixth cranial nerve improved spontaneously and has not required treatment. Two patients in the nonocular group underwent surgical release of a tight sternomastoid muscle. One had good results but the teenage girl required continuing physical therapy. Seven children responded to physical therapy alone. In 2 children, torticollis resolved spontaneously.

Conclusion.—Paralytic squint and nystagmus can lead to torticollis in children. When orthopedic evaluation reveals no structural cause of torticollis, an ocular origin should be considered and followed with an ophthalmic assessment.

▶ In my experience the frequency of torticollis in infancy has decreased. Close observation of an infant with torticollis usually fails to detect the mass in the sternocleidomastoid muscle that has been described in this condition.

Most infants with torticollis will spontaneously correct the asymmetry of the face and head and have normal motion by 1 year of age. Those that do not correct by age 1 should be considered for surgical release. Failure to detect limited motion or muscle tightness should raise the possibility of a visual etiology. If the infant is thought to have muscle tightness but fails to respond to surgical lengthening, an eye evaluation should be done.

P.P. Griffin, M.D.

Subacute Hematogenous Osteomyelitis: Are Biopsy and Surgery Always Indicated?

Hamdy RC, Lawton L, Carey T, et al (Children's Hosp of Eastern Ontario, Ottawa, Canada)
J Pediatr Orthop 16:220–223, 1996　　　　　　　　　　　　　　　8–19

Objective.—Whether subacute hematogenous osteomyelitis should be managed surgically or conservatively is controversial. The results of conservative vs. surgical management, the necessity of biopsy of the lesion, and indications for surgical débridement were retrospectively reviewed.

Methods.—The records of 44 consecutive patients (12 girls) aged 1–16 were reviewed. Lesions were most often found in the tibia (27%) and the pelvis (18%). An organism was isolated from 20 of 44 patients, and in 17 patients the pathogen was *Staphylococcus aureus.* Blood cultures were negative, but 15 of 20 intraoperative swabs and 56% of the bony aspirates were positive. Radiologic findings (Roberts classification) included 10 type I(a), 10 type I(b), 4 type II, 3 type IV, 3 type V, 4 type VI, and 10 unclassified. No patients had type III disease. Twenty patients were treated surgically with débridement and curettage of the lesion, followed by antibiotics for an average of 6 weeks, and 24 were treated conservatively with antistaphyloccocal antibiotics. Patients were monitored for an average of 18 months.

Results.—No failures or recurrences occurred in 23 of 24 patients receiving antibiotics. One patient who received insufficient antibiotic therapy required surgical débridement. All 20 patients treated surgically had no failures or recurrences. Radiologic evidence of healing appeared at 3–12 months.

Conclusion.—Conservative antibiotic therapy is as effective as surgical treatment for subacute hematogenous osteomyelitis.

▶ The diagnosis of subacute osteomyelitis can frequently be made by radiographs, with CT or MRI adding evidence when the orthopedic surgeon is not comfortable with the radiograph alone. When the lesion has the appearance of a benign lesion by having a well-defined sclerotic border or it is located in the epiphysis or crosses the physis, it is reasonable to make the diagnosis of subacute osteomyelitis. These patients will generally respond to antistaphylococcal antibiotic treatment without surgery. If the response to antibiotics is not satisfactory or the diagnosis by imaging is not sufficiently definitive, surgical treatment is necessary.

P.P. Griffin, M.D.

Intraoperative SSEP Monitoring During External Fixation Procedures in the Lower Extremities
Makarov MR, Delgado MR, Birch JG, et al (Texas Scottish Rite Hosp, Dallas; Univ of Texas, Dallas)
J Pediatr Orthop 16:155–160, 1996   8–20

Objective.—Acute peripheral nerve injury can occur during external fixation of the lower extremities. Although monitoring neural function during operative procedures via somatosensory evoked potentials (SSEPs) has been used to detect such injuries, its use has not been reported. A review of peripheral nerve injury associated with external fixation and its causes and outcome are presented.

Methods.—Ilizarov external fixator application was used to treat 42 short limbs (26 congenital and 14 acquired) in 40 children (10 girls) aged 6–17. Surgery was performed on the tibia in 22 patients, on the femur in 17, and on both in 3, and a bone corticotomy was performed on each treated segment. Additional procedures were performed on 13 patients. During the procedures SSEPs were monitored in both limbs.

Results.—Neurologic deficits developed in 2 patients postoperatively. Preoperative neuropathies worsened in 2 patients after surgery. The peroneal nerve was at greatest risk of injury.

> *Case 1.*—Girl, 8 years, with a clubfoot, tibial shortening, and a preoperative peroneal neuropathy experienced a deterioration of peroneal SSEPs after tibial corticotomy. After surgery she was found to have complete peroneal nerve palsy that partially resolved.
>
> *Case 2.*—Boy, 12 years, with a length difference and a varus deformity of the tibia had normal but lessened motor and sensory nerve conduction studies of the shortened leg before surgery. Somatosensory evoked potentials of the tibial and peroneal nerves disappeared when the tourniquet was applied, returned after its removal, but deteriorated after corticotomy. Dysesthesia and equinus contracture developed and necessitated cessation of limb lengthening. His foot was brought to neutral position via plantar fascia release with Achilles tendon lengthening.
>
> *Case 3.*—Boy, 13 years, with femoral and tibial shortening resulting from partial fibular hemimelia experienced partial tibial and complete loss of peroneal SSEPs. Nerve function recovery was incomplete after lengthening.
>
> *Case 4.*—Boy, 16 years, with tibial shortening as a result of partial fibular hemimelia experienced decreased peroneal ampli-

tude response and increased latency that did not resolve. The peroneal nerve palsy partially resolved but muscle strength has not been restored.

Conclusion.—Monitoring of SSEPs detected intraoperative nerve injury during external fixation procedures in the lower extremities.

▶ Nerve dysfunction after osteotomy and application of an Ilizarov apparatus can be devastating. The authors of this study suggest that SSEP monitoring during insertion of the wires and performance of the osteotomy may immediately detect nerve damage. Although immediate nerve damage during the procedure is not common, the use of SSEP monitoring while performing the procedure appears to be a good idea.

P.P. Griffin, M.D.

Bowlegs in Children

Hemiepiphyseal Stapling for Knee Deformities in Children Younger Than 10 Years: A Preliminary Report
Mielke CH, Stevens PM (Univ of Utah, Salt Lake City)
J Pediatr Orthop 16:423–429, 1996   8–21

Background.—Intervention is not usually required for angular deformity of the knee in children because it generally resolves spontaneously. When intervention is required, stapling is not generally recommended in children younger than 8 years because of fear of permanent growth arrest. A consecutive group of 25 children younger than 10 years treated with stapling for pathologic knee deformities is reported.

Patients.—Twenty-two children with pathologic genu valgum and 3 children with genu varum underwent hemiphyseal stapling to correct angular deformities of the knee. All patients had progressive, symptomatic deformity with significant displacement of the mechanical axis. The mean patient age at stapling was 6 years and 4 months; follow-up continued for an average of 3 years and 3 months.

> *Technique Overview.*—All growth plates are located fluoroscopically and the periosteum is carefully preserved while 1 or 2 Vitallium staples per physis are inserted and subsequently removed. Patients are evaluated every 3 or 4 months after insertion until staple removal is performed when the limb is straight clinically and radiographically (usually within 12–24 months after insertion.) Growth monitoring should be continued quarterly for the first year and then yearly until the patients are mature.

Results.—All patients experienced improvement of the mechanical axis and anatomical angle (tibiofemoral). Hardware failure, with the exception of 1 staple breaking at removal, did not occur. Patients with genu varum experienced a change from an average of 10.5 degrees of varus to 1.5 degrees of valgus with a neutral mechanical axis at follow-up. Patients with genu valgum underwent a change in average valgus from 20.4 degrees to 11.7 degrees postoperatively; their mechanical axes ratio changed from an average of 0.28 preoperatively to 0.11 at final follow-up. No premature physeal closure occurred. Further intervention was warranted in 7 patients, 6 of whom underwent further stapling.

Conclusions.—Despite empirical statements advising against stapling in children younger than 8 years, stapling is the only reversible means of manipulating growth, and in the authors' experience, a correctly performed stapling procedure can be reliable, predictable, and safe for children younger than 10 years. This technique is *not* intended for application with physiologic deformities that are likely to resolve spontaneously.

▶ Stapling can be a very effective method for correcting genu varum or valgum if the appropriate staple is used. Wire staples are not strong enough to resist the force of growth. The staple should be made of Vitallium. Meticulous placement without elevating the perichondrium or adjacent periosteum is important when inserting the staples, as well as when they are removed.

P.P. Griffin, M.D.

Physiological Bowlegs or Infantile Blount's Disease. Some New Aspects on an Old Problem
Eggert P, Viemann M (Universitäts-Kinderklinik, Kiel, Germany)
Pediatr Radiol 26:349–352, 1996   8–22

Background.—Differentiating between physiologic bowlegs and infantile Blount's disease is very difficult in children aged 11–30 months. The current study investigated whether the metaphyseal/diaphyseal angle is suitable for distinguishing one diagnosis from the other.

Methods.—Fourteen children with severe bowing of the legs were studied retrospectively. The patients were examined, and the tibiofemoral and metaphyseal/diaphyseal angles on radiographs obtained at the initial evaluations were measured.

Findings.—As expected, substantial variation of the tibiofemoral angle made it impossible to differentiate between Blount's disease and physiologic bowing with this parameter. The findings of metaphyseal/diaphyseal angle measurement were unexpected. Contrary to previous results by Levine and Drennan, measures of the metaphyseal/diaphyseal angle apparently do not differentiate between tibia vara and physiologic bowing. In the current series, some of these angles fell in a range that seemed to indicate physiologic bowleg according to Levine and Drennan, which was likely because the bowlegging disappeared in these children during the next months. However, many metaphyseal/diaphyseal angles fell in a range definitely indicating Blount's disease, which was clearly incorrect because

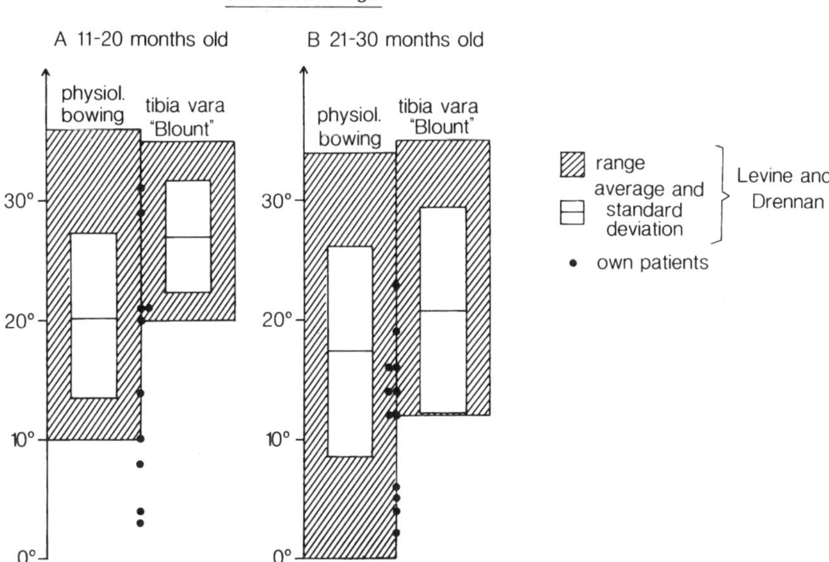

FIGURE 2.—A and B, A diagram showing the age-dependent tibiofemoral angle of our patients compared with data published by Levine and Drennan. (Courtesy of Eggert P, Viemann M: Physiological bowlegs or infantile Blount's disease: Some new aspects on an old problem. *Pediatr Radiol* 26:349–352, 1996. Copyright 1996 by Springer-Verlag.)

the bowlegging in these children also disappeared in the following months (Figs 2 and 3).

Conclusions.—Even with measurement of the metaphyscal/diaphyseal angle, it is impossible to safely differentiate physiologic bowlegging and early manifestations of infantile Blount's disease in 11- to 30-month-old children. The authors question whether infantile Blount's disease is a diagnosis in its own right.

▶ This study revisited Levine and Drennan's published criteria on the relationship of the femoral-tibial and the metaphyseal-diaphyseal angle to Blount's disease.[1] They were unable to differentiate Blount's disease and physiologic bowing by the recommended measurements. I agree that their measurements do not differentiate physiologic varus from Blount's disease. The radiographic changes of Blount's disease are more than beaking and bowing; rather it is the irregular ossification of the metaphyseal beaks that demonstrate the abnormal primary and secondary ossification in the medial metaphysis.

P.P. Griffin, M.D.

Reference

1. Levine AM, Drennan JC: Physiological bowing and tibia vara. *J Bone Joint Surg Am* 64:1158–1163, 1982.

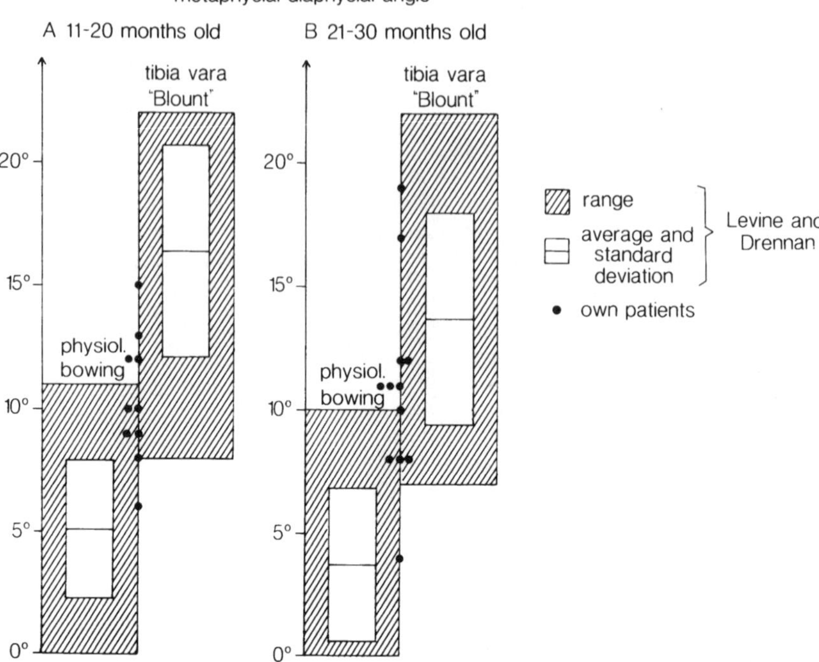

FIGURE 3.—A and **B.** A diagram showing the age-dependent metaphyseal/diaphyseal angle of our patients compared with data published by Levine and Drennan. (Courtesy of Eggert P, Viemann M: Physiological bowlegs or infantile Blount's disease: Some new aspects on an old problem. *Pediatr Radiol* 26:349–352, 1996. Copyright 1996 by Springer-Verlag.)

Dega Acetabuloplasty Combined With Intertrochanteric Osteotomies

Reichel H, Hein W (Martin-Luther-Univ Halle-Wittenberg, Germany)
Clin Orthop 323:234–242, 1996   8–23

Background.—Surgical treatment is sometimes needed in idiopathic developmental dysplasia of the hip. Factors that determine the operative method include the frequency of redislocation, rate of avascular necrosis of the femoral head, postoperative joint stiffness, influence on later joint development, and prevention of early osteoarthrosis. Combining acetabuloplasty with intertrochanteric osteotomy is controversial. It has been recommended that surgical correction of the acetabulum and open reduction of the hip joint be done simultaneously but that derotational varus osteotomy not be done. With this in mind a study was performed to investigate the long-term results of modified Dega acetabuloplasty with intertrochanteric osteotomy of the femur.

Methods.—A total of 70 modified Dega acetabuloplasties were performed simultaneously with intertrochanteric osteotomy of the femur in 51 patients with idiopathic developmental dysplasia of the hip. The mean patient age was 2.9 years. Mean follow-up was 15.2 years.

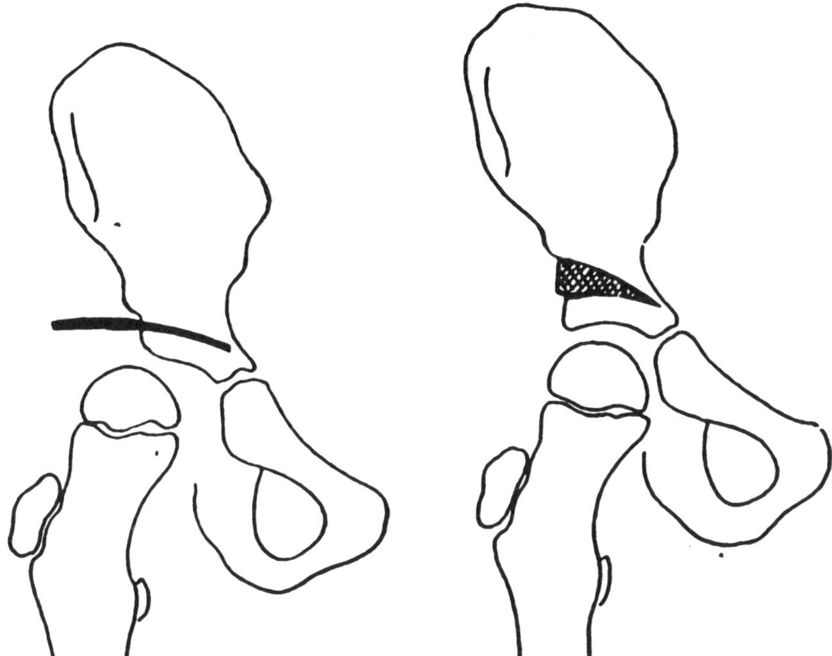

FIGURE 2.—Technique of modified Dega acetabuloplasty. The osteotomy of the ilium is done from a lateral position in the direction of the triradiate cartilage, and the medioposterior cortical corner remains intact (**left**). After levering down the entire acetabular roof, a bone wedge is interposed into the osteotomy gap to keep the acetabular roof in correct position (**right**). (Courtesy of Reichel H, Hein W: Dega acetabuloplasty combined with intertrochanteric osteotomies. *Clin Orthop* 323:234–242, 1996.)

Technique.—An anterolateral approach is used. After subperiosteal exposure of the lateral and medial surfaces of the ilium, the ilium is osteotomized in the direction of the triradiate cartilage from a lateral position above the anterior inferior iliac spine. The medioposterior cortical corner is left intact, and the acetabular roof is deflected into a lateral and anterior position (Fig 2).

Results.—The Severin classification and radiologic criteria of the Commission for the Study of Hip Dysplasia of the German Society of Orthopaedics and Traumatology were used. In 80% of the hips, results were good to very good. For difficult cases the Trendelenburg sign was useful. Radiographic measurements were categorized into deviation grades. In more than 80% of the hips, values for the acetabulum and the acetabulum-to-head relationship were normal or only slightly abnormal. Femoral head and neck measurements were in the low-normal range. Twenty-four cases of coxa valga occurred after acetabuloplasty with derotational varus osteotomy, and these had the lowest percentage of normal values. Poor outcome often resulted from avascular necrosis of the femoral head or recurring valgus deformity after derotational varus osteotomy. A 5.7% incidence of avascular necrosis caused by surgery was noted.

Discussion.—This combined surgical technique had generally good long-term results. The risk of avascular necrosis from derotational varus osteotomy is lower than the risk of deformities in the proximal portion of the femur. Longer follow-up is needed to study the development of osteoarthrosis.

▶ The Dega acetabuloplasty is effective in correcting the abnormal acetabular index and center edge angle and thus improving stability of the hip. I find that the Dega is easier to perform than the Pemberton osteotomy. It should be reserved for children under 4 years or so of age because of the remodeling required to give congruity in all degrees of motion. I have used it only in cerebral palsy patients and find it very effective in this group of patients.

P.P. Griffin, M.D.

Cuneiform Osteotomy of the Femoral Neck in Severe Slipped Capital Femoral Epiphysis

DeRosa GP, Mullins RC, Kling TF Jr (Indiana Univ, Indianapolis)
Clin Orthop 322:48–60, 1996   8–24

Objective.—Although cuneiform osteotomy of the femoral neck is the only procedure that restores anatomy to nearly normal, the safety and effectiveness of the procedure in children have not been established. Results of a retrospective evaluation of 27 grade III slipped epiphyses in 23 adolescent patients repaired by using a cuneiform osteotomy of the proximal neck of the femur are presented.

Methods.—Cuneiform osteotomies were performed on 15 boys and 8 girls aged 9.2–16.9 years, including bilateral procedures performed on 3 boys and 1 girl. Symptoms were present for an average of 10.4 months, and follow-up averaged 8.5 years. Pain, function, range of motion, and radiographic appearance were graded on the Southwick scale as good, fair, or poor.

Technique.—An anterior approach to the hip was used to release the femoral head. The hip joint capsule was incised with an H-shaped incision, the capsule was opened, and a wedge of femoral neck was resected. After the posterior cortex was removed, new bone formation was removed from the posteromedial neck and the osteotomy was fixed with 3 Knowles pins. Patients had limited activity for 8 weeks and were then given physical therapy.

Results.—All patients achieved good extension, flexion was 101 degrees, internal rotation was 23 degrees, external rotation was 47 degrees, final abduction was 40 degrees, and adduction was 30 degrees. When compared with preoperative results, flexion increased by 40 degrees, internal rotation by 40 degrees, and adduction by 17 degrees. External rotation decreased 8 degrees. There were 19 good, 4 fair, and 4 poor ratings. Partial or complete avascular necrosis developed in 4 hips (15%) of 3 patients, cartilage space narrowing occurred in 8 hips, fixation was lost in 2, and pin head exposure developed in 1. Joint flexion and internal rotation improved in patients with avascular necrosis. Joint space narrowing resolved by 20 months.

Conclusion.—Cuneiform osteotomy of the femoral neck is a suitable alternative treatment for severe slipped capital femoral epiphysis in adolescent patients.

▶ Osteotomy of the femoral neck to realign the capital epiphysis can be an effective procedure. The question one has to ask is whether the incidence of avascular necrosis (AVN) reported by most authors justifies this procedure as a treatment choice. I did approximately 30 of these from 1960 to 1978 and had 4 patients with severe chondrolysis and 2 of these 4 had AVN. It is a difficult operation because of the distorted anatomy and the proximity of the blood supply of the epiphysis. I believe that this procedure should be considered for the treatment of severe chronic slip if the surgeon who wants to use this procedure has observed the operation done by an experienced surgeon. The written description of the surgical procedure is not sufficient to learn the minutiae necessary to safely do this operation.

P.P. Griffin, M.D.

Infection

A Dynamic Biomechanical Analysis of the Etiology of Adolescent Tibia Vara

Davids JR, Huskamp M, Bagley AM (Shriners Hosp for Crippled Children, Greenville, SC)
J Pediatr Orthop 16:461–468, 1996   8–25

Background.—Although the etiology of infantile tibia vara or Blount's disease is well understood, the etiology of adolescent or late-onset tibia vara is more controversial. These authors propose that the gait deviations of obese adolescents used to compensate for increased thigh girth could lead to increased loading of the medial knee compartment and generate compressive forces that alter physeal growth. This dynamic process could cause the deformity characteristic of adolescent tibia vara. Three-dimensional motion analysis and an anthropometric model were used to examine the effects of excessive weight and gait on physeal development.

Methods.—Kinematic and kinetic analyses were performed on the gait of 6 normal adolescent boys. Their thigh radius was then increased by wrapping foam padding around each thigh to increase the girth by 75%. The subjects walked with neutral, internal and external foot progression angles. All reported that the external foot progression angle was the most natural in the padded condition. A fat-thigh gait kinematic/kinetic model was then generated. A mechanical model was also developed to quantify proximal tibial loading during gait.

Results.—Several gait deviations were associated with increased thigh girth, including dynamic stance-limb knee varus, increased stance-limb knee rotation, and swing-limb circumduction. When the fat-thigh gait deviation and excessive body weight parameters were applied to the anthropometric model, pathologic compressive forces were generated in the knee.

Conclusions.—This modeling study indicates that dynamic gait deviations used by obese adolescents to compensate for increased thigh girth can cause increased loading of the medial knee compartment. This increased dynamic loading coupled with excessive body weight can generate compressive forces sufficient to affect physeal growth and lead to the progressive proximal tibial deformity that is characteristic of adolescent tibia vara.

▶ Adolescents in whom bowing of the lower extremity develops and Blount's disease is diagnosed may have had perfectly normal-appearing lower extremities until adolescence. This study found that there is a dynamic varus force at the knee in gait. This force is found to be sufficient to retard growth on the medial side of the proximal tibial physis. I think that this force can also retard growth on the medial side of the distal tibial physis. I have found a varus deformity of the distal end of the femur that accounts for 30% to 70% of the varus deformity of the lower extremity in some patients with adolescent Blount's disease.

P.P. Griffin, M.D.

Prediction of Reduction in Developmental Dysplasia of the Hip by Magnetic Resonance Imaging

Kashiwagi N, Suzuki S, Kasahara Y, et al (Shiga Med Ctr for Children, Japan)
J Pediatr Orthop 16:254–258, 1996   8–26

Objective.—The contrast resolution of US is not always sufficient to allow evaluation of developmental dysplasia of the hip (DDH) and determine the extent of reduction accomplished with the Pavlik harness. Because recent evidence suggests that MRI may provide improved diagnostic imaging, MRI findings were analyzed for 33 hips in 29 patients with DDH, and the usefulness of MRI in predicting the probability of reduction with the Pavlik harness was assessed.

Methods.—Magnetic resonance imaging was performed on 33 hips in 29 patients (3 boys) aged 8 days to 8.6 months before application of the harness. Hips were classified into 3 groups: group 1, sharp acetabular rim with almost normal shape of the labrum and acetabular cartilage and possibly delayed ossification; group 2, rounded and dysplastic acetabular rim with a wide-open inlet; group 3, inverted acetabular rim with the inlet narrower than the diameter of the femoral head. The position of the femoral head in relation to the acetabulum was verified by US and classified as A, B, or C according to Suzuki.

Results.—According to MRI, there were 12 group 1, 13 group 2, and 8 group 3 hips. According to US, 9 group 1 hips were type A and 3 were type B. Three group 2 hips were type A, 7 were type B, and 3 were type C. Four group 3 hips were type B, and 4 were type C. All group 1 hips were reduced by the Pavlik harness, and type A and B hips in group 2 were reduced. No group 3 hips were reduced.

Conclusion.—All type C dislocations failed treatment with the Pavlik harness. Type B hips that displayed an inverted posterior labrum on MRI also failed treatment with the harness. Magnetic resonance imaging successfully predicted which patients with DDH would be helped by the Pavlik harness.

▶ This study of DDH using both MRI and US has shown us a method to select those patients who are not appropriate for treatment with the Pavlik harness. The harness does not successfully correct the deformity in 20% to 25% of these patients. According to this study we should use MRI on all patients who have a type B dislocation of the hip. If the MRI shows an inverted posterior labrum, the Pavlik harness will not be successful. The patients in this study who had a type "C" dislocation by US all failed treatment with the Pavlik harness. I believe that for now we should consider MRI for patients with type B US dislocations and, if the labrum is not inverted, recommend the harness. The harness will not be effective when the labrum is inverted and for type "C" dislocations.

P.P. Griffin, M.D.

Miscellaneous

Adductor Transfers in Cerebral Palsy: Long-term Results Studied by Gait Analysis

Scott AC, Chambers C, Cain TE (Shriners Hosp for Crippled Children, Houston; Univ of Texas, Houston; Baylor College of Medicine, Houston)
J Pediatr Orthop 16:741–746, 1996
8–27

Background.—Posterior transfer of the adductors to the ischium is used to improve hip range of motion and function in cerebral palsy patients. The long-term effects of these adductor transfers were examined both by conventional assessment and by gait analysis in a group of patients approaching skeletal maturity.

Methods.—Thirty-three ambulatory patients with spastic cerebral palsy involving the hip who underwent adductor transfer between 1978 and 1983 were included in this study. A chart review, physical therapist examination, and 3-dimensional motion analysis were performed for each patient. The average patient follow-up was over 10 years.

Findings.—Of 12 patients who were nonambulatory preoperatively, 9 were limited community ambulators with crutches or a walker. The other 3 were household or exercise ambulators. Of 12 patients who were exercise or household ambulators preoperatively, all progressed to community ambulators; 2 did not require aids. Of the 9 patients who were community ambulators preoperatively, 8 remained community ambulators and 1 became a household ambulator. Surgical complications were noted in 7 patients: 5 had local wound problems, 1 had synovitis of the knee, and 1 had sepsis. Seventeen patients had additional hip surgery. Hip range of motion demonstrated maintenance of abduction and extension. Seven patients had limited hip flexion. Unilateral hip subluxation occurred in 36%. Gait analysis demonstrated that 28 patients had pelvic obliquity, which was associated with adduction of the high hip and abduction of the low hip. In 20 patients this was also associated with knee extension on the high side and knee flexion on the low side.

Conclusions.—When ambulatory pediatric patients with cerebral palsy affecting the hip were treated with adductor transfer, hip range of motion and function were improved, but an abnormal gait developed in many of these patients because of pelvic obliquity. As a result of the development of this gait problem in these patients, adductor transfers are no longer performed at this institution.

▶ Pelvic obliquity in spastic cerebral palsy patients results from asymmetric forces on the hip. It occurs over time in *nonoperated* patients who have not had surgery of the adductors, but it is more common in those who have had a symmetric surgical procedure to reduce adductor strength. The patients in this study were thought to have had symmetric muscle function preoperatively. My experience has been different. I frequently find diplegic and quadriplegic patients with asymmetric active abduction and asymmetric strength in the hip abductors. The hip with the better abduction will generally have a greater hip flexion deformity and hamstrings that are not as tight. I think that one should attempt to identify asymmetry and do less surgery on the side with the best active abduction. The hamstrings have a role to play in hip subluxation and lengthening of the medial hamstrings (also asymmetrically) if the tightness is asymmetric and they should be considered in the treatment. I believe that the pelvic obliquity in the patients in this study resulted from asymmetry of the adductor/abductor or that the transfer pulled out on one side.

P.P. Griffin, M.D.

Protrusio Acetabuli: Its Occurrence in the Completely Expressed Marfan Syndrome and Its Musculoskeletal Component and a Procedure to Arrest the Course of Protrusion in the Growing Pelvis
Steel HH (Shriners Hosps for Crippled Children, Philadelphia)
J Pediatr Orthop 16:704–718, 1996   8–28

Background.—Protrusion of the acetabulum is common in Marfan's syndrome. Radiography is the most useful technique for diagnosis. This paper describes a surgical procedure to halt protrusion in children.

Surgical Technique.—With the patient supine, a skin incision is made over the iliac crest and extended inferiorly to end at the midportion of the os pubis. The oblique muscle is dissected and the cartilage split to expose the bone. The hip is flexed to release tension. The triradiate physis is then carefully obliterated. A small cortical graft harvested from the ilium crest is slotted in to bridge each of the limbs of the physis. No immobilization is necessary.

Results.—The triradiate physis was closed surgically in 21 hips of 11 patients aged 8–12 years with classic Marfan's disease and protrusio acetabuli. Nineteen of these hips were monitored to maturity. Hip architecture was restored to normal in 12 and reduced from protrusio to acetabular deepening in 4. Three were unchanged. All of the unchanged hips were in children operated on at the older end of the age spectrum.

Conclusions.—Protrusio acetabuli is frequently associated with Marfan's syndrome. A technique has been developed for surgical closure of the triradiate physis to halt the protrusio. It can be successfully performed on children with Marfan's syndrome and protrusio who are 8–10 years of age. For these children, progression can be halted, correction achieved, and symptoms alleviated.

▶ This report describes and defines the anatomy of the hip with protrusio as seen in routine radiographs. Protrusio of the acetabulum is common in patients with Marfan's syndrome. Because surgical closure of the triradiate cartilage is effective in stopping progression of the protrusio, abnormal growth of the triradiate cartilage must be the cause of the deformity.

This is a classic article that should be read by all who are interested in hip pathology.

P.P. Griffin, M.D.

Pediatric Lumbar Disc Surgery: 20 Patients Under 15 Years of Age

Shillito J Jr (Harvard Med School, Cambridge, Mass)
Surg Neurol 46:14–18, 1996

8–29

Background.—Central lumbar disk protrusions have been documented in children and young adults with back pain and a sciatica or with painless scoliosis. Differences between pediatric and adult disk symptomatology as well as surgical findings and results were compared.

Methods.—Sixty patients younger than 20 years of age who underwent lumbar diskectomy were identified in a review of Children's Hospital and office medical records from 1958 through 1995. Twenty patients were younger than 15 years. The youngest patient was 10 years, 8 months at the time of surgery. All but 3 patients were monitored for up to 20 years.

Findings.—At the initial assessment, only 20% of the patients reported sciatic pain. Sixty percent had such pain by the time of surgery, and the remaining 20% never had it. In 75% of the patients, the offending disk was at L5-S1. Disk protrusion was central in 75%. None of the disks had ruptured. In 40% of the patients, the posterior spinal ligament had ossified in the protruded position. Computed tomography provided especially useful information. Forty-five percent of the patients had significant antecedent trauma, and 60% had a family history of disk disease.

Conclusions.—Because sciatica is often absent, lumbar disk disease in the first 2 decades of life may be overlooked. In this series, lumbar diskectomy was safe in children younger than 15 years and was successful in 88%.

▶ In children who have back pain, a herniated disk may be present. This author, a very well known and busy pediatric neurosurgeon, reports on 20 children under 15 years of age with disk disease. Symptoms in this group were different from those in adults. Rapid onset of lumbar or thoracolumbar scoliosis with or without back pain should call our attention to the possibility of a disk problem or tumor and requires appropriate evaluation with CT or MRI. Sciatica is not always present. Pain on flexion and/or a positive straight-leg test was positive in virtually all patients. Many orthopedic surgeons see large numbers of children with back pain. We must look for the clinical signs, i.e., scoliosis of rapid onset, pain on flexion, and a positive straight-leg raise test, and in these patients do the appropriate workup. The author found that patients with a herniated disk do not respond to conservative treatment.

P.P. Griffin, M.D.

Long-term Results After Realignment Operations for Slipped Upper Femoral Epiphysis

Jerre R, Hansson G, Wallin J, et al (Gothenburg Univ, Sweden; Östra Hosp, Gothenburg, Sweden; Central Hosp, Halmstad, Sweden)
J Bone Joint Surg Br 78:745–750, 1996   8–30

Objective.—There is disagreement about the appropriate realignment procedure for moderate or severe slips of the upper femoral epiphysis (SUFE) because of unsatisfactory long- and short-term results and the increased risk of osteoarthritis. The clinical and radiologic long-term results of manipulative reduction and subcapital or intertrochanteric osteotomy for the treatment of SUFE are reviewed and reported.

Methods.—Realignment procedures were performed on 41 patients with SUFE between 1946 and 1959. The 36 patients (37 hips) who agreed to participate had been monitored for an average of 33.8 years and were divided into 3 treatment groups: group I (n = 22 hips), subcapital osteotomy; group II (n = 11 hips), intertrochanteric osteotomy; and group III (n = 4 hips), manipulative reduction. Clinical results were assessed by using the Harris hip score (HHS). Radiographic results were evaluated. Joint space degenerative changes were classified as normal, mild, or severe. Outcomes based on combined HHS and radiologic results were categorized as excellent, good, fair, or poor.

Results.—Seven (32%) group I, 3 (27%) group II and 3 (27% group III patients had short-term complications. Avascular necrosis developed in 5 group I, 1 group II, and 2 group III patients. Excellent or good results were achieved in 41% of the hips treated by subcapital osteotomy, 36% of the hips after intertrochanteric osteotomy, and no hips after manipulative reduction. Seven hips required arthrodesis or total hip replacement.

Conclusion.—Subcapital and intertrochanteric osteotomy and manipulative reduction did not appear to improve the natural history of SUFE.

▶ The results of surgical correction of the deformity present in a slipped capital femoral epiphysis have been poor in the hands of most orthopedic surgeons. Fish, in 1984, published a series of patients treated by cuneiform osteotomy of the femoral neck with good results.[1] Most others have experienced a high rate of avascular necrosis and chondrolysis in excess of the natural history. The results of an untreated slipped epiphysis, as stated in 1941 by Howorth,[2] can be better than a poorly treated slip. If one is tempted to correct the deformity by a cuneiform osteotomy, the risk should be carefully weighed and the technique described by Fish followed closely. However, only a few patients are in need of correction.

P.P. Griffin, M.D.

References

1. Fish JB: Cuneiform osteotomy of the femoral neck in the treatment of slipped capital femoral epiphysis. *J Bone Joint Surg Am* 66:1153–1168, 1984.
2. Howorth MB: Slipping off the upper femoral epiphysis. *Surg Gynecol Obstet* 73:723–732, 1941.

Infantile Blount Disease: Long-term Follow-up of Surgically Treated Patients at Skeletal Maturity
Doyle BS, Volk AG, Smith CF (Southern California Permanente Med Group, Fontana; Univ of Southern California, Los Angeles; Orthopaedic Hosp, Los Angeles)
J Pediatr Orthop 16:469–476, 1996

8–31

Background.—The correct timing of surgery in the treatment of patients with infantile Blount's disease has not been well defined. This study analyzed a large group of skeletally mature patients who had infantile Blount's disease treated by surgery during childhood to determine the appropriate age and stage for surgical treatment.

Study Design.—The medical records from 1952 to 1980 at Orthopedic Hospital in Los Angeles were reviewed, and 104 patients with infantile Blount's disease were identified. Of these 104 patients, 51 were treated surgically. Three male and 14 female skeletally mature patients from this series could be located and participated in this study. Of these 17 patients, 9 were black, 6 were Hispanic, and 2 were white. The mean age at initial osteotomy was 5.6 years, with a mean follow-up of 14.8 years. The mean initial varus deformity was 22 degrees, and after surgery the average correction was 12 degrees' valgus angulation. When the patients were recontacted, they were queried about pain, swelling, stiffness, instability, function, and satisfaction. Range of motion and stability were assessed. Radiographs were obtained. Patients with significant pain or instability had MRI, and 4 underwent arthroscopy.

Findings.—In this study, 13 limbs had a single osteotomy, and 13 had at least 2 surgical procedures. On average, there were more than 2 procedures on each affected limb. Repeat osteotomies were more common in children who had their initial osteotomy after the age of 4 years or at Langenskiöld stage III or greater. Those patients who had required only 1 osteotomy had significantly less pain at maturity than did those who required multiple procedures. All symptomatic or unstable knees were associated with abnormal ligamentous, meniscal, or bony changes that were confirmed by MRI and arthroscopy.

Conclusions.—Seventeen skeletally mature patients who had been treated surgically for infantile Blount's disease were extensively evaluated. The results of this evaluation demonstrated that operative treatment before the age of 4 or Langenskiöld stage III should reduce the need for repeated osteotomy and significantly reduce pain, instability, and knee pathology at maturity.

▶ This article emphasizes the importance of age in the success rate of tibial osteotomies in infantile Blount's disease. In this study patients averaged 2½ osteotomies. We must continue to ask why repeated osteotomies are so common. I believe that there are 3 reasons to consider. One, the osteotomy is done too low. The best way to avoid this is to do a reversed dome osteotomy so that the center of rotation of the correction is nearer the site of deformity. Second, the tibial joint angle must be corrected to slight valgus. Third, if the physis is not likely to respond to the change in mechanical forces (older children or grade III or more), the lateral physis should be stapled until there is radiographic evidence that the medial physis is growing and then the staple removed.

P.P. Griffin, M.D.

Avascular Necrosis and the Pavlik Harness: The Incidence of Avascular Necrosis in Three Types of Congenital Dislocation of the Hip as Classified by Ultrasound
Suzuki S, Kashiwagi N, Kasahara Y, et al (Shiga Med Centre for Children, Japan)
J Bone Joint Surg Br 78:631–635, 1996   8–32

Background.—The Pavlik harness is used to treat congenital dislocation of the hip (CDH) because it permits easy infant care and allows spontaneous reduction of the femoral head without forcible manipulation. Not all hips are successfully reduced by this device, and a serious complication, avascular necrosis, may occur during its use. In 1993, Suzuki described a

US classification system for CDH. With this classification system a series of CDH patients were analyzed to determine whether avascular necrosis was associated with a particular type of CDH classification.

Methods.—From December 1988 to October 1993, 101 congenitally dislocated hips in 9 boys and 81 girls were treated with the Pavlik harness and monitored for at least 1 year. The age of the patients when they joined the study group ranged from 8 days to 10 months. Patients who had previous treatment or who had teratologic or neuromuscular dislocation were excluded from the study group. The hips were classified into type A, with the femoral head posteriorly displaced but within the socket and contact between the head and the posterior inner wall of the acetabulum; type B, with the femoral head in contact with the posterior acetabulum margin and the center at this level or anterior; and type C, with the head displaced from the socket. There were 69 type A hips, 23 type B hips, and 9 type C hips. After US the child was placed in traction for an average of 16 days. Then the Pavlik harness was applied with the hip in 100 degrees of flexion. Ultrasonography was performed daily to check on the progress of reduction. If dislocation persisted for more than 2 weeks, use of the Pavlik harness was discontinued. If reduction occurred, the harness was left in place for approximately 2 months and then progressively removed. The extent of avascular necrosis was recorded for all classes of CDH.

Results.—Of the 101 hips included in this study, 87 were reduced by the Pavlik harness. Of these, avascular necrosis developed in 7. All 69 of the hips with type A CDH were reduced, and only 1 case of mild avascular necrosis developed. Of the 23 hips with type B CDH, 18 were reduced and avascular necrosis developed in 6. In 1 of these patients the femoral head was severely damaged. None of the 9 hips with type C CDH were reduced by the Pavlik harness.

Conclusions.—The US classification of hips with congenital hip dislocation is useful and has demonstrated that although the Pavlik harness is effective in the reduction of type A CDH hips, it should not be used to treat type B or type C CDH.

▶ The stage or position of the femoral head in relation to the acetabulum affects the difficulty of obtaining reduction, the development of the acetabulum in those that on routine radiography appear to be reduced, and the development of avascular necrosis. The deformed labrum and pulvinar partially fill the anterior superior part of the acetabulum and prevent adequate contact of the head with the triradiate cartilage, which is necessary for normal acetabular development when the head is subluxed and adjacent to the inner table of the posterior wall of the acetabulum. These structures can cause pressure on the femoral head when the hip is abducted. This pressure may cause ischemia involving the head.

P.P. Griffin, M.D.

Talocalcaneal Coalition Resection: A 10-Year Follow-up

McCormack TJ, Olney B, Asher M (Univ of Kansas, Kansas City)
J Pediatr Orthop 17:13–15, 1997   8–33

Background.—Some authors have found good initial outcomes in patients undergoing resection of the talocalcaneal bar, whereas others believe that it is rarely indicated. A 10-year follow-up study of patients undergoing talocalcaneal coalition resection for persistently symptomatic coalitions of the talocalcaneal joint was reported.

Methods and Findings.—Nine patients underwent 10 resections between 1977 and 1984. One patient was lost to follow-up. The mean length of follow-up was 11.5 years, with a range of 10–16 years. The 8 patients (with 9 treated feet) re-examined had virtually no decrease in range of motion on physical assessment. None of the patients needed repeat surgery. No evidence of degenerative change or joint space narrowing was seen on radiography. Ratings on the Painful Foot Center questionnaire indicated excellent outcomes in 6 patients, fair in 1, and poor in 1. Two patients had preoperative talar beaking. In the patient with a poor outcome, talar beaking developed after the initial operation.

Conclusions.—Resection of symptomatic talocalcaneal coalition appears to yield satisfactory outcomes in most patients. The benefits of this treatment are maintained for 10 years or longer.

▶ This important study shows that in a painful talocalcaneal coalition, pain can be allievated and motion regained by adequate resection of the coalition. Those attempting this difficult procedure should follow the surgical technique described by the authors.

P.P. Griffin, M.D.

Deficiencies of Current Methods for the Timing of Epiphysiodesis

Little DG, Nigo L, Aiona MD (Shriners Hosp for Crippled Children, Portland, Ore)
J Pediatr Orthop 16:173–179, 1996   8–34

Objective.—The methods of Anderson and Green, Menelaus, and Moseley, when used to determine the timing for epiphysiodesis, have resulted in less predictable or discouraging outcomes. The accuracy of predicting outcomes for these methods was investigated in a retrospective review of epiphysiodeses.

Methods.—A roentgenographic review was performed on 71 epiphysiodesis patients (29 boys) aged 8.9–16.2 years. The number of patients falling 2.0 and 1.5 cm outside the prediction for each method was recorded, and the results were compared statistically.

Results.—Forty-one Phemister and 30 percutaneous epiphysiodeses were performed. The mean discrepancy before surgery was 3.12 cm, and the mean discrepancy after surgery was 1.05 cm. Nineteen patients had been undercorrected by greater than 2.0 cm and 24 by greater than 1.5 cm. One patient was overcorrected by 2.0 cm. Although all methods tested had limited accuracy, the Moseley method was significantly less accurate than the others, with computer-generated graphs deviating more than 2.0 cm in 61% of the patients. The Menelaus method, based on chronologic age, is recommended because it is the easiest to use. None of the methods factor in qualitative elements.

Conclusion.—All the methods tested had limited accuracy in timing epiphysiodesis, but the Menelaus method is recommended because of its simplicity. Parents and patients should be advised of the discrepancies in the results.

▶ To achieve effective results of epiphysiodesis to equalize leg length, many parameters are involved: the stage of maturity (skeletal age), the percentage of inhibition, and whether the discrepancy is constant static or progressive. If skeletal age is interpreted closely, the results of both the Green and Mosely charts should be more accurate than the results by chronologic age. However, in my experience, few radiologists or orthopedic surgeons will use all 21 bones of the hand and wrist recommended to determine the average bone age. Margaret Anderson, who worked with W.T. Green, Sr., on the growth-remaining charts, read bone age in 3-month intervals, whereas many radiologists read them at plus or minus 10–12 months. This later is useless in the timing of an epiphysiodesis. If the skeletal age is used to time an epiphysiodesis, the interpreter must be capable of determining the skeletal age to within 3 to 6 month intervals as Margaret Anderson did in the study that developed through growth-remaining charts.[1]

P.P. Griffin, M.D.

Reference

1. Anderson M, Green WT, Messner WB: Growth and predictions of growth in the lower extremities. *J Bone Joint Surg Am* 45:1–14, 1963.

9 Hand

Introduction

One of the tonics for the "print-black blood" of the information broker is "profiling" the annual collection of topics in our interest niche that surface in the 50-odd journals that are reviewed for YEAR BOOK purposes. Driven by a multitude of forces, fundings, and interests, they nevertheless display the concentrate of our profession better than the pulses of professionalism, the ballistics of business, the grossness of government, the seductions of societies, or the currents of cultures. A barely perceptible blip on the profile chart may rise over time to be the dominant column, then slowly or even precipitously wane and be replaced. This year's profile leader is the continuing preoccupation with nerves, particularly as they pertain to pain problems and particularly as elements in the raging controversy about their relationships to occupational syndromes, repetitive pain syndromes, and the like. It is a good battle, fully joined and world-wide. Like many medical controversies, it is quite likely that its legal determinations will be made quite independently of medical opinion of physiological fact. But, for the nonce, it is fun to observe the battle, and I predict that it will continue into the next millennium.

And what other blips will we see in the near millennium years? We are due something new and exciting. Microsurgery, with its many dramatic additions to our management armamentarium, is still contributing and advancing, but the thrill is gone. The same is true of external fixation with its many variations of distraction, compression, transport, stretching, three-dimensional correction, etc. We find ourselves asking, "Well, what have you done for us lately?" and looking for some new direction or some development that will mainstream approaches that are currently but a mote in the eye. Will endoscopic diagnosis and treatment wax, until almost all our procedures can be done that way, or wane, as we find ways to make open procedures equally well tolerated? Will imaging techniques improve until we can read both anatomy and physiology in action? And with that assistance will we become able to pinpoint laser or other energies at the treatment site without opening or damaging the "surround" tissues? What of DNA and the possibilities of altering pathology by altering cellular structure or function? And what role will tropism play in tissue repair, particularly of nerve and vessels? And when will we learn to fix fractures and muscle-tendon injuries for immediate function and also speed up the healing processes? And where will the breakthrough studies of spinal cord healing and the interfacing of biologic and mechanical systems lead us in the new millennium? Ah, there is so much on hand as well as just inside tomorrow's doorway. Happy are you who will live to see the millennial potpourri of progress, and even happier are you who will be able to avoid the cul-de-sacs of the same.

James H. Dobyns, M.D.

Elbow, Forearm and Wrist

Coronal Shear Fractures of the Distal End of the Humerus

McKee MD, Jupiter JB, Bamberger HB (Massachusetts Gen Hosp, Boston; Ohio Univ, Dayton)
J Bone Joint Surg (Am) 78A:49–54, 1996

9–1

Introduction.—Identification of distal end osteochondral shearing fractures of the humerus using standard radiographs may be difficult. Operative management may also be problematic. The capitellum is involved in most of these osteochondral fractures, which have been classified into 3 groups, based on the extent of involvement of the capitellum. The operative course and recovery of 6 patients with distal end coronal shear fractures of the humerus were retrospectively reviewed.

Methods.—During a 3-year period, 6 patients were treated for distal end coronal shear fractures of the humerus. Computed tomography before surgery in 2 patients and direct visualization at the time of surgery in 4 patients were used to make the diagnosis. All patients had closed fractures resulting from a fall. At the time of surgery, it was noted that the fracture line extended into the coronal plane and included most of the trochlear

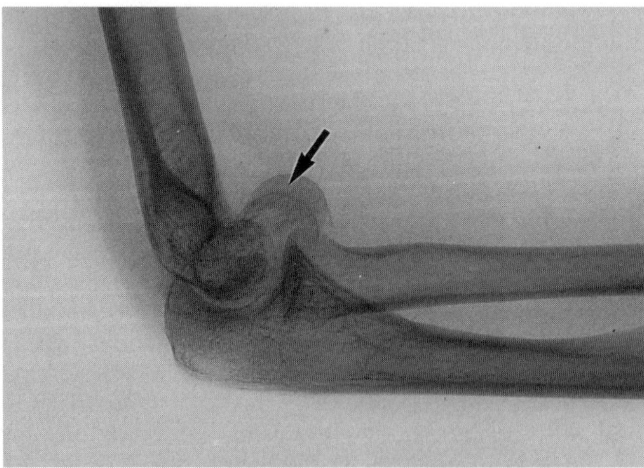

FIGURE 2.—Lateral radiograph showing the characteristic double-arc sign (*arrow*). One arc represents the subchondral bone of the capitellum and the other, the lateral ridge of the trochlea. (Courtesy of McKee MD, Jupiter JB, Bamberger HB. Coronal shear fractures of the distal end of the humerus. *J Bone Joint Surg [Am]* 78A:49–54, 1996.)

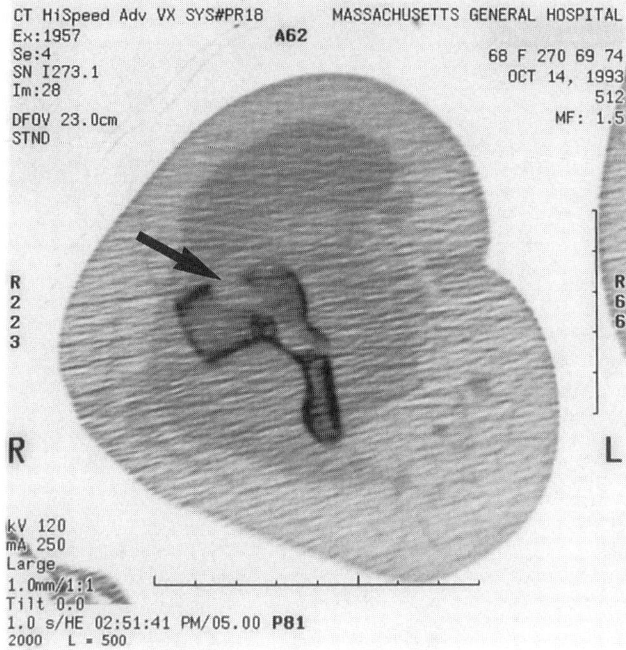

FIGURE 3.—Preoperative CT scan, made through the distal end of the humerus in an axial fashion in another patient. Shown are the coronal fracture line (*arrow*) and involvement of both the capitellum and the lateral ridge of the trochlea. (Courtesy of McKee MD, Jupiter JB, Bamberger HB. Coronal shear fractures of the distal end of the humerus. *J Bone Joint Surg [Am]* 78A:49–54, 1996.)

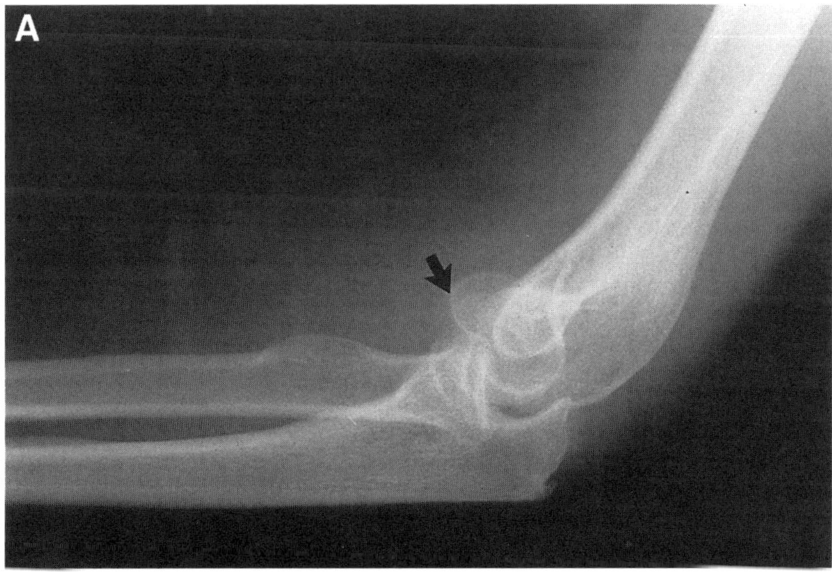

FIGURE 4 (cont.)

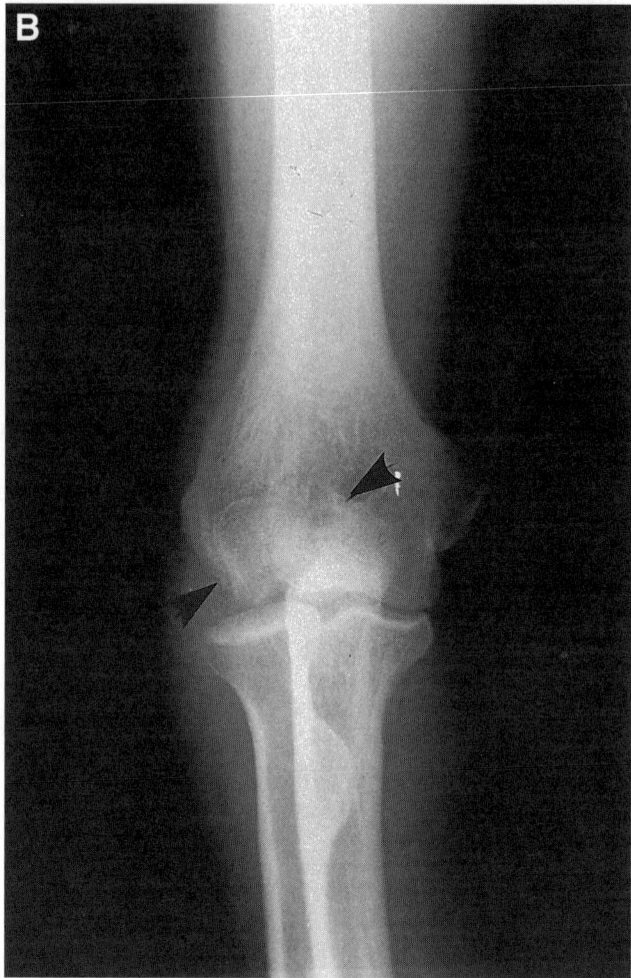

(Continued)

ridge as well as the lateral half of the trochlea. Radiography revealed the double-arc sign, with 1 arc for the subchondral bone of the displaced capitellum and the second arc indicating the lateral ridge of the trochlea (Fig 2). Axial or transverse plane CT also showed the coronal fracture line, with capitellum and lateral ridge involvement (Fig 3). Open reduction was performed on all patients, with internal fixation using standard Herbert screws or cancellous-bone AO screws (Fig 4). Two patients required the addition of a short plate along the posterolateral aspect of the condyle. Postoperative management included the use of a thermoplastic orthosis and motion, muscle-strengthening, and endurance exercises. Follow-up

FIGURE 4 (cont.)

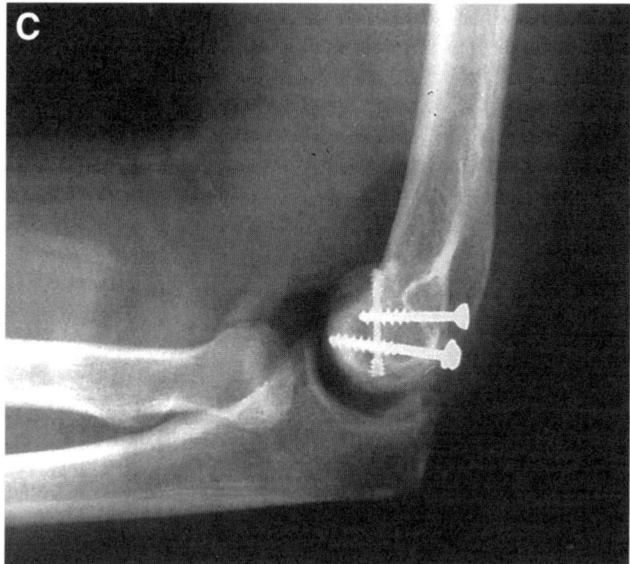

(*Continued*)

evaluation included physical examination, radiography, and elbow function assessment.

Results.—No operative complications were noted and all fractures healed in an average of 6 weeks. Only 2 patients reported pain with strenuous activity at follow-up. The average elbow flexion was 111 degrees with a 15-degree average flexion contracture. No patient complained of any functional difficulties or elbow instability. Five of the 6 patients regained rotation equal to that of the uninjured side, whereas 1 patient had pronation and supination of 50 degrees and 55 degrees, respectively—less than that of the contralateral side.

Conclusion.—In this series of patients with coronal shear fractures, the fracture was found to extend across the trochlea. Arc of flexion, elbow extension, and elbow stability may be adversely affected if reduction of this injury is not achieved. Good results were achieved in all patients who underwent open reduction and fixation of this injury.

▶ This short article features a fracture that is difficult to diagnose and analyze but is critical to identify because open reduction to align fragments and articular surfaces is necessary for good results.

J.H. Dobyns, M.D.

FIGURE 4 (cont.)

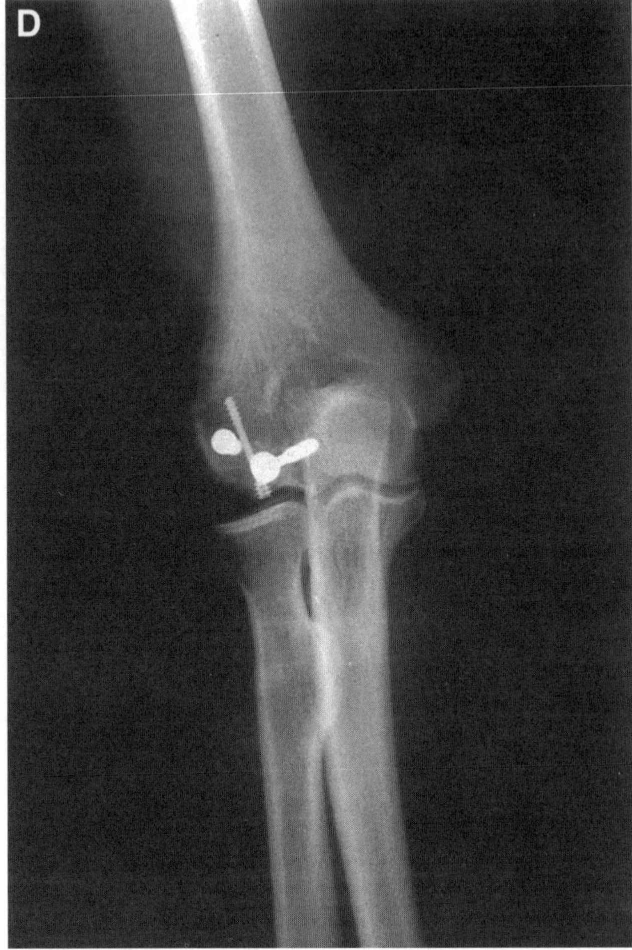

FIGURE 4.—Case 4. **A**, preoperative lateral radiograph showing the so-called double-arc sign (*arrow*) in a third patient. **B**, preoperative anteroposterior radiograph. Close inspection reveals the lateral and medial borders of the fracture (*arrows*). **C** and **D**, postoperative lateral and anteroposterior radiographs showing the anatomical reduction and internal reduction obtained with Herbert and 4.0-mm AO screws. The patient had a good result, with an elbow score of 92 points at 1-year follow-up. (Courtesy of McKee MD, Jupiter JB, Bamberger HB. Coronal shear fractures of the distal end of the humerus. *J Bone Joint Surg (Am)* 78A:49–54, 1996.)

Plate Osteosynthesis of Diaphyseal Fractures of the Radius and Ulna

Hertel R, Pisan M, Lambert S, et al (Univ of Berne, Switzerland)
Injury 27:545–548, 1996
9–2

Introduction.—The "gold standard" for fractures of the forearm is currently open reduction and internal fixation using compression plates.

Controlled trials will be needed to evaluate new implants and techniques being developed. A single implant system used during a 10-year period in patients with forearm fractures was evaluated retrospectively by assessing union, infection, and refracture outcomes in the patients. A secondary purpose was to provide a definitively documented historical control group to compare the new implants under development.

Methods.—One hundred thirty-two forearm fractures in 131 patients were reviewed. All patients were managed by plate osteosynthesis of 1 or both forearm bones. One hundred twenty-two patients were available for telephone questionnaire at a mean long-term follow-up of 122.5 months. Most patients had been injured because of motor vehicle accidents. Thirty-seven patients had multiple injuries. Twenty-nine patients had open fractures, and 103 patients had closed fractures. All fractures were stabilized using 3.5-mm stainless-steel dynamic compression plates. Patients underwent internal fixation at a mean of 1.8 days after injury. Patients with closed fractures usually received at least 2 postoperative doses of IV antibiotics, and patients with open fractures received selected antibiotics until wound closure.

Results.—Of 122 forearms, 112 fractures united before 4 months and 15 of 17 without further intervention within 6 months. Six of 17 delayed fractures occurred in patients with open fractures. There were 2 nonunion fractures and 2 delayed union fractures that were treated with reoperation. One patient with a closed fracture had a superficial wound infection that was treated effectively. One patient with a head injury subsequently had a radioulnar synostosis that he chose not to have reoperated. There were no failures of initial fixation or refractures in patients who did not undergo reoperation to have plates removed. At long-term follow-up, 70 of 122 respondents (57%) had their plates removed at a mean of 33 months after initial operation. Three patients who underwent plate removal had a refracture at a mean of 4.3 months after plate removal. One patient was considered to have a true refracture.

Conclusions.—To date, this report has the longest and highest rate of follow-up on use of a single implant system in a single institution with a sufficient number of patients. The 3.5-mm stainless-steel dynamic compression plate is a satisfactory implant in the treatment of diaphyseal fractures of the radius and/or ulna. The rate of problem-free union was 96.3%. The infection rate was 0.8%. The true refracture rate was 1.4% in patients who had plates removed and 0% in patients whose plates were left in place. Routine plate removal is not recommended.

▶ This is a short, sweet, significant paper, that should be in every upper limb surgeon's reference file. As the authors say, it gives the longest and highest rate of follow-up of a sufficient number of patients, using a single implant system in a single institution. Would that all of our favorite procedures were equally reviewed and supported.

J.H. Dobyns, M.D.

A Comparison of Early and Late Reconstruction of Malunited Fractures of the Distal End of the Radius

Jupiter JB, Ring D (Massachusetts Gen Hosp, Boston)
J Bone Joint Surg [Am] 78A:739–748, 1996   9–3

Background.—The decision to reconstruct a malunited fracture of the distal end of the radius is based primarily on impaired wrist function, pain, or cosmetic deformity assessed long after the injury. Many patients function adequately after delayed intervention, despite residual deformity. However, a delay in intervention may also result in soft-tissue maladaptation and dysfunction of the radioulnar joint. Reconstructing malunion at an earlier stage may facilitate definition, and correction of malalignment through the original site of the fracture may enable avoidance of maladaptive soft-tissue contracture and the development of distal radioulnar joint dysfunction, and may reduce the period of disability.

Methods.—The outcomes of 10 patients with a malaligned fracture of the distal end of the radius treated with early reconstruction were compared retrospectively with the outcomes of 10 patients undergoing late reconstruction for functional limitation after complete healing of a fracture of the distal end of the radius in a malreduced position. Early reconstruction, performed a mean of 8 weeks after injury, consisted of an osteotomy through the site of the fracture, autogenous cancellous iliac-crest bone-grafting, and internal fixation. Late reconstruction, done a mean of 40 weeks after injury, consisted of an osteotomy, corticocancellous bone-grafting, and internal fixation. The early and late treatment groups were followed for an average of 48 and 34 months, respectively.

Findings.—After early reconstruction, average wrist flexion was 45 degrees; wrist extension, 52 degrees; forearm pronation, 79 degrees; and forearm supination, 77 degrees. The corresponding values for the late treatment group were 42, 45, 77, and 68 degrees. Grip strength after early and late reconstructions was 42 kg and 25 kg, respectively. One patient in each group reported mild pain in the radiocarpal joint. Outcomes were excellent in 7 patients and good in 3 patients after early reconstruction. After late reconstructions, outcomes were excellent in 1 patient, good in 7, and fair in 2. One patient undergoing early reconstruction had a complication—rupture of the extensor pollicis longus tendon 12 weeks after treatment. Two patients in the late treatment group had complications—persistent pain at the donor site of the iliac-crest bone graft in 1 and a delayed union requiring a second procedure in the other (Figs 1 and 2).

Conclusions.—Early and late reconstructions of malunited fractures of the distal end of the radius appear to produce similar outcomes. Early reconstruction is technically easier and decreases the length of disability in patients with radiographic signs predicting persistent functional limitation.

► Although 10 of this and 10 of that is not a big bunch of anything, we need all the help we can get in making the commonly needed decision about

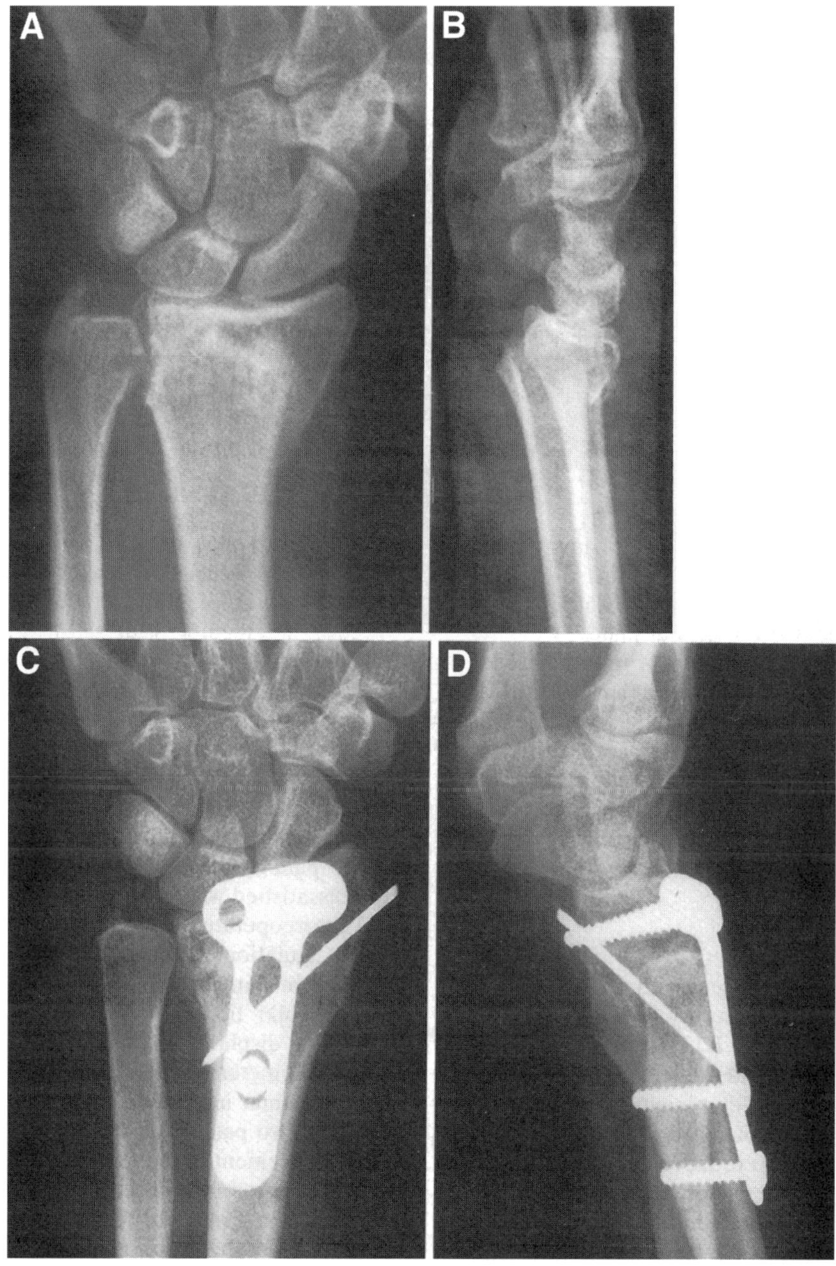

(*Continued*)

FIGURE 1 (cont.)

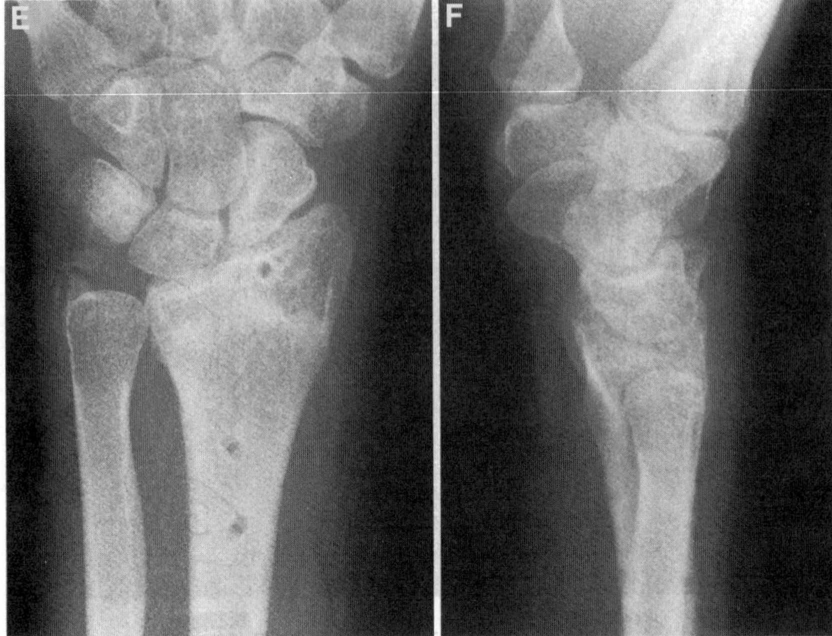

FIGURE 1.—A–F, a 20-year-old woman who sustained a fracture of the distal end of the left radius in a motor-vehicle accident and was initially managed with a cast after attempted closed reduction. A and B, anteroposterior and lateral radiographs showing early malunion of the distal end of the radius. E and F, anteroposterior and lateral radiographs obtained after removal of the plate because of synovitis of the overlying extensor tendons. (Courtesy of Jupiter JB, Ring D: A comparison of early and late reconstruction of malunited fractures of the distal end of the radius. *J Bone Joint Surg [Am]* 78A:739–748, 1996.)

whether and when to reconstruct malformed fractures of the distal radius. My colleagues and I agree with the author's suggestion that reconstruction should be done whenever the opportunity presents and that it is easier to do early than late. Best of all, of course, is to rebuild the damaged distal radius well at the initial treatment phase.

J.H. Dobyns, M.D.

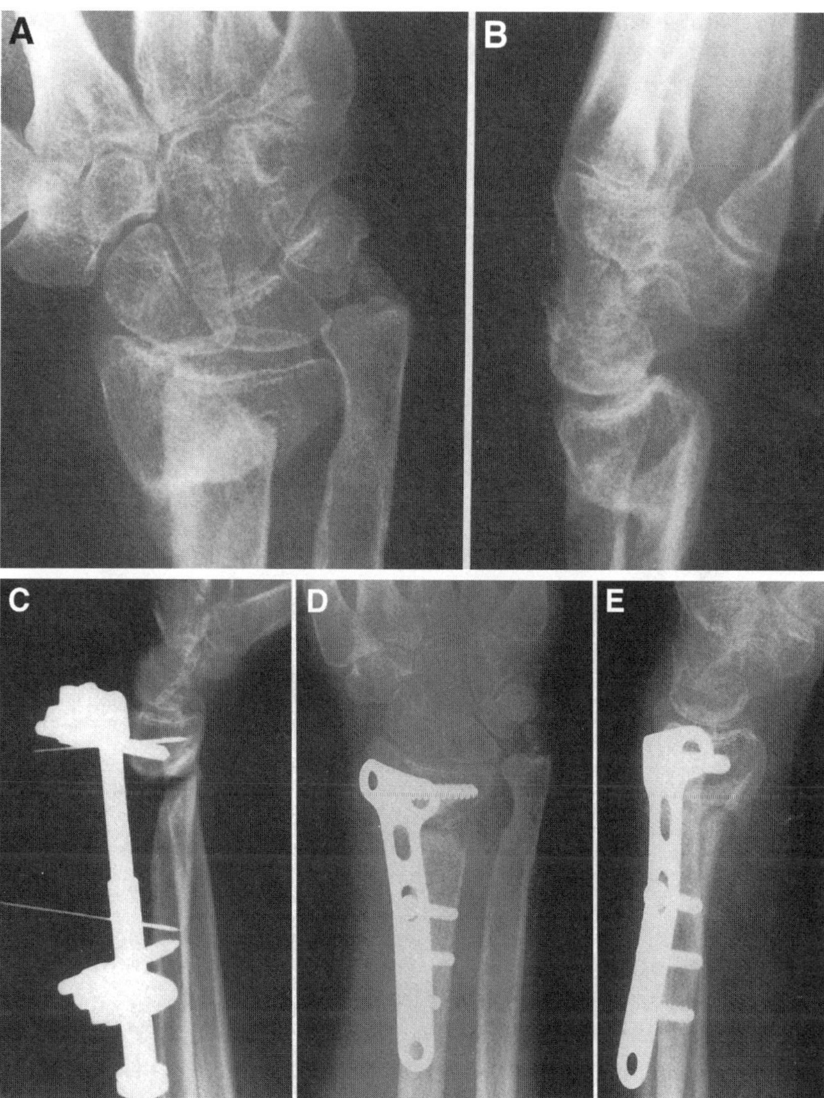

FIGURE 2.—A–E, a 26-year-old woman who fell from a height and sustained an open fracture of the distal end of the right radius. The fracture and subsequent infection were treated in an external fixator. A and B, anteroposterior and lateral radiographs showing the distal radial malunion 36 weeks after injury. C, lateral radiograph showing use of a distractor to realign the distal end of the radius. There is a resultant defect. D and E, anteroposterior and lateral radiographs obtained 3 weeks after surgery, showing the realignment of the distal end of the radius. (Courtesy of Jupiter JB, Ring D: A comparison of early and late reconstruction of malunited fractures of the distal end of the radius. *J Bone Joint Surg [Am]* 78A:739–748, 1996.)

Arthroscopic-Assisted Reduction of Distal Radius Fractures

Wolfe SW, Easterling KJ, Yoo HH (Yale Univ, New Haven, Conn)
Arthroscopy 11:706–714, 1995

9–4

Background.—Comminuted intra-articular fractures of the distal radius represent a unique subgroup of injuries that are difficult to diagnose and treat. Authorities have demonstrated the importance of anatomically restoring and maintaining the articular surface, advocating surgical reconstruction with open reduction, and internal fixation to prevent posttraumatic arthritis. However, the capsular and ligamentous dissection needed to provide sufficient exposure of the articular surface during open reduc-

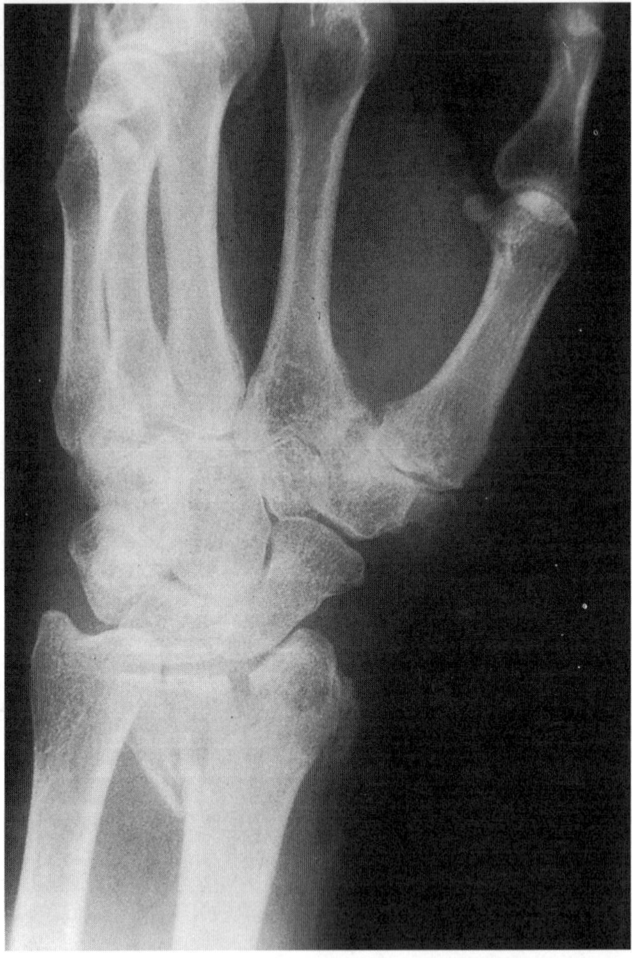

FIGURE 2.—Markedly comminuted intra-articular distal radius fracture. (Courtesy of Wolfe SW, Easterling KJ, Yoo HH: Arthroscopic-assisted reduction of distal radius fractures. *Arthroscopy* 11:706–714, 1995.)

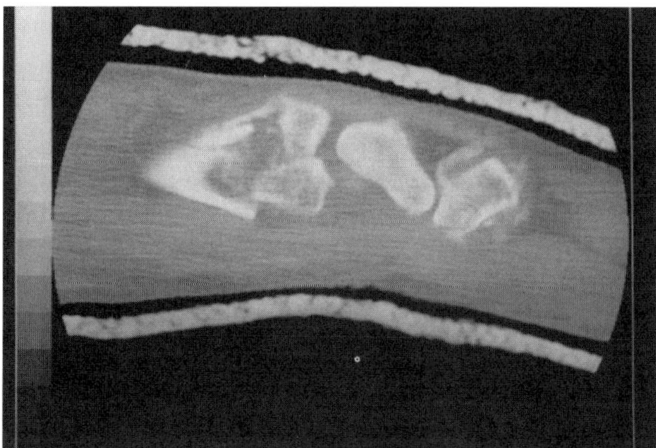

FIGURE 3.—Postreduction CT scan documents residual articular surface impaction. (Courtesy of Wolfe SW, Easterling KJ, Yoo HH: Arthroscopic-assisted reduction of distal radius fractures. *Arthroscopy* 11:706–714, 1995.)

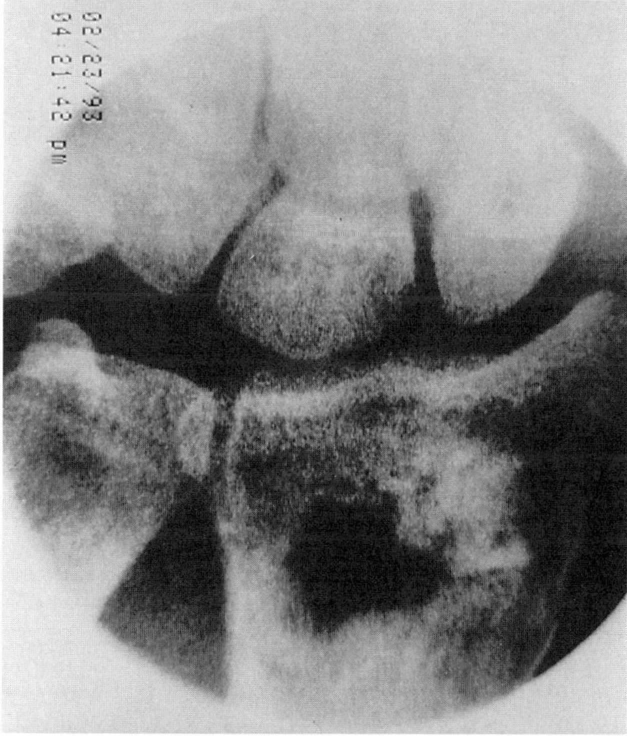

FIGURE 8.—Metaphyseal defect partially filled with autogenous graft. (Courtesy of Wolfe SW, Easterling KJ, Yoo HH: Arthroscopic-assisted reduction of distal radius fractures. *Arthroscopy* 11:706–714, 1995.)

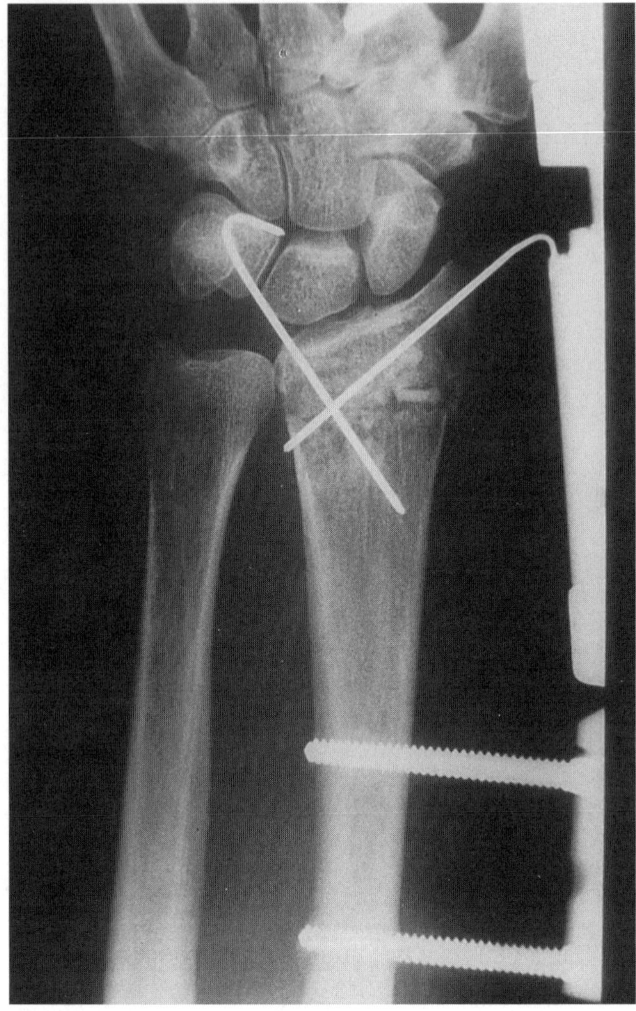

FIGURE 9.—Immediate postoperative postanterior radiograph showing placement of supplementary percutaneous K-wires and external fixation in neutral alignment. (Courtesy of Wolfe SW, Easterling KJ, Yoo HH: Arthroscopic-assisted reduction of distal radius fractures. *Arthroscopy* 11:706–714, 1995.)

tion is extensive and may result in postoperative stiffness. A technique of arthroscope-assisted reduction and percutaneous fixation of distal radius fractures (ARPEF) was developed.

Methods and Findings.—Seven patients with severe comminuted intra-articular fractures of the distal radius undergoing ARPEF were included in the retrospective review. All had C3-type fractures according to the AO classification scheme. Patients were followed for 12 to 45 months. All patients were free of pain and had returned to work. None of the patients had articular incongruency of more than 1 mm. No evidence of radiocarpal degenerative change was observed. Active range of motion was a mean

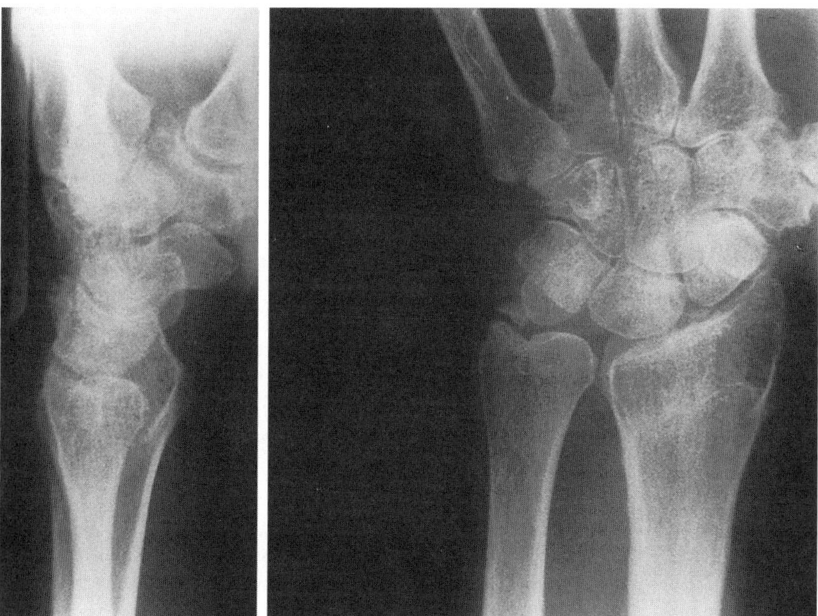

FIGURE 10.—One-year follow-up radiographs demonstrate maintenance of articular alignment but 3-mm radial subsidence. (Courtesy of Wolfe SW, Easterling KJ, Yoo HH: Arthroscopic-assisted reduction of distal radius fractures. *Arthroscopy* 11:706–714, 1995.)

of 92% of that of the uninjured wrist and maximal strength was 98% (Figs 2, 3, 8, 9, and 10).

Conclusions.—In this small group of patients with severe comminuted intra-articular fractures of the distal radius, ARPEF yielded excellent results. Complications were minimal.

▶ Although the numbers were small (7 cases) and the follow-up period was short (mean 27 months), this report is an excellent representation of an advance in the treatment of comminuted, articular fractures of the distal radius. This advance is occurring in multiple centers around the world. The pace of change in the management of these fractures has accelerated in the past decade. Much of the world is still pondering the emphasis on near-complete reduction, aided if necessary by fixation; others are convinced but still experiment with the types of fixation: The cutting edge is now the investigators who accept the need for full reduction and its maintenance by fixation devices and bone replacement if needed but are also concerned about ways to minimize additional trauma to the damaged tissues.

J.H. Dobyns, M.D.

Ulnar Lengthening and Radial Recession Procedures for Kienböck's Disease: Long-term Clinical and Radiographic Follow-up

Trail IA, Linscheid RL, Quenzer DE, et al (Mayo Clinic, Rochester, Minn)
J Hand Surg (Br) 21B:169–176, 1996   9–5

Objective.—The long-term clinical and radiologic outcome was reviewed for 20 patients who underwent ulnar lengthening or radial recession for treatment of Kienböck's disease. These joint-leveling procedures were found to yield good subjective clinical results at earlier follow-up.

Methods.—Sixteen patients had undergone ulnar-lengthening procedures and 4 were treated with radial recession. The average age at diagnosis was 26.9 years, and the average follow-up was 11 years. Preoperative tomograms were available for 14 patients; all 20 had new trispiral tomograms of the wrist in anteroposterior and lateral projections. Follow-up x-ray evaluation included analysis of ulnar variance, radiologic staging, and determination of radioscaphoid and radiolunate angles and carpal height.

Results.—Ulnar lengthening averaged 4 mm and radial recession, 2 mm. There were 14 additional procedures, including 11 simple late removals. Earlier follow-up (average, 28.5 months) had shown 19 of 20 patients to be subjectively improved. Eleven years after the procedures, 15 were able to work full-time without restrictions at their original jobs. All reported less pain in the surgically treated wrist than before surgery, 17 believed that the surgically treated wrist was stronger, and 16 believed that the range of motion was improved. Clinical examination confirmed significant increases in the arc of wrist extension and flexion and in grip strength. Thirteen patients had new bone formation at the lunate fossa of the radius, a finding not present in any cases preoperatively, and 12 showed osteoarthritic changes. Four of 9 patients with lunate bone fragmentation before surgery had partial resolution at long-term follow-up. Ulnar variance averaged +0.6 mm at follow-up, compared with +1.9 mm postoperatively. Carpal height did not change significantly.

Conclusion.—All 20 patients who underwent a joint leveling procedure for Kienböck's disease reported subjective improvement at an average of 11 years postoperatively. There appeared to be no deterioration in results compared with earlier follow-up. Radiologic examination, however, indicated continuing fragmentation, cysts, and non-union of the lunate fractures.

▶ The basic joint-leveling procedures for Kienböck's disease have been time-tested before, but seldom with the wealth of detail provided here. Clinically, most patients do well despite lunate healing problems (nonhealing or healing with deformity), osteoarthritic problems (mostly in the radioscaphoid joint), and new bone formation (mostly radiolunate fossa). The observations are made that current staging is inadequate for appropriate treatment selection, primarily because standard x-ray films, the basis for currently used staging, do not show the lunate status adequately. Better, more prolonged methods of protecting the fragmented, deformed, and vascularly compromised lunate are needed until healing is advanced enough to cope with the central column stresses.

J.H. Dobyns, M.D.

Total Wrist Fusion: A Functional Assessment
Field J, Herbert TJ, Prosser R (St Luke's Hosp, Sydney, Australia)
J Hand Surg (Br) 21B:429–433, 1996   9–6

Background.—Wrist fusion is indicated primarily for post-traumatic wrist problems and rheumatoid arthritis. The procedure appears to be effective in patients with rheumatoid wrist, who often have gross instability and a low functional demand. Wrist fusion also is performed in younger patients with high functional demand, especially for the SLAC wrist after late scaphoid collapse and as a salvage procedure after limited carpal fusion. A functional assessment of total wrist fusion was done.

Methods and Findings.—Twenty patients underwent total wrist fusion performed for posttraumatic conditions. All reported good pain relief and were satisfied with the position of the fused wrist. All patients said they would have had the procedure sooner. Before fusion, a mean of 3 operations had been attempted. Forty-five percent of the patients had complications. Assessment by means of the Jebsen and Purdue tests indicated that hand function was poor, possibly because of a decreased range of finger movements. Position of fusion, carpal height, and number of joints fused radiologically were not correlated with pain score, grip strength, and Buck-Gramcko score.

Conclusions.—Overall, patients were very satisfied with the outcomes of wrist function, though hand function was significantly decreased. A period of immobilization before surgery in an unremovable splint is recommended to determine the best fusion position and to allow patients to get used to the immobile wrist.

▶ The dust of carpal investigations with its plethora of new findings from lab to lyceum is still swirling, and the "bottom line" will be some time in emerging. In this whirlwind, new treatments abound—and so does confusion about the old treatments. The authors offer considerable encouragement about 1 of the oldest of all surgical treatments for the painful post-traumatic wrist, the total wrist fusion. Their bias against partial wrist fusions notwithstanding, they make a good case for continued and earlier use of total wrist fusion. They also confirm my concern about the need to observe patients closely after total wrist fusion for carpal tunnel syndrome (approximately half of the patients identified with carpal tunnel syndrome will need release) and for extensor tendon irritation (more than half of the cases will need plate removal). A similar report[1] is supportive.

J.H. Dobyns, M.D.

Reference

1. Sagerman SD, Palmer AK: Wrist arthodesis using a dynamic compression plate. *J Hand Surg (Br)* 21B:437–441, 1996.

Herbert Screw Fixation of Scaphoid Fractures

Filan SL, Herbert TJ (St Luke's Hosp, Sydney, Australia)
J Bone Joint Surg Br 78B:519–529, 1996   9–7

Objective.—The Herbert bone screw is widely accepted as an effective method of internal fixation, but most reports of the technique advocate additional plaster immobilization. A review of 431 cases of screw fixation of the scaphoid examined whether rigid internal fixation provided adequate fixation, encouraged acceleration of healing and wrist function, or improved the prognosis for scaphoid fractures.

Methods.—The study included 431 patients, 90% of whom were male. A standard Herbert bone screw was used in 409 patients and a mini Herbert screw was used in 22. There were 82 acute fractures and 349 fracture nonunions, which included 48 revision operations. Kirschner wires were also required in 30 patients. Plaster immobilization was not used. Patients were reviewed radiographically at 2 weeks, 6 weeks, 3 months, and 1 year. Clinical, radiologic, and operative findings were scored (Fig 1). Fractures were classified (Fig 2). Specific types of fractures required specialized treatment (Fig 3).

Results.—The correlation between clinical and radiologic findings for acute type-B fractures was poor. Most were completely unstable. Late nonhealing was observed in some conservatively treated acute fractures (Fig 6). A minimum of 6 months of follow-up data were available on 304 patients. Wrist function, with the exception of wrist extension, and grip strength had improved. At an average of 4.7 weeks after surgery, 277 patients were able to return to preinjury work, 27 were not working, and 15 were collecting workers' compensation. The rates of union for acute fractures was 88%. The review showed that the Herbert bone screw provided sufficient stability to allow normal wrist function and symptomatic relief even when the scaphoid did not heal (Fig 7). Stabilization of the scaphoid allowed normal wrist function (Fig 8).

Conclusion.—Although Herbert screw fixation is technically difficult, it provides sufficient fixation to allow healing without plaster immobilization and improves healing and function of acute fractures; in established nonunion the technique reduces the progress of osteoarthritis and speeds functional recovery. There is poor correlation between clinical and radiologic findings of scaphoid fractures.

▶ If all were as skilled in case selection, surgical approach, and device utilization as Dr. Herbert, this article of many subtleties and abundant experience could serve as the template for scaphoid injury management. How-

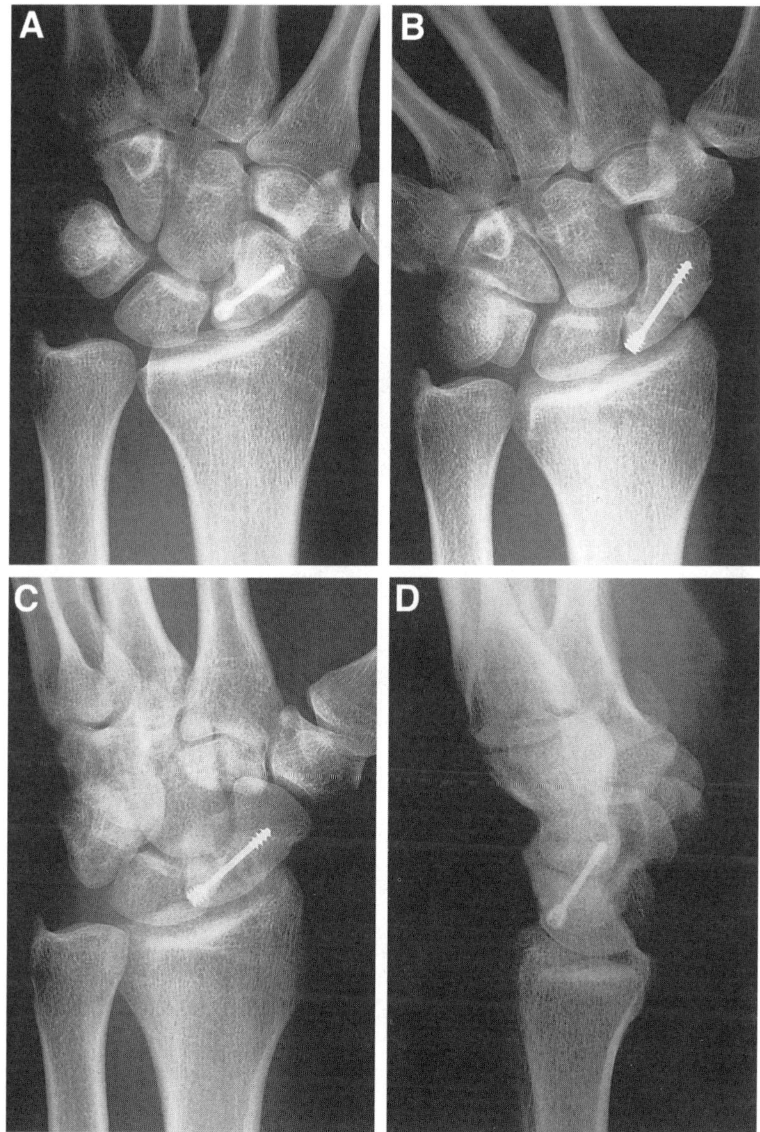

FIGURE 1.—The standard 4-view radiographs: posteroanterior radial (**A**) and ulnar (**B**) deviation, 45 degrees oblique (**C**) and true lateral (**D**). The lucency seen in the radial deviation film (*arrow*) indicates nonunion by the criteria used in our study. (Courtesy of Filan SL, Herbert TJ: Herbert screw fixation of scaphoid fractures. *J Bone Joint Surg [Br]* 78B:519–529, 1996.)

ever, all who treat these injuries are not as skilled, and cases of poor selection or technical incompetence litter the landscape. The article sidesteps a rather high incidence of 'lost-to-follow-up,' which slyly implies that type A as well as type B fractures might also be best treated by the

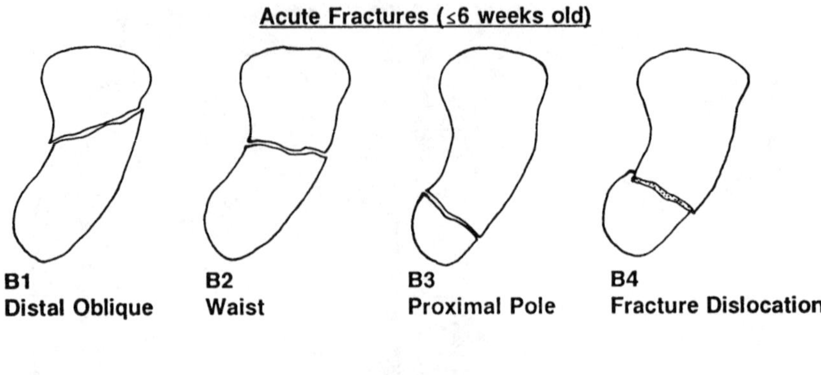

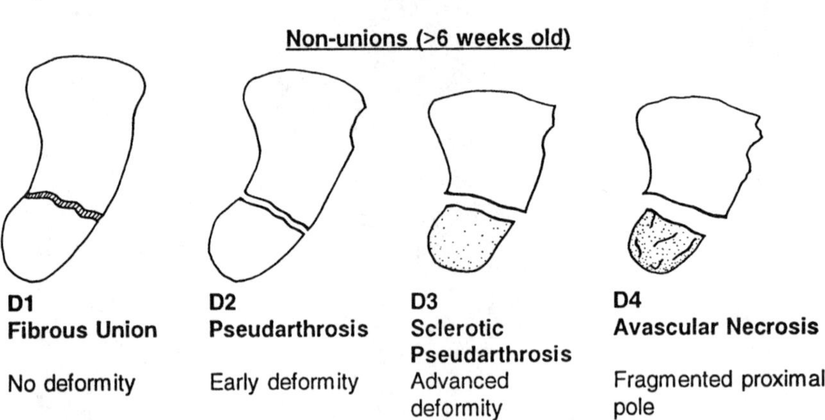

FIGURE 2.—Modified staging system for scaphoid fractures. Type A fractures are not illustrated. Types B5 (comminuted) and C (delayed union) have been omitted from the classification because they did not form natural groups. (Courtesy of Filan SL, Herbert TJ: Herbert screw fixation of scaphoid fractures. *J Bone Joint Surg [Br]* 78B:519–529, 1996.)

recommended method, and skimps such difficult problems as the B4 fracture with significant dislocation of a fragment, the B5 comminuted fragment, and the D3–D4 group. Furthermore, the x-ray analysis is dependent on high quality standard views that may be unavailable or insufficient. Nevertheless, the experience, insights, and conclusions shared are pure gold and any practitioner with high exposure to the scaphoid injury problem should develop the same expertise, not necessarily with the same device, but with the same goals in mind. Many other articles over the past decade, including one in the same journal issue,[1] have been generally favorable to the techniques and device espoused by Herbert, although with some variation in regard to selection. There are, in fact, a variety of internal fixation devices (some as good as or perhaps even better than the Herbert screw) for support of the fractured scaphoid with/without bone graft as needed. There is little doubt, however, that the Herbert screw was a step forward from the devices previously used, and that the dedicated investigation of its potential by Dr.

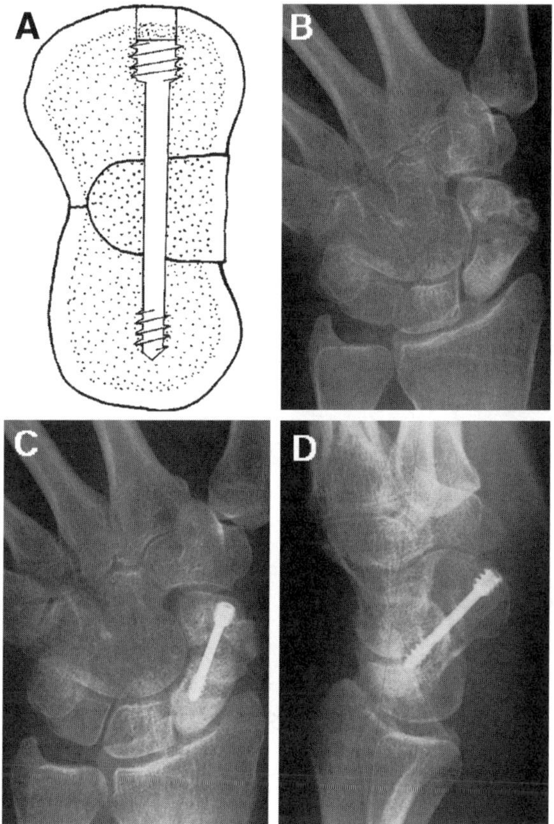

FIGURE 3.—A corticocancellous graft (**A**) gives stability to compression after the complete excision of a scaphoid pseudoarthrosis. The preoperative collapse and shortening (**B**) have been corrected by a successful reconstruction (**C**). In the lateral view (**D**) the cortical element of the graft is visible. (Courtesy of Filan SL, Herbert TJ: Herbert screw fixation of scaphoid fractures. *J Bone Joint Surg Br* 78B:519–529, 1996.)

Herbert continues to lead and invigorate the management of humankind's most common carpal fracture.

J.H. Dobyns, M.D.

Reference

1. Established non-union of the scaphoid treated by volar wedge grafting and Herbert screw fixation. (Daly K, Gill P, Magnussen PA, et al, *J Bone Joint Surg* 78B:530–53) 1996.)

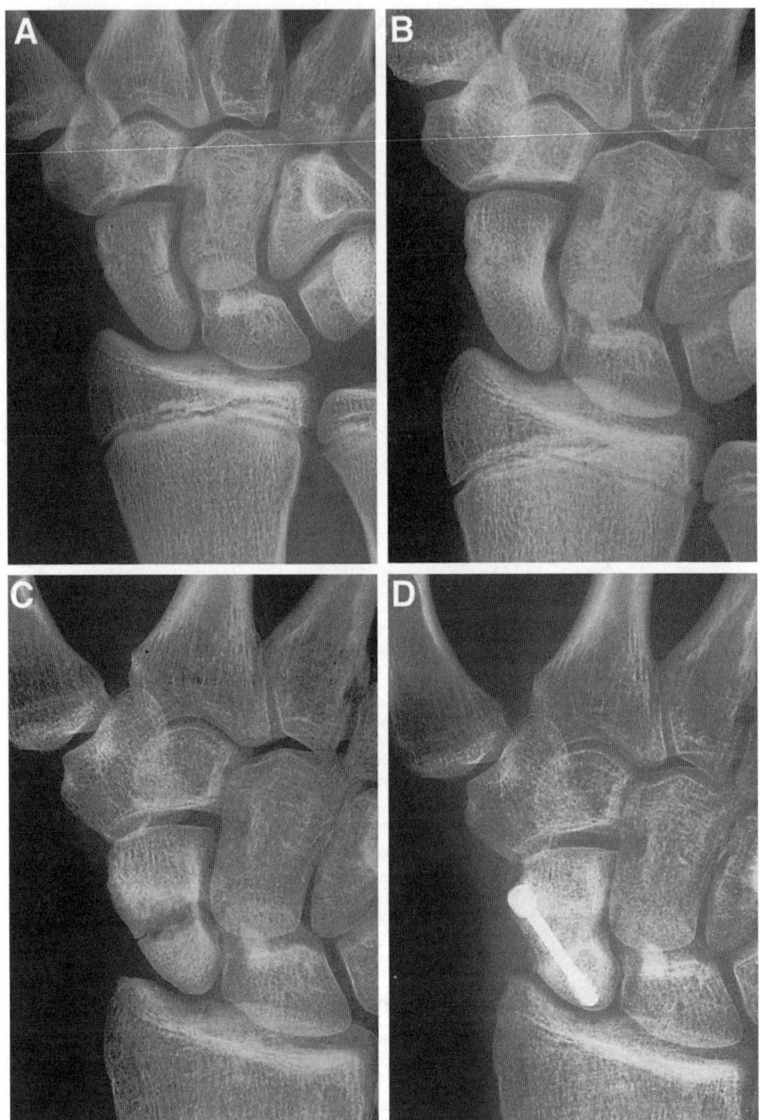

FIGURE 6.—A 15-year-old boy with an acute scaphoid fracture (**A**) treated by plaster immobilization. Two months later the fracture appeared to have united (**B**). The patient failed to attend for follow-up, but returned 6 years later complaining of slowly deteriorating wrist function. Radiographs showed the classical signs of late failure after fibrous nonunion (**C**). After reconstruction and Herbert screw fixation, the nonunion healed (**D**) and the patient had returned to work as a motor mechanic. (Courtesy of Filan SL, Herbert TJ: Herbert screw fixation of scaphoid fractures. *J Bone Joint Surg Br* 78B:519–529, 1996.)

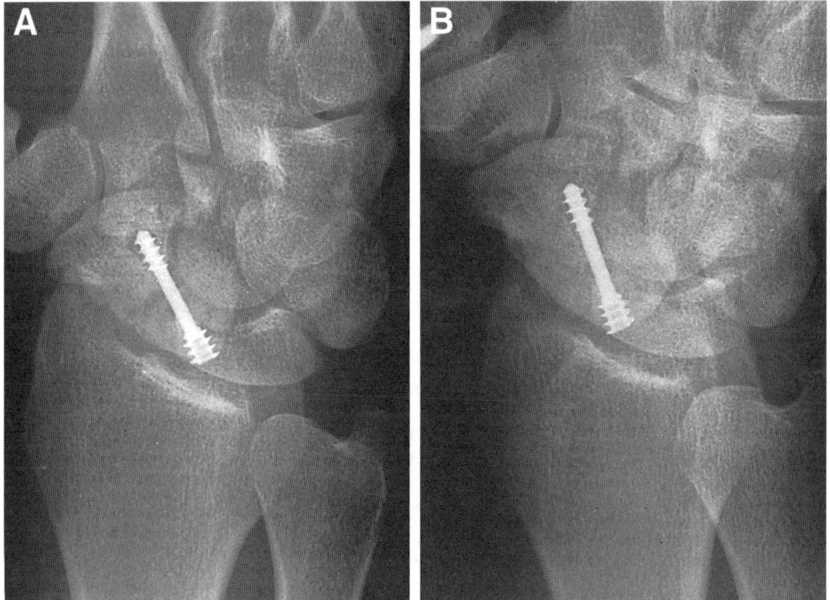

FIGURE 7.—A 21-year-old football player fractured his right scaphoid, but the diagnosis was delayed and a D2 proximal pole nonunion was reconstructed after 8 months. Sixteen months after surgery the fracture line was still visible (**A**). At 33 months, after he had sustained a Bennett's fracture that was also fixed, the fracture had finally united (**B**). (Courtesy of Filan SL, Herbert TJ: Herbert screw fixation of scaphoid fractures. *J Bone Joint Surg Br* 78B:519–529, 1996.)

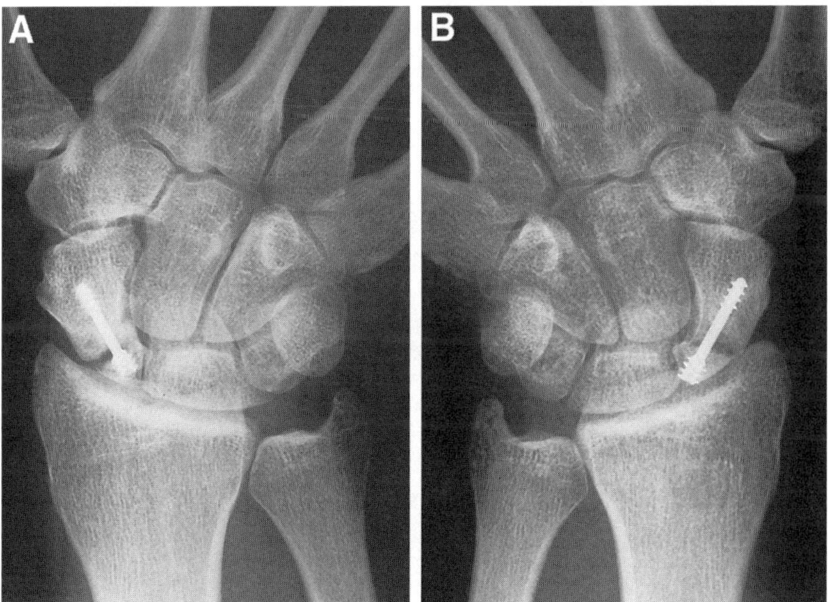

FIGURE 8.—An active sportsman and shearer/wool buyer fractured his *right* scaphoid playing football. The fracture was not diagnosed until 6 months after injury and at 13 months a D3 proximal pole fracture was reconstructed, but failed to unite. He then fractured his *left* scaphoid and a D2 proximal pole fracture was grafted and fixed. At 5 years (**A**) and 3 years (**B**) after operation, both wrists were asymptomatic with no restriction of movement or use (Courtesy of Filan SL, Herbert TJ: Herbert screw fixation of scaphoid fractures. *J Bone Joint Surg Br* 78B:519–529, 1996.)

Hand

Characteristics of Patients With Hypoplastic Thumbs
James MA, McCarroll HR Jr, Manske PR (Univ of California, San Francisco; Washington Univ, St Louis; Shriners Hosp, St Louis)
J Hand Surg (Am) 21A:104–113, 1996   9–8

Objective.—Thumb hypoplasia is a complex congenital disorder that is sometimes associated with other congenital anomalies and syndromes (Figs 1–3). Reported estimates of the prevalence of these syndromes vary considerably. It is important to classify thumb hypoplasia according to the modified Blauth classification; some types are amenable to reconstruction, whereas others are not. To assess the associated pathologic findings and to

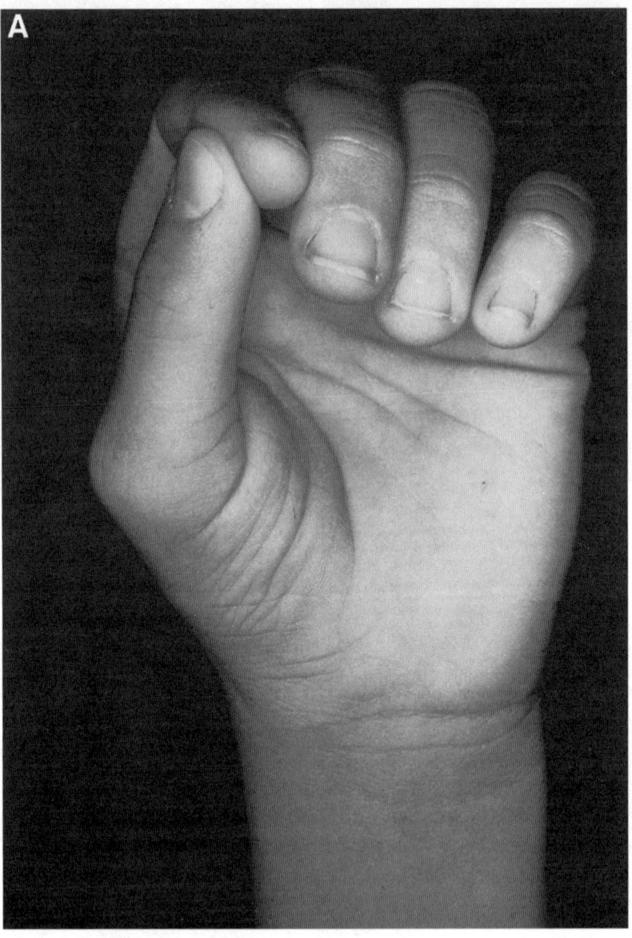

(Continued)

FIGURE 1 (cont.)

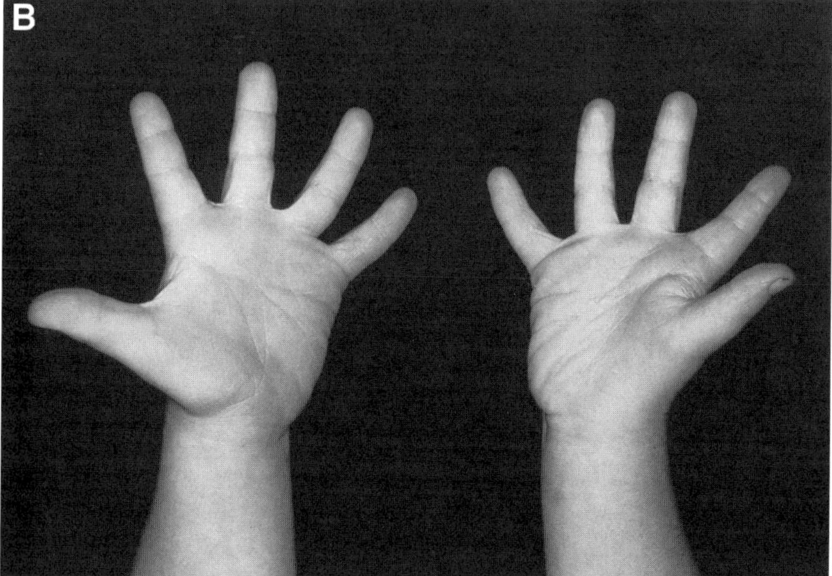

FIGURE 1.—**A,** type 1 thumb hypoplasia, with hypoplastic thenar muscle mass. **B,** type 2 thumb hypoplasia, with distal and tight web space (right hand). (Courtesy of James MA, McCarroll HR Jr, Manske PR: Characteristics of patients with hypopolastic thumbs. *J Hand Surg (Am)* 21A:104–113, 1996.)

determine the prevalence of the various types according to the modified Blauth classification, a large series of patients with hypoplastic thumbs was reviewed.

Findings.—The review included 160 hypoplastic thumbs of 98 patients seen between 1923 and 1993. The patients were 62 males and 36 females; 62 patients had both thumbs affected. Of 139 thumbs that were classifiable according to the modified Blauth classification, 19% were types 1 and 2, 23% were type 3, and 58% were types 4 and 5.

Fifty-nine percent of the patients had radial dysplasia and 86% has associated anomalies. Forty-four percent of the patients had an associated syndrome, the most common of which were the VATER (vertebral, anal, tracheoesophageal, renal) with its radial limb anomalies association and the Holt-Oram syndrome. The vertebral, anal, tracheoesophageal, renal, and radial limb anomalies association was most frequent in patients with spine, genitourinary, or gastrointestinal anomalies, whereas the Holt-Oram syndrome was more likely in patients with cardiac anomalies. Other syndromes were likely to be present in patients with lower-extremity anomalies. A total of 107 operations—including 24 thumb reconstructions and 35 pollicizations—were done in 63 upper extremities.

Conclusions.—Associated anomalies and syndromes are common in patients with hypoplastic thumbs. All patients with hypoplastic thumbs

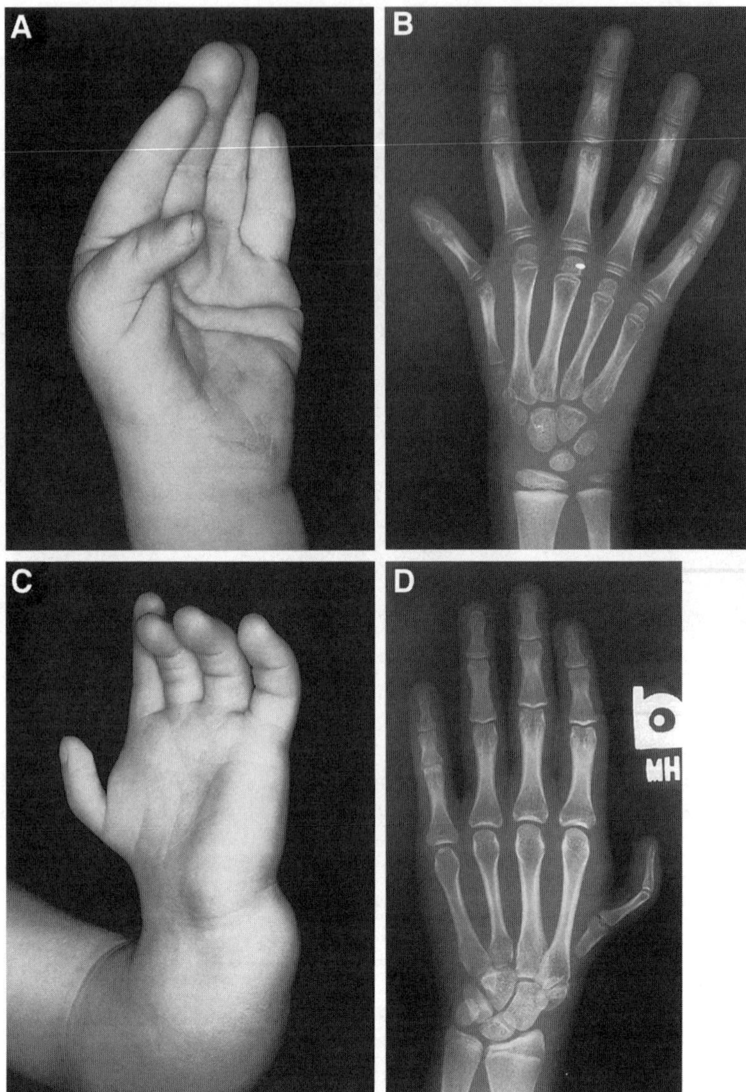

FIGURE 2.—**A,** type 3A thumb hypoplasia, with absent interphalangeal flexion (resulting from absent or anomalous flexor pollicis longus). **B,** type 3A thumb hypoplasia; x-ray film shows hypoplastic metacarpal. **C,** type 3B thumb hypoplasia; basal joint is unstable because of absence of proximal metacarpal. **D,** type 3B thumb hypoplasia; x-ray film shows proximal metacarpal is absent. (Courtesy of James MA, McCarroll HR Jr, Manske PR: Characteristics of patients with hypopolastic thumbs. *J Hand Surg (Am)* 21A:104–113, 1996.)

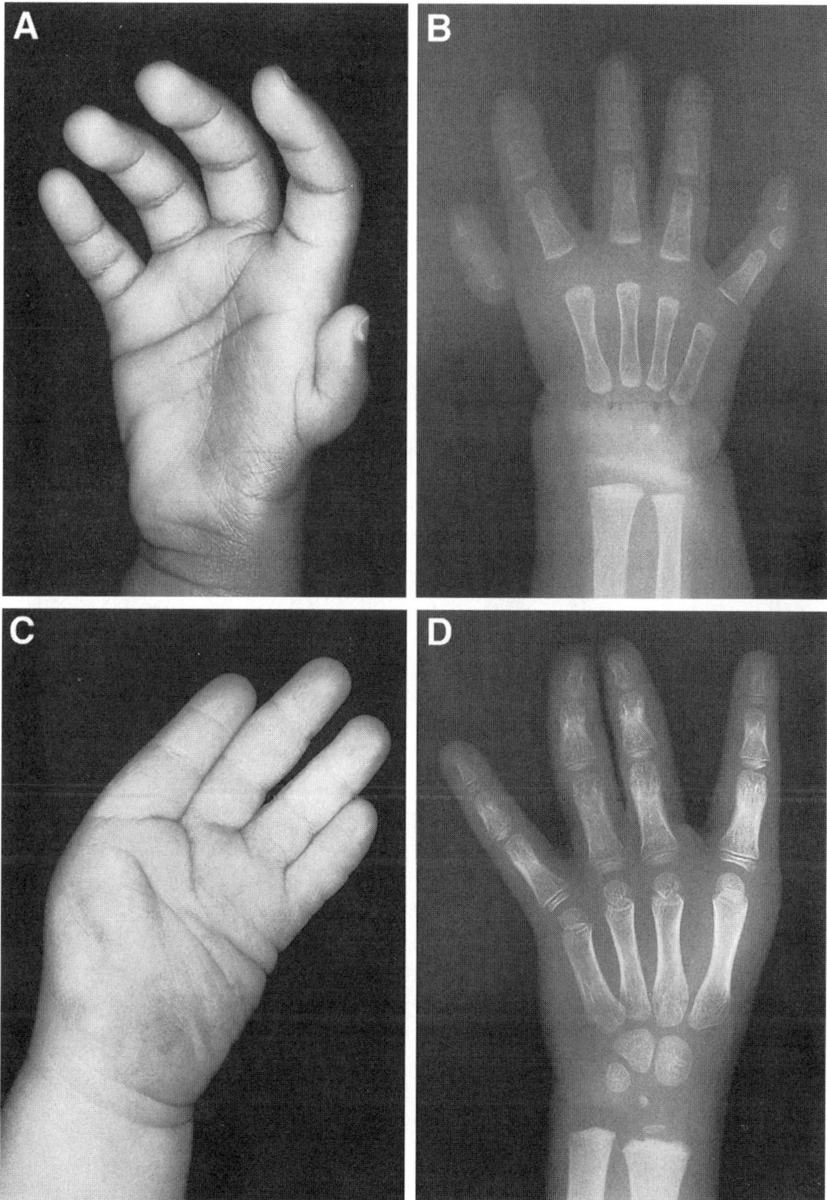

FIGURE 3.—**A,** type 4 thumb hypoplasia; thumb is connected to hand by soft tissue only. **B,** type 4 thumb hypoplasia; x-ray film shows no bony connection between thumb and hand. **C,** type 5 thumb hypoplasia; thumb is absent. **D,** type 5 thumb hypoplasia; x-ray film shows no thumb development. (Courtesy of James MA, McCarroll HR Jr, Manske PR: Characteristics of patients with hypopolastic thumbs. *J Hand Surg (Am)* 1A:104–113, 1996.)

need a careful evaluation for these associated conditions, as well as for bilaterality. The modified Blauth classification aids in treatment planning.

▶ Hypoplastic thumbs are common problems in white and Asiatic populations, and most of them are seen by clinicians who are not hand surgeons. This article does a favor for all such clinicians by not hiding away the spectrum of thumb hypoplasia in multiple and often confusing categories. The associations, particularly the syndromes, often require special precautions, but the straightforward presentation of the thumb problems and their usual management in clear, concise, and understandable terms is a boon to all.

J.H. Dobyns, M.D.

Magnetic Resonance Imaging Scanning in the Diagnosis of Zone II Flexor Tendon Rupture

Matloub HS, Dzwierzynski WW, Erickson S, et al (Med College of Wisconsin, Milwaukee; Med College of Seattle)
J Hand Surg [Am] 21A:451–455, 1996   9–9

Background.—Magnetic resonance imaging is useful for demonstrating the fine anatomy of the hand. Although MRI has been widely used to diagnose tendon and ligament rupture in the shoulder and lower extremities, its value in the diagnosis of tendon disorders in the hand has not been fully determined.

Methods and Findings.—Nine patients, aged 16 to 37 years, suspected of having flexor tendon rupture were studied. All had a difficult or uncer-

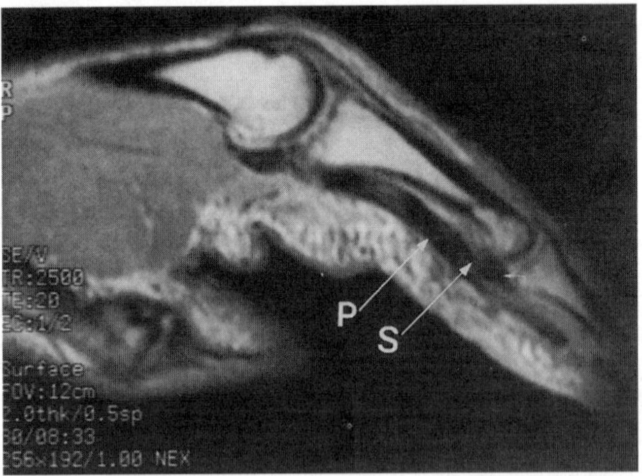

FIGURE 1.—Sagittal MRI showing delineation of flexor digitorum superficialis (*S*) and flexor digitorum profundus (*P*) tendons in a normal finger. The palmarplate (*small arrow*) is also visualized as a dark structure separate from the flexor tendons. (Courtesy of Matloub HS, Dzierzynski WW, Erickson S, et al: Magnetic resonance imaging scanning in the diagnosis of zone II flexor tendon rupture. *J Hand Surg [Am]* 21A:451–455, 1996.)

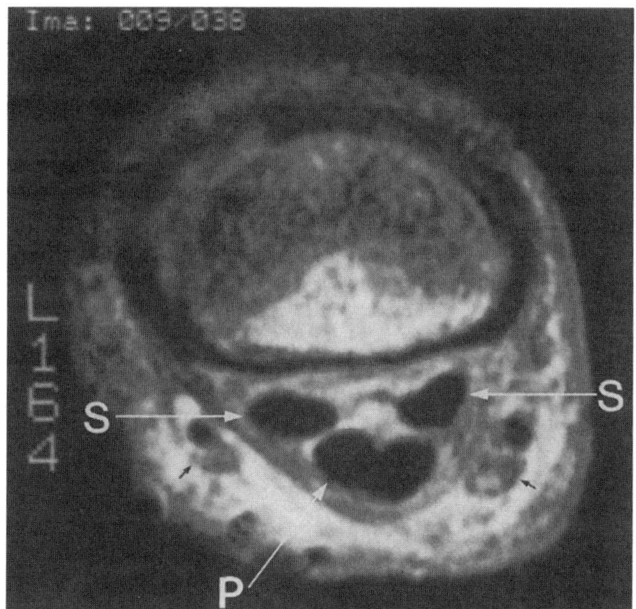

FIGURE 2.—Axial MRI at the level of the proximal phalanx shows normal flexor digitorum profundus (*P*) tendon and separate slips of the FDS (*S*) tendons. The neurovascular bundles (*small arrows*) can also be seen lateral to the tendons. (Courtesy of Matloub HS, Dzierzynski WW, Erickson S, et al: Magnetic resonance imaging scanning in the diagnosis of zone II flexor tendon rupture. *J Hand Surg [Am]* 21A:451–455, 1996.)

tain diagnosis. Eleven digits with a total of 16 tendons underwent MRI. Flexor tendons were clearly seen on all MRI scans (Figs 1 and 2). Clinical suspicion was correlated with MRI and operative results. The diagnostic accuracy of clinical diagnosis was 60%. On MRI, ruptures were differentiated from adhesions with 100% accuracy (Figs 3, 4, and 5).

Conclusions.—Magnetic resonance imaging, a noninvasive technique that provides good delineation of soft-tissue structures, is valuable in the early and differential diagnosis of tendon repair. It clearly demonstrates the anatomy of the flexor tendons in the hand and demonstrates tendon rupture, usually providing a clear differentiation from adhesions.

▶ Inadequate performance of repaired flexor tendons is a universal and common problem with hand surgery that has well-established protocols for management, including quick surgical re-entry for definite rupture. Although history and clinical examination are usually adequate for the diagnosis of rupture, questions remain about a substantial number of cases. Exponents of both ultrasound and MRI techniques propose to give us aid; on the basis of published work to date, MRI seems to have the edge.

J.H. Dobyns, M.D.

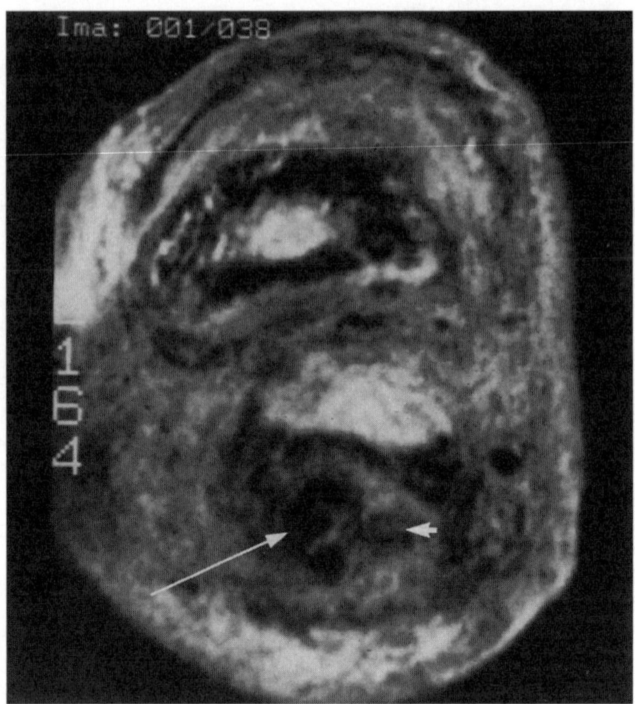

FIGURE 3.—Axial MRI at the level of the proximal interphalangeal joint shows flexor digitorum profundus tendon (*long arrow*) with an interstitial tear (*short arrow*). Flexor digitorum superficialis tendons are not visualized. (Courtesy of Matloub HS, Dzierzynski WW, Erickson S, et al: Magnetic resonance imaging scanning in the diagnosis of zone II flexor tendon rupture. *J Hand Surg [Am]* 21A:451–455, 1996.)

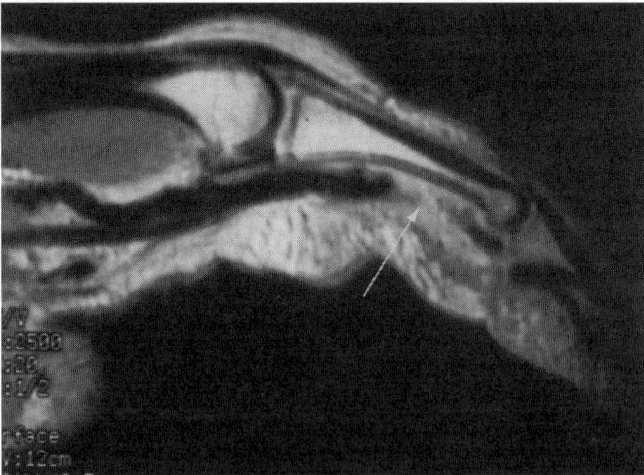

FIGURE 4.—Area of discontinuity (*arrow*) in both the flexor digitorum superficialis and flexor digitorum profundus tendons of the long finger at the level of the proximal phalanx. (Courtesy of Matloub HS, Dzierzynski WW, Erickson S, et al: Magnetic resonance imaging scanning in the diagnosis of zone II flexor tendon rupture. *J Hand Surg [Am]* 21A:451–455, 1996.)

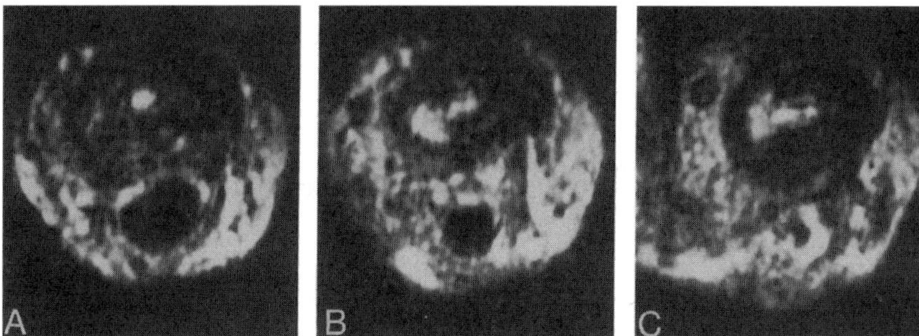

FIGURE 5.—Serial axial images of the ring finger showing flexor digitorum profundus tendon: **A,** level of proximal phalanx; **B,** 9 mm proximal to A; **C,** 6 mm proximal to B. Marked attenuation with partial tendon continuity can be appreciated. Scan was read as inconclusive for tendon rupture. (Courtesy of Matloub HS, Dzierzynski WW, Erickson S, et al: Magnetic resonance imaging scanning in the diagnosis of zone II flexor tendon rupture. *J Hand Surg [Am]* 21A:451–455, 1996.)

Effect of Motion and Tension on Injured Flexor Tendons in Chickens

Kubota H, Manske PR, Aoki M, et al (Washington Univ, St Louis, Mo)
J Hand Surg [Am] 21A:456–463, 1996   9–10

Background.—After primary tendon repair, mobilization improves the gliding function and tensile properties of the repair site. In vitro studies have shown that tension may affect the intrinsic repair response of the tendon. However, previous in vivo experiments have not examined the specific roles of motion and tension in enhancing tendon healing. The

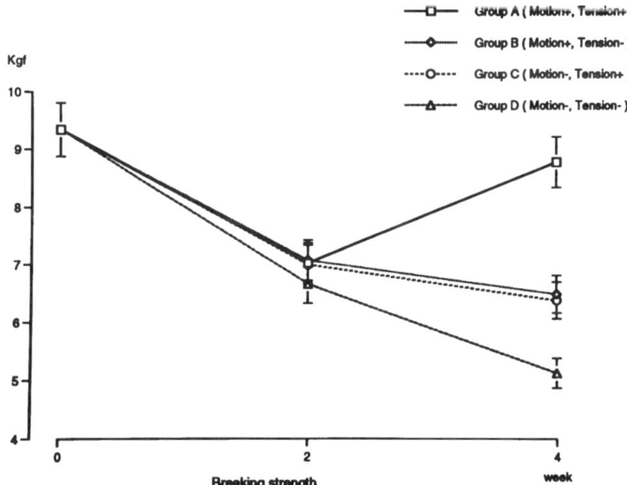

FIGURE 3.—Comparison of breaking strength of all experimental groups (10 tendons in each group). Data represent mean ± SD. Motion (−), elimination of the injured tendon's movement by cast; tension (−), elimination of the tensile force by flexor muscles. (Courtesy of Kubota H, Manske PR, Aoki M, et al: Effect of motion and tension on injured flexor tendons in chickens. *J Hand Surg [Am]* 21A:456–463, 1996.)

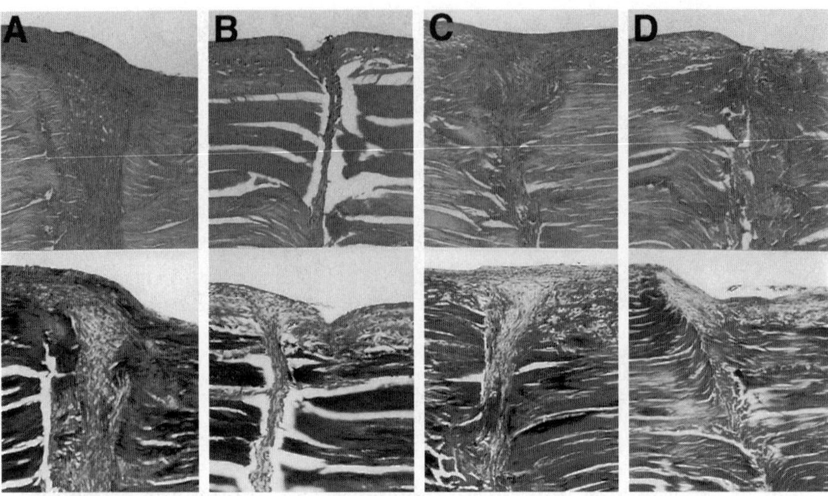

FIGURE 4.—Longitudinal section of chicken flexor tendon perpendicular to the laceration site, excluding the intact marginal fibers at 2 weeks stained with hematoxylin and eosin (*above*) and Masson's trichrome (*below*). **A,** group A; **B,** group B; **C,** group C; **D,** group D (original magnification × 100). Note clear blue-stained fiber formation with Masson's stain in group A and lesser response in group C, followed by group B in the original color picture. (Courtesy of Kubota H, Manske PR, Aoki M, et al: Effect of motion and tension on injured flexor tendons in chickens. *J Hand Surg [Am]* 21A:456–463, 1996.)

individual effects of motion and tension on the healing response of injured flexor profundus tendons were studied in chickens.

Methods and Findings.—Fifty-three chickens were subjected to partial midsection transverse lacerations of the profundus tendons. After surgery, the chickens were randomly assigned to 1 of 4 treatments: motion and tension, motion only, tension only, and neither motion nor tension. At 4 weeks, biomechanical assessment demonstrated that breaking strength was significantly increased with both motion and tension, significantly reduced with neither, and intermediate with only motion or tension. Histologically, cellular activity was generally greatest with both motion and tension, the least with neither, and intermediate with motion or tension only. Increases in collagen fiber staining were primarily seen in the tension groups (Figs 3 and 4).

Conclusions.—Both motion and tension contribute to the tendon's response to injury, affirming the notion that active tendon mobilization is important in postoperative tendon rehabilitation. The current findings support the use of previously described active mobilization protocols, assuming that active forces do not exceed the breaking strength of the repair.

▶ By now, we should surely have a formula that translates chicken tendon results to human tendon results. Despite the absence of such a formula and despite the modifications necessary to transfer the data about half-tendon severance to whole-tendon severance, we should be able to accept the conclusions drawn in this paper—that both motion and tension within safety ranges are useful in rebuilding damaged flexor tendon substance.

J.H. Dobyns, M.D.

Splint Immobilization of Gamekeeper's Thumb
Landsman JC, Seitz WH Jr, Froimson AI, et al (Case Western Reserve Univ, Cleveland, Ohio)
Orthopedics 18:1161–1165, 1995   9–11

Introduction.—Gamekeeper's thumb, a term used to describe instability of the metacarpophalangeal joint, results from acute and chronic injuries to the ulnar collateral ligament. There is little controversy regarding the closed treatment of incomplete ruptures of the ligament. However, closed management of complete ruptures of the ulnar collateral ligament have been reported to result in failure rates as high as 50%. It has also been reported that early surgical intervention produces better results than delayed surgery. The nonsurgical treatment of acute complete rupture of the ulnar collateral ligament of the thumb metacarpophalangeal joint was evaluated in a retrospective study.

Methods.—Thirty-nine patients were included in the trial, with complete rupture of the ulnar collateral ligament in 40 thumbs. The diagnosis of ligament rupture was made using radiography and clinical stress testing. The thumb was immobilized with a thumb spica splint worn 24 hours a day; a hand-based thermoplastic splint was worn during daytime hours and a forearm-based splint was used during the night. Treatment lasted between 8 and 12 weeks. During that time, radiographs were obtained every 2 weeks to confirm proper alignment during healing. Patients who did not respond to treatment at the end of 12 weeks were referred for surgical reconstruction. Patients were followed for an average of 2.4 years (range, 1–5 years).

Results.—Thirty-four of the 40 injured thumbs were considered healed with splint immobilization. Range of motion from 60% to 100% of the contralateral hand was achieved. Six of the 34 patients complained of occasional discomfort with strenuous activities. An average pinch strength of 82% was achieved, with a range of 80% to 100%. Radiography showed all bony avulsion lesions to be healed. Surgical reconstruction was performed in the remaining 6 thumbs, achieving a range of motion of 69% and a pinch strength of 75% of the contralateral hand. One patient complained of persistent pain and required additional treatment.

Conclusion.—Splint immobilization was successful in treating 85% of thumbs with complete rupture of the ulnar collateral ligament. Surgical treatment was effective in those patients who failed to respond to 12 weeks of splint immobilization.

▶ Ancient names ("gamekeeper's thumb") and ancient ways (splint treatment of skier's thumb) are not just for the history books. The orthopedist's evolution from nonsurgical specialist to nearly 100% surgical specialist demeans the capabilities of our physiology and exceeds the needs of our patients. For who would "quietus make with a bare bodkin" if 'twere unnecessary? Although I have yielded to temptation more than the authors, my experience parallels theirs, and I join them in recommending that the option of nonsurgical treatment be considered for this as well as other items on our trauma agenda.

J.H. Dobyns, M.D.

Isolated Injuries to the Dorsoradial Capsule of the Thumb Metacarpophalangeal Joint

Krause JO, Manske PR, Mirly HL, et al (Washington Univ, St Louis)
J Hand Surg [Am] 21A:428–433, 1996   9–12

Background.—The most common injury to the metacarpophalangeal (MP) joint of the thumb involves the ulnar collateral ligament. Radial collateral ligament injuries are less common. Little attention has been given to isolated dorsal capsular injuries. A series of patients with dorsoradial capsular injuries of the thumb MP joint without clinical radial collateral ligament or ulnar collateral ligament laxity was described.

Methods and Findings.—Eleven patients, aged 10 to 45 years, with injuries to the dorsoradial capsule of the thumb MP joints were seen between 1989 and 1993. The mechanism of injury was breaking a fall (5 patients), a direct blow (3 patients), and a sports-related injury (3 patients). Seven injuries were confirmed at surgical exploration and repaired by imbrication or a direct technique (Fig 2). No complications resulted from surgery. Six of the 7 patients later returned to unrestricted

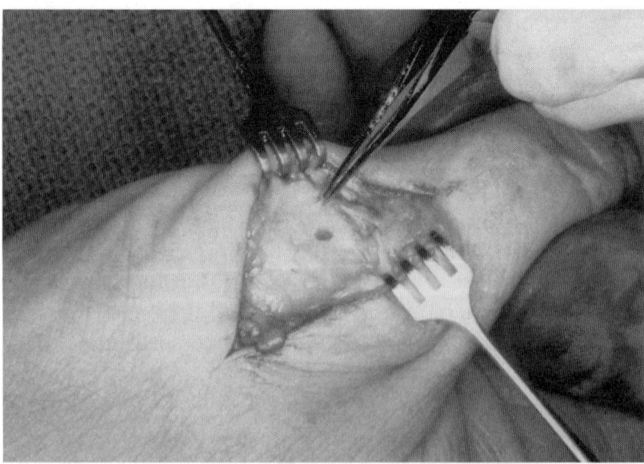

FIGURE 2.—Intraoperative photograph showing defect in dorsoradial capsule of the metacarpophalangeal joint of the thumb. (Courtesy of Krause JO, Manske PR, Mirly HL, et al: Isolated injuries to the dorsoradial capsule of the thumb metacarpophalangeal joint. *J Hand Surg* [Am] 21A:428–433, 1996.)

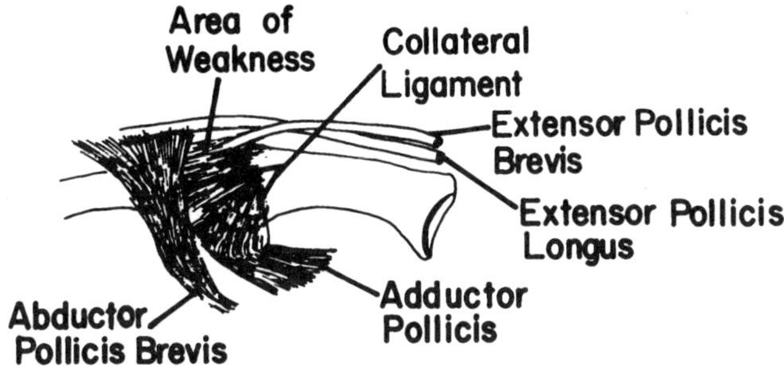

FIGURE 5.—Drawing of metacarpophalangeal joint of the thumb demonstrating the area of potential weakness in the dorsoradial capsule. (Courtesy of Krause JO, Manske PR, Mirly HL, et al: Isolated injuries to the dorsoradial capsule of the thumb metacarpophalangeal joint. *J Hand Surg [Am]* 21A:428–433, 1996.)

activity with no need for analgesics. One patient continued to report tenderness over the dorsoradial capsule and minor pain (Fig 5).

Conclusions.—Although much less common than collateral ligament injuries, isolated injuries to the dorsoradial capsule of the thumb MP joint do occur. Patients with palmar subluxation of the proximal phalanx will probably need surgical exploration and repair. Nonoperative treatment was ineffective in the patients in this series who had palmar subluxation and extensor lag.

▶ At long last, the dorsal and radial aspects of the MP joint of the thumb are getting their due, and the injuries there are as intriguing as those of the better known "skier's thumb." We have long recognized that some radial collateral ligament ruptures require repair for best results and that most of them are associated with dorsal capsular injury. The authors of this paper give good evidence that in certain patients (they postulate that those of us with increased thumb MP flexion are at risk), tear of the dorsal capsule alone can result in chronic pain or palmer subluxation or limited extension. Early adequate splinting in full extension may control the problems of these patients, but this is not always done; even if it is done, persistent pain may occur. Most patients in this series were treated with surgical repair for chronic symptoms, but recognition of the syndrome may lead to better early management. It is of interest that an article in the same issue[1] discusses another little-known aspect of injury to the radial aspect of the thumb MP joint, that is, combined radial collateral ligament tear, dorsal MP capsular tear, and rupture of the extensor pollicus brevis. With this combination, surgery is even more necessary.

J.H. Dobyns, M.D.

Reference

1. Failla JM: Combined extensor pollicis brevis and radial collateral ligament injury. Three case reports. *J Hand Surg [Am]* 21A:434–437, 1996.

A Comparison of Methods of Treatment of PIP Joint Contractures in Dupuytren's Disease

Breed CM, Smith PJ (Mount Vernon Hosp, Northwood, Middlesex, England)
J Hand Surg (Br) 21B:246–251, 1996   9–13

Background.—Proximal interphalangeal (PIP) joint contracture caused by Dupuytren's disease is difficult to treat. Authorities disagree on how to best manage the residual PIP joint contracture when digital fasciectomy does not result in full extension. Procedures recommended include release of the volar plate, accessory collateral ligament, check-rein ligaments, arthroplasty, and amputation. Few studies have compared conservative treatment by manipulation and splintage with more aggressive operative management. Different treatments used in 1 series were compared.

Methods and Findings.—Seventy-five severely contracted PIP joints were treated with some form of release because of a residual flexion contracture after a release of all the Dupuytren's tissue in the digit. These represented 40% of 188 PIP joints in hands affected by Dupuytren's disease treated between 1980 and 1992. Thus, 2 broad groups were identified: 113 PIP joints responding with full correction after digital fasciectomy, and 75 requiring a PIP joint release after digital fasciectomy. The patients needing PIP joint procedures had PIP joint contracture for twice as long as those who did not. There was a 10.9-year difference between the average age of Dupuytren's disease onset and the average age at which a PIP procedure was performed. Treatments were gentle passive manipulation only in 22 fingers, surgical release of the PIP in 31, PIP joint release with extensor tendon repair in 10, and no further PIP treatment in 7. Gentle passive manipulation alone yielded better outcomes with fewer complications than did more aggressive surgical intervention.

Conclusions.—In this series, the outcomes of manipulation differed significantly from those of surgical treatment of the PIP joint after digital fasciectomy in patients with residual flexion deformity at the PIP joint level associated with Dupuytren's disease. Gentle passive manipulation alone is more effective and safer than more aggressive surgical intervention.

▶ For adding disaster to disease my 2 nominees are the surgical treatment of camptodactyly in the child and Dupuytren's in the adult. For that reason I am delighted to see and to agree with the central theme of this paper, i.e., that gentle, sustained stretch of contracted PIP joints in the Dupuytren's afflicted digit is preferable, IF POSSIBLE. There are some cases, only 7 documented in this paper but somewhat more in my experience, that are fixed in the flexed deformity (more often those where previous surgery has been done, but not all) and will not yield to gentle suasion.

J.H. Dobyns, M.D.

Corrective Osteotomy for Post-traumatic Malunion of the Phalanges in the Hand
Büchler U, Gupta A, Ruf S (Univ of Bern, Switzerland)
J Hand Surg (Br) 21B:33–42, 1996
9–14

Background.—Phalangeal malunion can result in rotation, angulation, deviation, shortening, or a combination of deformities, impairing hand function. Corrective osteotomy was done for posttraumatic malunion of the phalanges in 1 series of patients.

Patients.—Fifty-seven patients, aged 5 to 61 years, had phalangeal corrective osteotomies for posttraumatic malunion between 1978 and 1990. A total of 59 rotational, radial/ulnar deviation, flexion/extension, length adjustment and combination procedures were done. Rigid internal fixation was used. Half of the patients underwent concurrent tenocapsulolysis.

Outcomes.—Surgical correction was satisfactory in 76% of the patients. In all, bony union was achieved. Eighty-nine percent of the patients had a net gain in active range of motion. Surgical outcomes were excellent or good in 96% of patients undergoing corrective osteotomies for malunion involving the bone only and in 64% of those undergoing corrections for malunion with multiple structure involvement (OR4).

Conclusions.—With comprehensive planning, meticulous technique, and intensive aftercare, corrective osteotomy of the phalanges can yield very satisfactory results. In patients with complex, multistructural involvement, capsulotomy, tenolysis, nerve grafting, and skin flap, applications are important and may be performed safely in 1 stage when rigid internal fixation is used. The best functional outcomes are not associated with type and degree of bony deformity or procedure complexity but are associated with the nature of the initial injury.

▶ It is difficult to present a treatment series and a mini-instructional course at the same time, but I believe that these authors have succeeded. The fine details of surgical technique for bone fixation and for treatment of associated soft-tissue problems are not included, but I have not seen a better overview of bony phalangeal deformity, its assessment, and its management.

J.H. Dobyns, M.D.

Basal Joint Arthritis: Trapeziectomy With Ligament Reconstruction and Tendon Interposition Arthroplasty
Lins RE, Gelberman RH, McKeown L, et al (Massachusetts Gen Hosp, Boston; Washington Univ, St Louis, Mo; Brigham and Women's Hosp, Boston)
J Hand Surg [Am] 21A:202–209, 1996
9–15

Objective.—Excisional arthroplasty has been effective in the relief of pain and preservation of thumb motion, but recent surgical techniques have focused on ligament reconstruction to improve thumb function.

Results of a retrospective qualitative and quantitative assessment of thumb function in patients who underwent ligament reconstruction and tendon interposition (LRTI) were presented.

Methods.—At an average of 43 months after surgery, a survey was sent to 27 patients (30 thumbs), 43 to 77 years of age, who underwent LRTI between 1987 and 1993 to evaluate satisfaction; pain frequency, severity, and duration; and ability to perform activities of daily life. Radiographic studies evaluated the trapezial space ratio for thumbs before and immediately after surgery and at least 12 months after surgery (Fig 2).

Technique.—With the Burton method, an incision is made in the thumb, the trapezium is excised, and 12 cm of the flexor carpi radialis is drawn through a metacarpal drill hole and sutured to itself and to the periosteum. The trapezial space is preserved and the thumb is stabilized in the abducted fist position. The remaining tendon is rolled to act as a spacer and secured. The wound is closed, and the thumb is splinted. Movement is allowed at 12 weeks.

Results.—The average pain frequency rating was 3 on a scale of 1 to 10, and pain severity rating averaged 2. Pain frequency improved greatly or resolved in 85% of patients and duration and severity improved in 89%. Ability to perform activities of daily life improved in 18 thumbs. Web space measurements, grip strength, and pinch strength improved significantly. The trapezial space ratio decreased from 0.33 before surgery to

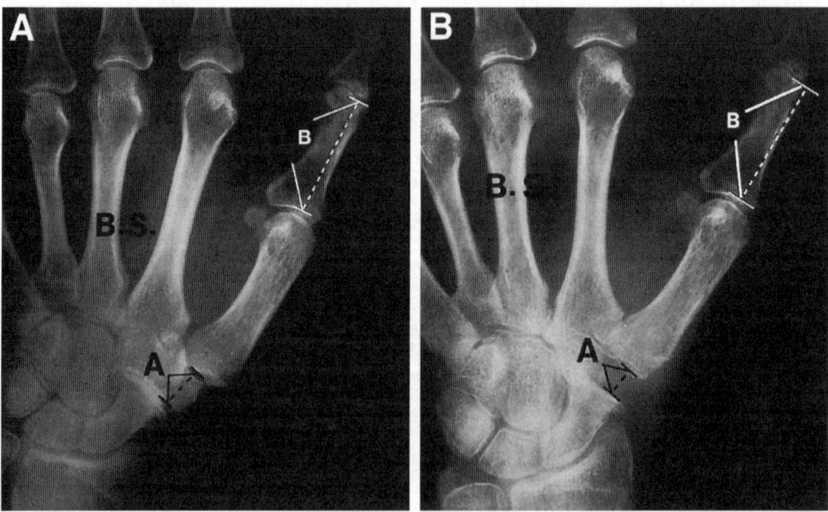

FIGURE 2.—X-ray films of an arthritic thumb taken (A) before and (B) after basal joint arthroplasty. The trapezial space and proximal phalanx height are marked *A* and *B*, respectively. (Courtesy of Lins RE, Gelberman RH, McKeown L, et al: Basal joint arthritis: Trapeziectomy with ligament reconstruction and tendon interposition arthroplasty. *J Hand Surg [Am]* 21A:202–209, 1996).

0.23 after surgery and remained unchanged 36 months later. A major postoperative complication that necessitated resection arthroplasty developed in 1 patient and tendinitis developed in 2 patients.

Conclusion.—Patients were generally very satisfied with the results of LRTI. Ability to perform activities of daily life improved significantly and pain decreased significantly. Trapezial space ratios decreased significantly after surgery but did not appear to interfere with function or to increase discomfort.

▶ Another premier hand service confirms the value of the standard and well-accepted "suspension interposition arthroplasty" for the thumb carpometacarpal joint, as popularized by Burton and colleagues. The authors include an excellent method for documentation of the trapezial space changes, whether from the arthritic process or from the surgical method, although the consistent loss of two thirds of that space does not seem to affect the generally good results. These results, along with a low level of complication, make this procedure the current standard for symptomatic degenerative or posttraumatic arthritis of the thumb carpometacarpal joint. Although increased comfort led to a satisfaction rate of nearly 90%, functional improvement was only around 70%—a standard that may not be good enough.

J.H. Dobyns, M.D.

Benefits and Use of Digital Prostheses
Pereira BP, Kour A-K, Leow E-L, et al (Natl Univ Hosp, Singapore, Japan)
J Hand Surg [Am] 21A:222–228, 1996   9–16

Background.—In patients with digital amputations, the loss of form and cosmetic appearance may be so psychologically damaging that active hand function is inhibited. Fitting a socially acceptable, custom-made prosthesis can augment microsurgical reconstruction. One clinical experience with such prostheses was reported.

Methods and Findings.—One hundred thirty-six digital prostheses were fitted in 90 patients. Thirty patients were followed for at least 2 years. Seventy-three percent reported using their prostheses daily, and 23% reported using them intermittently. Twenty-three percent of the patients using their prostheses occasionally had technical problems, such as loose fit and perspiration (Figs 1, 2, 3, and 4).

Conclusions.—High-quality digital prostheses can provide near-normal appearance and form, improve body image, and contribute to better physical outcomes in patients with digital amputations. Careful patient selection, with special attention to patient expectations, is crucial.

▶ Patients are often unaware of the availability and uncertain of the value of digital prostheses. Too often, their physicians adopt a laissez-faire attitude and neglect to inform them of the possibilities. We owe these authors a debt

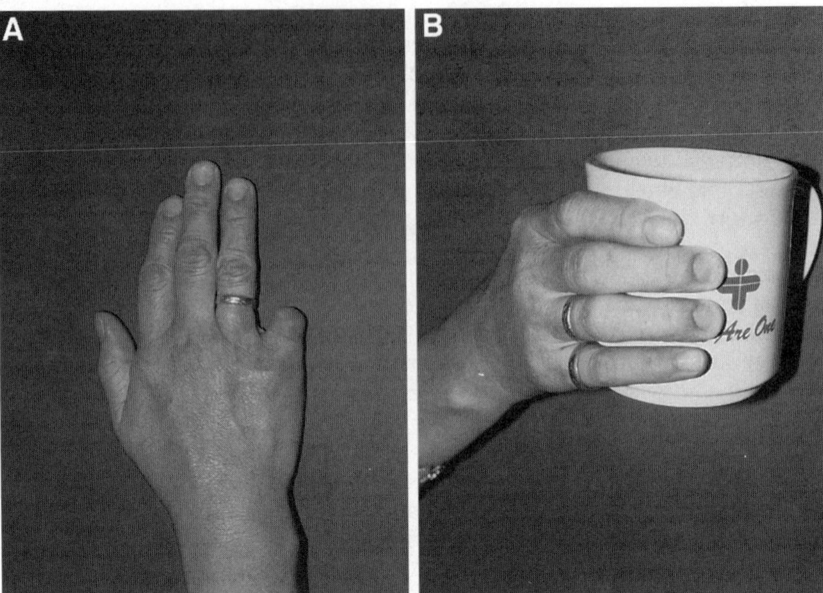

FIGURE 1.—A patient with a single digital amputation through the proximal phalanx of the little finger (**A**) before fitting and (**B**) after fitting a prosthesis. (Courtesy of Pereira BP, Kour A-K, Leow E-L, et al: Benefits and Use of Digital Prostheses. *J Hand Surg [Am]* 21A:222-228, 1996.)

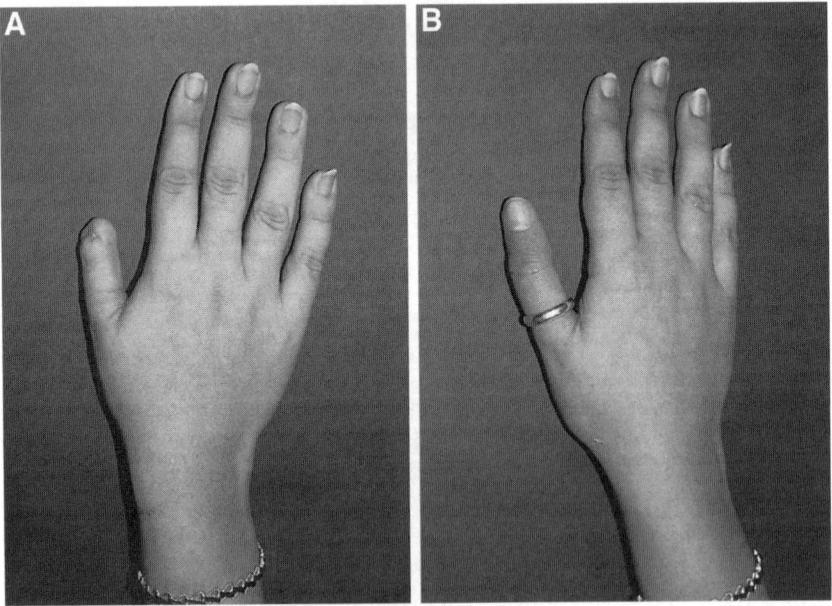

FIGURE 2.—Another patient with a single digit amputation through the distal interphalangeal joint of the thumb (**A**) before fitting and (**B**) after fitting. (Courtesy of Pereira BP, Kour A-K, Leow E-L, et al: Benefits and Use of Digital Prostheses. *J Hand Surg [Am]* 21A:222-228, 1996.)

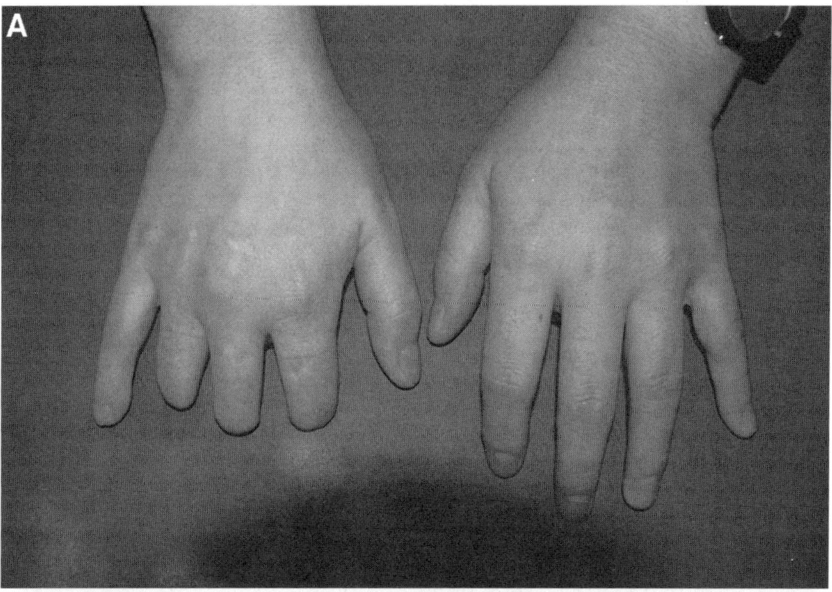

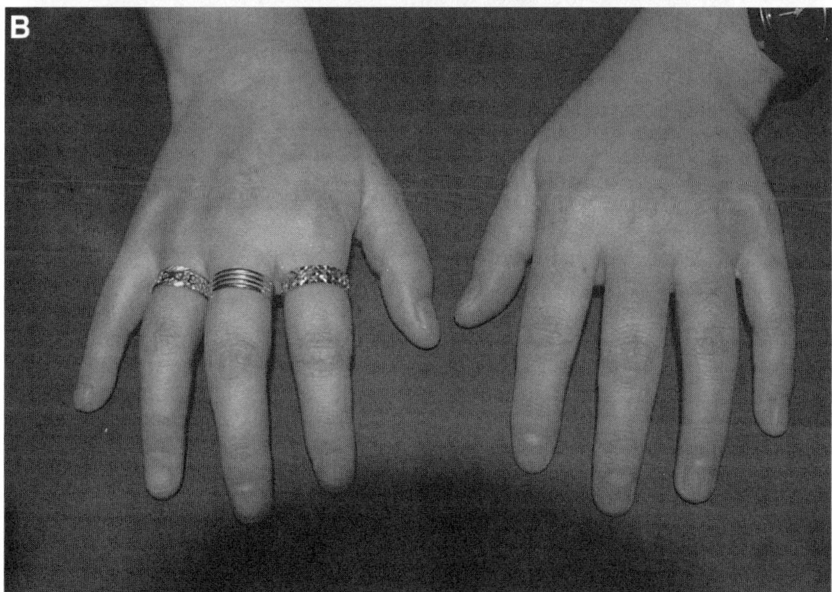

FIGURE 3.—A patient with multiple-digit amputations of the index, middle, and ring fingers at the proximal interphalangeal joint (**A**) before fitting and (**B**) after fitting. (Courtesy of Pereira BP, Kour A-K, Leow E-L, et al: Benefits and Use of Digital Prostheses. *J Hand Surg [Am]* 21A:222-228, 1996.)

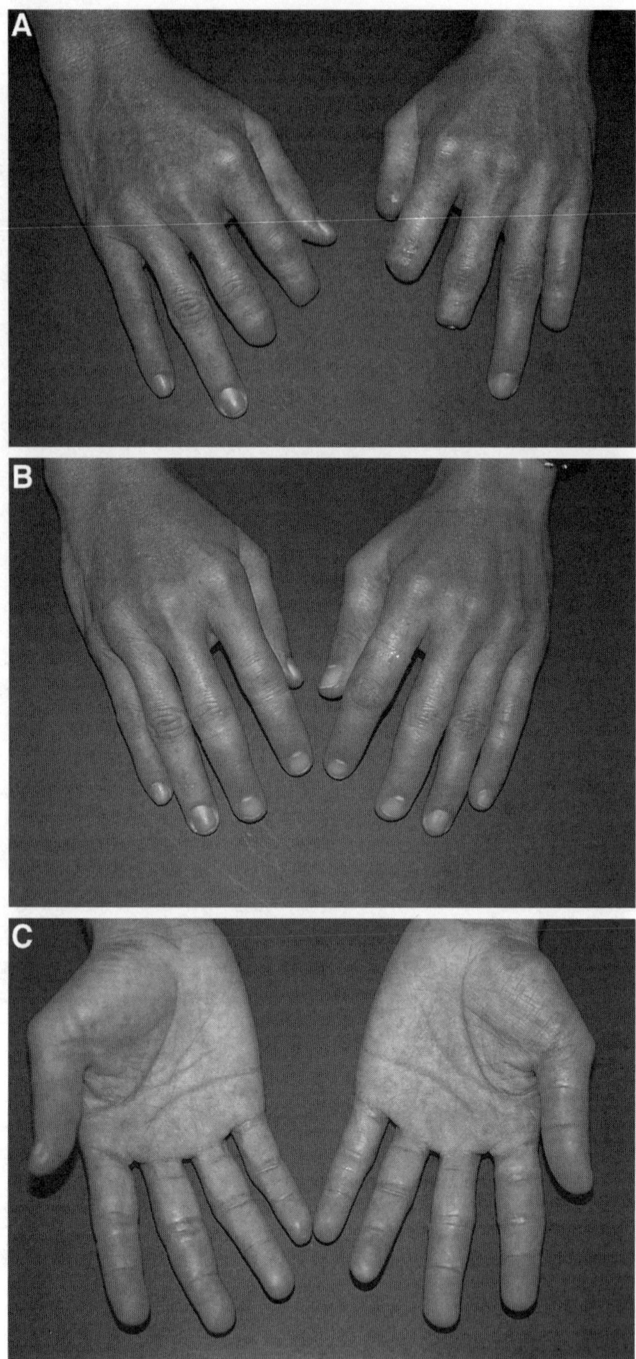

FIGURE 4.—Bilateral involvement with multiple-digit amputations due to a pathologic condition (Buerger's disease): **A**, before fitting and, **B**, after fitting of prosthesis, dorsal side and, **C**, palmar side. (Courtesy of Pereira BP, Kour A-K, Leow E-L, et al: Benefits and Use of Digital Prostheses. *J Hand Surg [Am]* 21A:222-228, 1996.)

of gratitude for reminding and encouraging us about the benefits of digital prostheses.

J.H. Dobyns, M.D.

Neurovascular

Medial Epicondylectomy or Ulnar-Nerve Transposition for Ulnar Neuropathy at the Elbow?
Geutjens GG, Langstaff RJ, Smith NJ, et al (Queen's Med Centre, Nottingham, England)
J Bone Joint Surg (Br) 78B:777–779, 1996   9–17

Background.—A variety of procedures have been recommended for the treatment of ulnar nerve lesions at the elbow. Medial epicondylectomy and anterior transposition for such lesions were compared in a prospective, randomized study.

Methods.—Fifty-two patients underwent surgery for ulnar neuropathy between 1985 and 1992. Forty-three were available for follow-up assessment. Patients were assessed neurologically and orthopedically. Mean follow-up time was 4.5 years.

Findings.—None of the patients reported spontaneous pain in the elbow. Hand pain was significantly more common after nerve transposition, but such pain was only mild. Considerably fewer patients undergoing medial epicondylectomy reported that they were no better or worse postoperatively than those undergoing anterior transposition. Almost all the patients undergoing the former procedure said they would be willing to have the procedure again, compared to about half of those undergoing anterior transposition.

Conclusions.—The outcomes of medial epicondylectomy were better than those of anterior transposition, patient satisfaction being higher after the former than the latter. However, motor power or nerve conduction rates did not differ significantly. Sensory fibers may be more vulnerable to devascularization after anterior transposition. Neither procedure seemed to affect elbow function significantly.

▶ A simple question, simply answered, qualifies in my opinion for the much-desired outcomes study. We may all be using this type of study for all our treatments before very long. I would have anticipated the result here, i.e., that medial epicondylectomy, carefully done, is a little easier on the ulnar nerve. Perhaps the only more gentle ulnar nerve decompression is the next one the authors promise to investigate, i.e., simple decompression.

J.H. Dobyns, M.D.

A Comparison of Traditional Electrodiagnostic Studies, Electroneurometry, and Vibrometry in the Diagnosis of Carpal Tunnel Syndrome

Cherniack MG, Moalli D, Viscolli C (Yale Univ, New Haven, Conn; Lawrence and Mem Hosp, New London, Conn)
J Hand Surg (Am) 21A:122–131, 1996

9–18

Background.—Forearm electrodiagnostic studies have long been relied on for the diagnosis of peripheral nerve injuries of the upper limb, particularly nerve entrapment syndromes. However, some have questioned whether the cost and discomfort of these tests justify using them for conditions that must ultimately be diagnosed clinically. New portable devices, such as the digital electroneurometer, now offer alternatives for the quantitative assessment of these conditions. Vibrometry is regarded as an essential part of qualitative sensory testing. The results of electroneurometry, vibrometry, and traditional nerve conduction studies were compared in the same series of patients and controls.

Methods.—Ninety-eight hands of 49 patients referred to a hospital-based electrodiagnostic laboratory were studied. Each extremity was tested by conventional nerve conduction studies; electroneurometry, with skin-surface electrical stimulation of the motor nerve; and 120-Hz, single-frequency vibrometry. Both the median and ulnar nerves were tested. A separate group of asymptomatic controls was tested as well.

Results.—Correlations with the results of motor nerve conduction studies of the median nerve were $r = 0.81$ for electroneurometry and $r = 0.48$ for vibrometry. The relation with electroneurometry showed high sensitivity but low specificity when the diagnosis of carpal tunnel syndrome was made on the sole basis of clinical criteria or a nerve conduction abnormality. For vibrometry, the relation was the opposite. All of the associations were greatly influenced by the way in which normal values were selected from a reference population. Good predictability, with thresholds corresponding to the results of nerve conduction studies, was achieved using the manufacturer's recommended normal values. However, the associations were much weaker using normal values generated by standard techniques.

Conclusions.—The choice of a screening test for entrapment neuropathies and other peripheral nerve injuries depends on the prevalence and seriousness of the disease being sought, as well as the consequences of overdiagnosis and underdiagnosis. More extensive study is needed before vibrometry and electroneurometry come into routine use in screening for entrapment neuropathies.

▶ Convenience and cost are driving the profession toward relying on office-type screening tests, and manufacturers are happy to provide the tools and to supply continual upgrades. There is always a limit to what can be reliably achieved in this way; experienced clinical examination and laboratory-type electrodiagnostic studies are still more reliable, although there are occasions when the portable assessments are appropriate. As the authors say in their abstract, "The selection of an appropriate electrical screening test for peripheral nerve injury, such as entrapment neuropathy, depends on the prevalence and seriousness of the target disease and the relative consequences of over- and underdiagnosis." That the whole issue of what constitutes adequate electrodiagnostic testing may be moot is suggested by findings in *The Journal of Hand Surgery.*[1] Symptom outcome after carpal tunnel release was found to be essentially the same in groups that were electrodiagnostically positive, that were electrodiagnostically negative, and that received no electrodiagnostic workup at all.

J.H. Dobyns, M.D.

References

1. Glowacki KA, Breen CJ, Sachar K, et al: Electrodiagnostic testing and carpal tunnel release outcome. *J Hand Surg (Am)* 21A:117–122, 1996.

Diagnosis and Staging of Carpal Tunnel Syndrome: Comparison of Magnetic Resonance Imaging and Intra-operative Findings
Kleindienst A, Hamm B, Hildebrandt G, et al (Univ of Cologne, Germany; Humboldt-Universität zu Berlin)
Acta Neurochir (Wien) 138:228–233, 1996   9–19

Background.—There is much interest in the use of MRI for the diagnosis of carpal tunnel syndrome (CTS) because it produces high contrast of

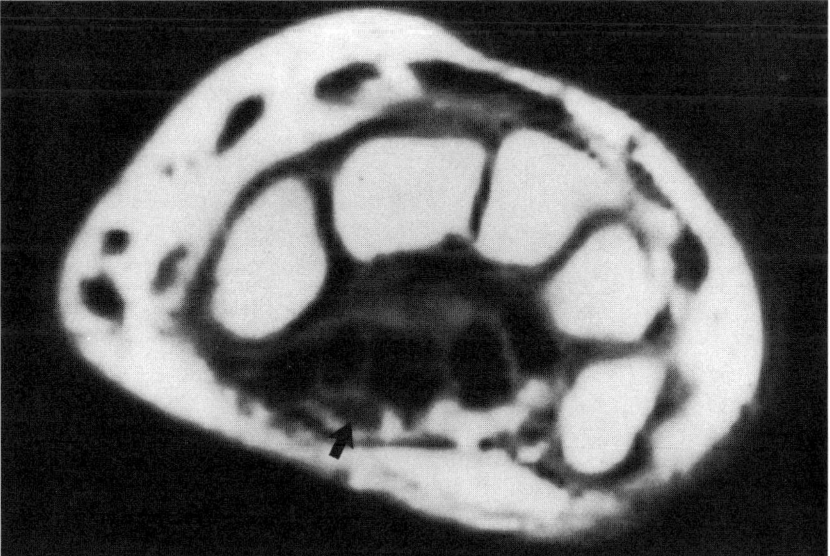

FIGURE 1.—Normal median nerve at the proximal part of the carpal tunnel. Axial slice at the level of the pisiform bone. T1-weighted spin echo sequence (TR = 500 ms, TE = 15 ms). The median nerve can be easily identified (*arrow*). (Courtesy of Kleindienst A, Hamm B, Hildebrandt G, et al: Diagnosis and staging of carpal tunnel syndrome: Comparison of magnetic resonance imaging and intra-operative findings. *Acta Neurochir (Wien)* 138:228–233, 1996.)

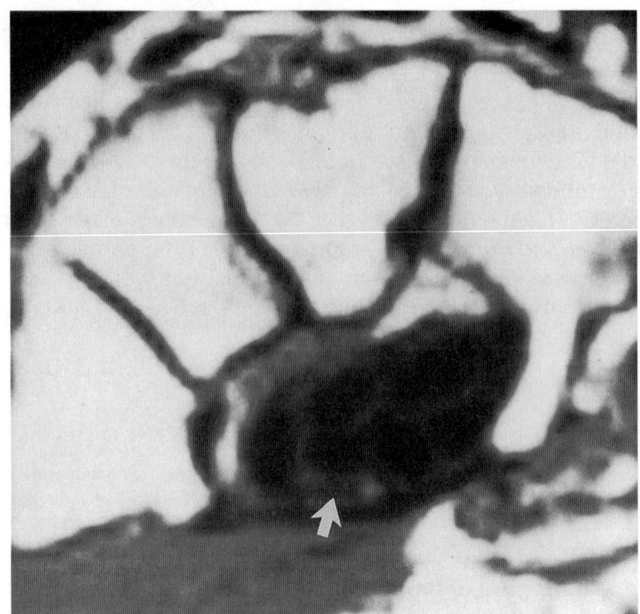

FIGURE 2.—Normal median nerve at the distal part of the carpal tunnel. Axial slice at the level of the hamate bone, T1-weighted spin-echo sequence (TR = 500 ms, TE = 15 ms). The nerve flattening (*arrow*) can also be identified in normal control subjects. (Courtesy of Kleindienst A, Hamm B, Hildebrandt G, et al: Diagnosis and staging of carpal tunnel syndrome: Comparison of magnetic resonance imaging and intra-operative findings. *Acta Neurochir (Wien)* 138:228–233, 1996.)

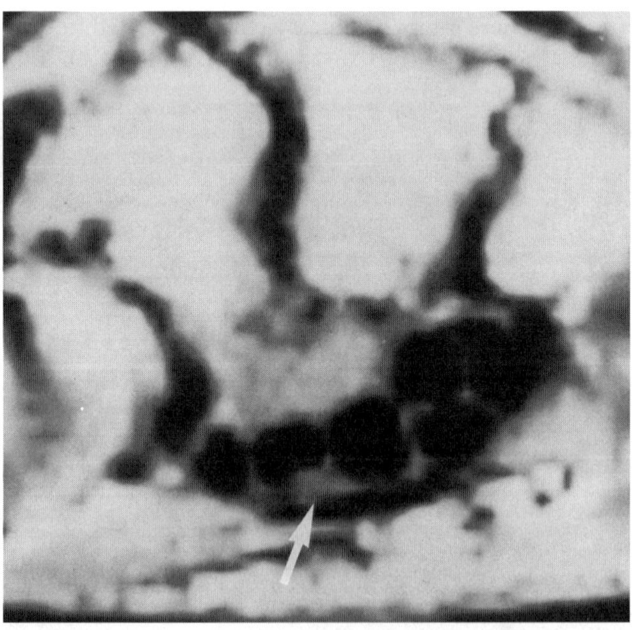

FIGURE 3.—Median nerve compression in a patient with rheumatoid arthritis. Axial slice at the level of the pisiform bone, proton-density-weighted spin-echo sequence (TR = 2,000 ms, TE = 15 ms). Synovial hypertrophy can be identified by MRI as a cause of median nerve compression (*arrow*). (Courtesy of Kleindienst A, Hamm B, Hildebrandt G, et al: Diagnosis and staging of carpal tunnel syndrome: Comparison of magnetic resonance imaging and intra-operative findings. *Acta Neurochir (Wien)* 138:228–233, 1996.)

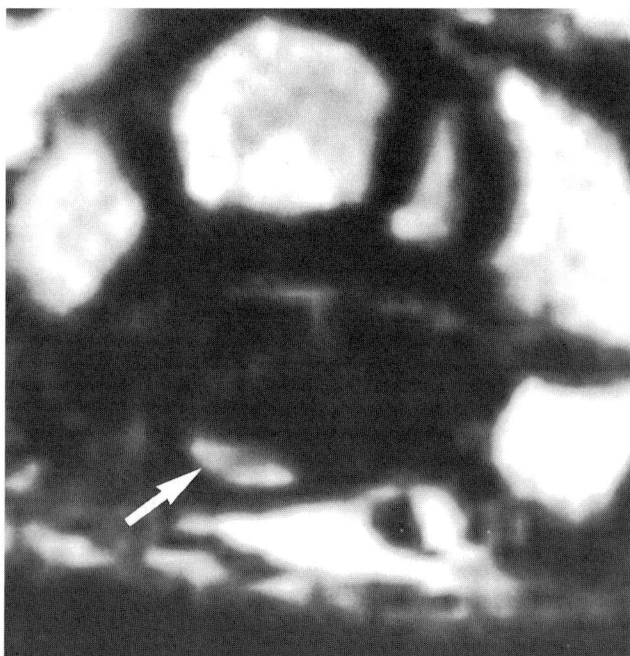

FIGURE 4.—Early carpal tunnel syndrome. T2-weighted spin-echo sequence (TR = 2,000 ms, TE = 90 ms). Epineural edema of the median nerve is seen in MRI as hyperintense contour around the nerve (*arrow*). (Courtesy of Kleindienst A, Hamm B, Hildebrandt G, et al: Diagnosis and staging of carpal tunnel syndrome: Comparison of magnetic resonance imaging and intra-operative findings. *Acta Neurochir (Wien)* 138:228–233, 1996.)

soft-tissue structures. Because MRI makes it possible to visualize the median nerve within the carpal tunnel, it may be a valuable tool in the assessment of the extent of CTS. The accuracy of MRI in the diagnosis and staging of CTS was determined in a prospective study by comparing imaging results to intraoperative findings.

Methods.—An MRI was performed in 55 patients with CTS in 58 wrists. The mean age of patients was 54 years, and 45 patients were women. Physical examination and electrodiagnostic studies were performed before MRI and surgical release of the transverse ligament.

Results.—The median nerve can be visualized in MRI scans both in patients with CTS and in normal control subjects (Fig 1). The flattening, swelling, and signal intensity of the median nerve are significantly different in early and advanced CTS. Flattening has not been proved to be significant (Fig 2). After surgical findings were compared with findings from MRI, it was determined that median nerve compression was correctly diagnosed in 91% of cases. The MRI correctly established the presence of additional lesions in the carpal tunnel (Fig 3). These were confirmed by surgery.

Discussion.—Because MRI produces high soft-tissue contrast, it is the only valuable imaging method in the diagnosis of CTS. Proton-density-

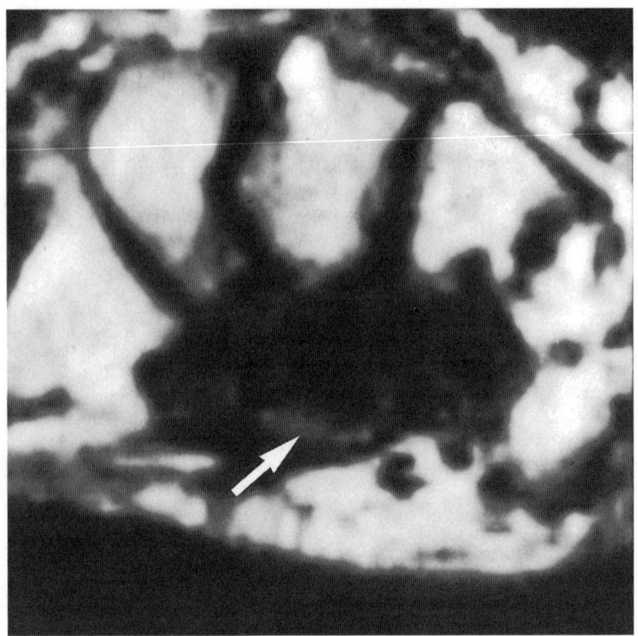

FIGURE 5.—Advanced carpal tunnel syndrome. T2-weighted spin-echo sequence (TR = 2,000 ms, TE = 90 ms). Fibrotic degeneration of the median nerve is manifested in MRI by decreased signal intensity, inhomogeneous structure, and impaired demarcation of the nerve (*arrow*). (Courtesy of Kleindienst A, Hamm B, Hildebrandt G, et al: Diagnosis and staging of carpal tunnel syndrome: Comparison of magnetic resonance imaging and intra-operative findings. *Acta Neurochir (Wien)* 138:228–233, 1996.)

weighted and T2-weighted spin-echo sequences are recommended for imaging the wrist in patients with suspected CTS. Early CTS can be recognized by a hyperintense contour of the nerve from epineural edema (Fig 4). Advanced CTS is seen as decreased signal intensity, inhomogeneous structure, and impaired demarcation of the nerve (Fig 5). This technique is not meant to replace standard ways to diagnose CTS.

▶ The conclusions of this article rest upon a rather frail assumption, that there are always demonstrable gross abnormalities of the median nerve at surgery for CTS. Nevertheless, clinical diagnostic features and postoperative symptom abatement should suffice to support the thesis. Cost, availability, and expertise in interpretation are current limitations that will disappear in time, and the availability of a non-invasive confirmation of suspected CTS will become increasingly attractive. However, additional support for this thesis is needed.

J.H. Dobyns, M.D.

Carpal Tunnel Surgery Outcomes in Workers: Effect of Workers' Compensation Status

Higgs PE, Edwards D, Martin DS, et al (Washington Univ, St Louis, Mo)
J Hand Surg [Am] 20A:354–360, 1995   9–20

Background.—Previous studies have had difficulty determining whether less favorable outcomes after surgery for occupational carpal tunnel syndrome (CTS) are due to the task of work itself, the enticement of financial gain from workers' compensation or litigation, or some combination. Outcomes in patients with CTS covered by a workers' compensation program were compared with those of working patients whose CTS was not covered.

Methods.—One hundred thirteen patients with workers' compensation and 53 without workers' compensation who had had open carpal tunnel release were interviewed a mean of 42 months after surgery. Data on job status and the presence of residual symptoms of numbness, pain, or nocturnal waking were obtained.

Findings.—Fifty-three patients with and 39 without workers' compensation were still at their original jobs at the time of the follow-up interview. Seventeen patients with and 2 without workers' compensation were unemployed. These between-group differences were significant. Residual symptoms were significantly more common in patients with workers' compensation than in patients without workers' compensation. Ninety-two of the former and 26 of the latter patients reported such symptoms.

Conclusions.—Although a causal association between workers' compensation and poor outcomes could not be established, they are related. Compared with patients without workers' compensation, those with workers' compensation have more residual symptoms and a lower rate of return to gainful employment.

▶ Selection was careful, numbers were adequate, outcomes review was meticulous, but did we need another retrospective review to tell us that patients with workers' compensation do worse than working patients who do not have compensation. We really didn't, but the authors' frustration, their speculations as to cause, and their call for *prospective* studies is a clarion call. Industry, workers, government, physicians, rehabilitation specialists, and even lawyers should listen.

J.H. Dobyns, M.D.

The Hypothenar Fat Pad Flap for Management of Recalcitrant Carpal Tunnel Syndrome

Strickland JW, Idler RS, Lourie GM, et al (St Vincent Hosp, Indianapolis, Ind; Indiana Hand Ctr, Indianapolis; Hand Treatment Ctr, Atlanta, Ga; et al)
J Hand Surg (Am) 21A:840–848, 1996
9–21

Background.—Open carpal tunnel decompression is unsuccessful in 10% to 25% of patients. Recurrence often results from the tethering of a median nerve in the carpal canal. Soft-tissue flaps have been used to alleviate residual compression and adherence of the median nerve in the carpal canal. However, many of the procedures described are technically demanding and involve the use of tissue that may be inadequate in dimension or poorly positioned to sufficiently cover the median nerve. The outcomes of a procedure using the hypothenar fat pad flap (HTFPF), which interposes tissue from the hypothenar eminence between the median nerve and overlying transverse carpal ligament and surgical scar, were assessed.

Methods.—Fifty-eight patients with recurrent symptoms after failed open carpal tunnel release were included in the review. Revision carpal tunnel decompression with a HTFPF flap was performed on a total of 62 affected hands. Mean follow-up was 33 months.

Findings.—At the final follow-up assessment, 95% of the patients said they were satisfied. Mean time to return to work was 12 weeks for the patients without workers' compensation and 37 weeks for those with workers' compensation. The outcomes of the HTFPF procedure were equal to or better than those of other soft-tissue flaps used for revision decompression in patients with recurrent symptoms after failed open carpal tunnel release.

Conclusions.—The HTFPF yields excellent outcomes in patients with recalcitrant idiopathic carpal tunnel syndrome. A prospective study comparing HTFPF surgery with other surgical approaches in patients with recurrent carpal tunnel syndrome would be useful.

▶ Along with direct injury to the median nerve, the steep escalation of carpal tunnel release surgery has resulted in frequent need for secondary surgery for a painful nerve in a scarred environment. Localized lysis, extended lysis, and early nerve excursion exercises (Hunter) and various types of tissue cover have been applied to this problem. The technique described here is usually successful in improving (seldom in curing) the problem and is within the risk level and expertise level of most surgeons who perform carpal tunnel release surgery. If the area of nerve and scar involvement is too great for the tissue available in this manner, a recent paper by Tham et al.[1] gives a reasonable alternative option, as do free flaps such as the temporalis fascia flap (according to my associate Dr. W. Chris Pederson).

J.H. Dobyns, M.D.

References

1. Tham SKY, Ireland DCR, Riccio M, et al: Reverse radial artery fascial flap: A treatment for the chronically scarred median nerve in recurrent carpal tunnel syndrome. *J Hand Surg (Am)* 21A:849–854, 1996.

Non-traumatic Paralysis of the Posterior Interosseous Nerve

Hashizume H, Nishida K, Nanba Y, et al (Okayama Univ, Japan)
J Bone Joint Surg (Br) 78B:771–776, 1996   9–22

Background.—Nontraumatic paralysis of the posterior interosseous nerve is a rare condition associated with a variety of disorders, including entrapment by the edge of the supinator, a space-occupying lesion, inflammatory changes, and neuralgic amyotrophy. The best management for this condition is unclear. One experience with patients with moderate to severe symptoms was reviewed.

Patients and Findings.—Thirty-one patients with nontraumatic paralysis of the posterior interosseous nerve were treated during 15 years. They were 21 women and 10 men aged 17–71 years. Surgery was performed in 25 patients (Fig 2). In the remaining 6, treatment was conservative. Entrapment occurred at the supinator in 14 patients. Three of those patients had double compression at the entrance and exit from the muscle. Entrapment was caused by a ganglion in 4 patients, a lipoma in 1, a dislocated radial head in 1, and marked constriction in the nerve of unknown cause in 2. In the remaining 3 patients diagnosis was made retrospectively of neuralgic amyotrophy, the only observable change at surgery being slight nerve edema. The paralysis resolved 2–18 months postoperatively in 24 of the 25 patients. The last patient subsequently had a tendon transfer.

Conclusions.—Patients with entrapment neuropathy may recover spontaneously. However, if recovery has not occurred within 6 weeks, decompression should be performed. Surgery may be delayed for up to 6 months if neuralgic amyotrophy is suspected. Surgery may also be done early, as the risk to the patient is minimal, and release of the arcade of Frohse may provide improvement in some patients.

▶ There is still controversy over the nonparalytic posterior interosseous nerve syndrome, but there can be little doubt about that group in the syndrome that has progressed to palsy. The authors give a good differential between entrapment neuropathy, which surgery can benefit, and neuralgic amyotrophy. They also give good evidence for the efficacy of surgery for the entrapment variety, if recovery is not occurring in 6 weeks. These authors report 2 cases of a marked constriction in the nerve of unknown cause; four similar cases reported by Inoue and Shionoya[1] required neurolysis and epineurotomy in 1 case, excision of the damaged area in 3 cases with 2 repaired by neurorrhaphy (with good motor return within 1 year) and 1 with too large a gap for neurorrhaphy, treated by tendon transfers. Quarrel as we

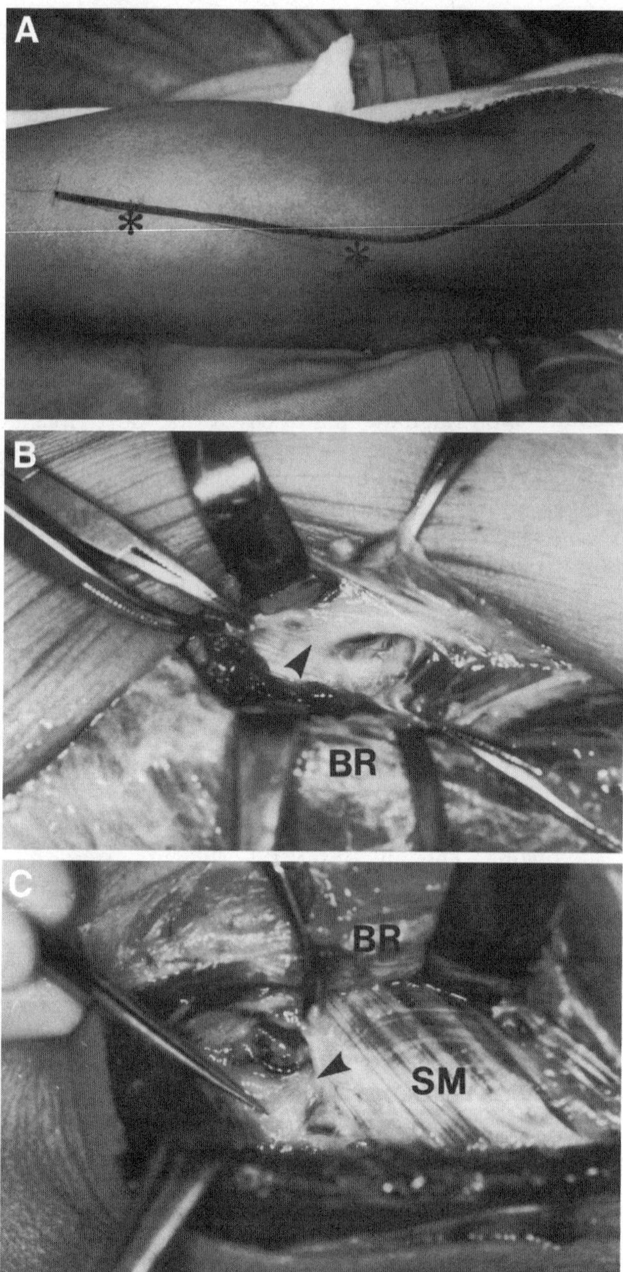

FIGURE 2.—Long lateral approach. **A,** a line is drawn from the lateral epicondlye (*) to Lister's tubercle and divided into 3 equal parts. The skin incision starts at least 3 cm beyond the probable exit (*) of the posterior interosseous nerve from the supinator and is traced on the proximal part of this line. A slightly curved line of the same length is then drawn from the lateral epicondyle up between the biceps and triceps muscle. **B,** nerve compression at the arcade of Frohse (*black arrow*). Brachioradialis (*BR*) is retracted laterally for exploration of the arcade and the area proximal to the arcade. **C,** nerve compression at the exit of supinator (*black arrow*). Brachioradialis (*BR*) is retracted medially for exploration of the supinator muscle (*SM*) and its exit. (Courtesy of Hashizume H, Nishida K, Nanba Y, et al: Non-traumatic paralysis of the posterior interosseous nerve. *J Bone Joint Surg [Br]* 78B:771–776, 1996.)

may about the causes, no evidence of return after 3 months is sufficient reason for exploration and such treatment as may be indicated.

J.H. Dobyns, M.D.

Reference

1. Inoue C, Shionoya K: Constructive paralysis of the posterior interosseous nerve without external compression. *J Hand Surg* 21B:164–168, 1996.

Correction of Severe Spastic Flexion Contractures in the Nonfunctional Hand
Pomerance JF, Keenan MAE (Hand Surgery Associates, SC, Arlington Heights, Ill; Albert Einstein Med Ctr, Philadelphia)
J Hand Surg (Am) 21A:828–833, 1996   9–23

Background.—The main surgical treatment of spasticity in nonfunctional hands is directed at the extrinsic flexors of the hand and wrist, the major goal being improved hygiene. However, long-term follow-up of such patients has indicated that recurrence of the wrist deformity and incomplete digital correction from unaddressed intrinsic abnormalities can occur. The use of a single-stage procedure to provide comprehensive correction of the severely spastic hand was described.

Methods.—Fourteen patients underwent a total of 15 procedures to alleviate severe flexion contractures of the hand and wrist during a 3-year period. All patients had had unsuccessful nonsurgical treatment or had chronic skin problems. The single-stage, comprehensive procedure consisted of superficialis to profundus transfer, wrist flexor release, flexor pollicis longus lengthening, wrist arthrodesis, carpal tunnel release, and ulnar motor branch neurectomy or intrinsic release. The mean follow-up period was 1 year.

Findings.—Wrist fusion (proximal row carpectomy) was needed in two patients after the index procedure occurred in 13 patients. One patient needed replating and another needed prolonged casting to achieve union. In 2 patients, a residual claw hand resulted, with only partial correction of a thumb-in-palm deformity. All hygiene problems and infections seen before surgery resolved after surgery (Figs 1 and 2).

Conclusions.—The comprehensive protocol used in these patients enabled correction of severe hand and wrist contractures by a single operation. Improved care and appearance of the hand resulted. This protocol is recommended for all nonfunctional hands.

▶ The requirements for orthopedists to manage a severe, spastic, nonfunctional hand are increasing. It is comforting to know how much can be done in such an efficient manner at 1 surgical operation. The recipe is straightforward and relatively simple, but there are a few options that must be decided during the procedure, all nicely detailed by the authors.

J.H. Dobyns, M.D.

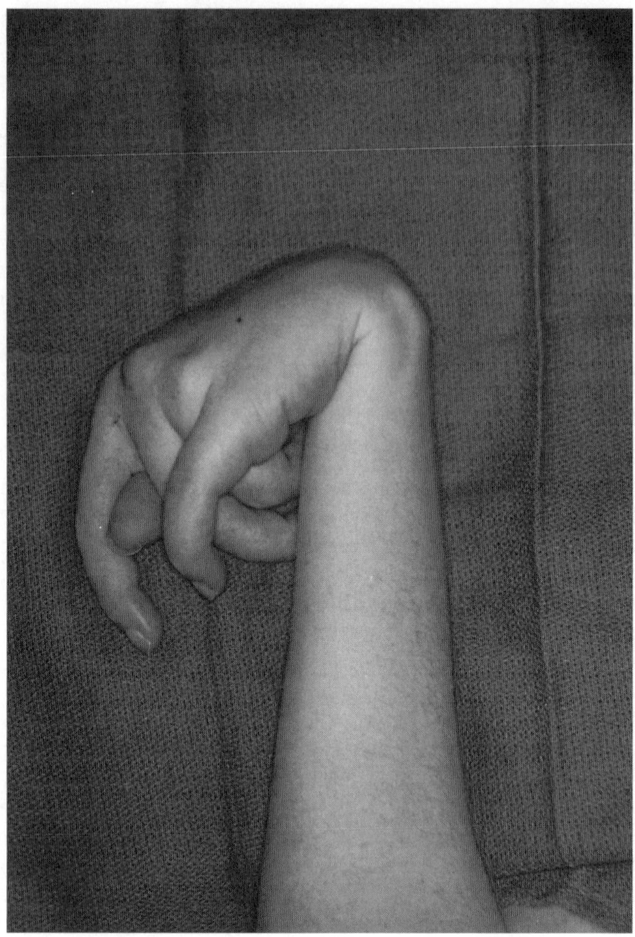

FIGURE 1.—Preoperative flexion deformities in the hand and wrist in a 29-year-old woman 29 months after traumatic brain injury. (Courtesy of Pomerance JF, Keenan MAE: Correction of severe spastic flexion contractures in the nonfunctional hand. *J Hand Surg [Am]* 21A:828–833, 1996.)

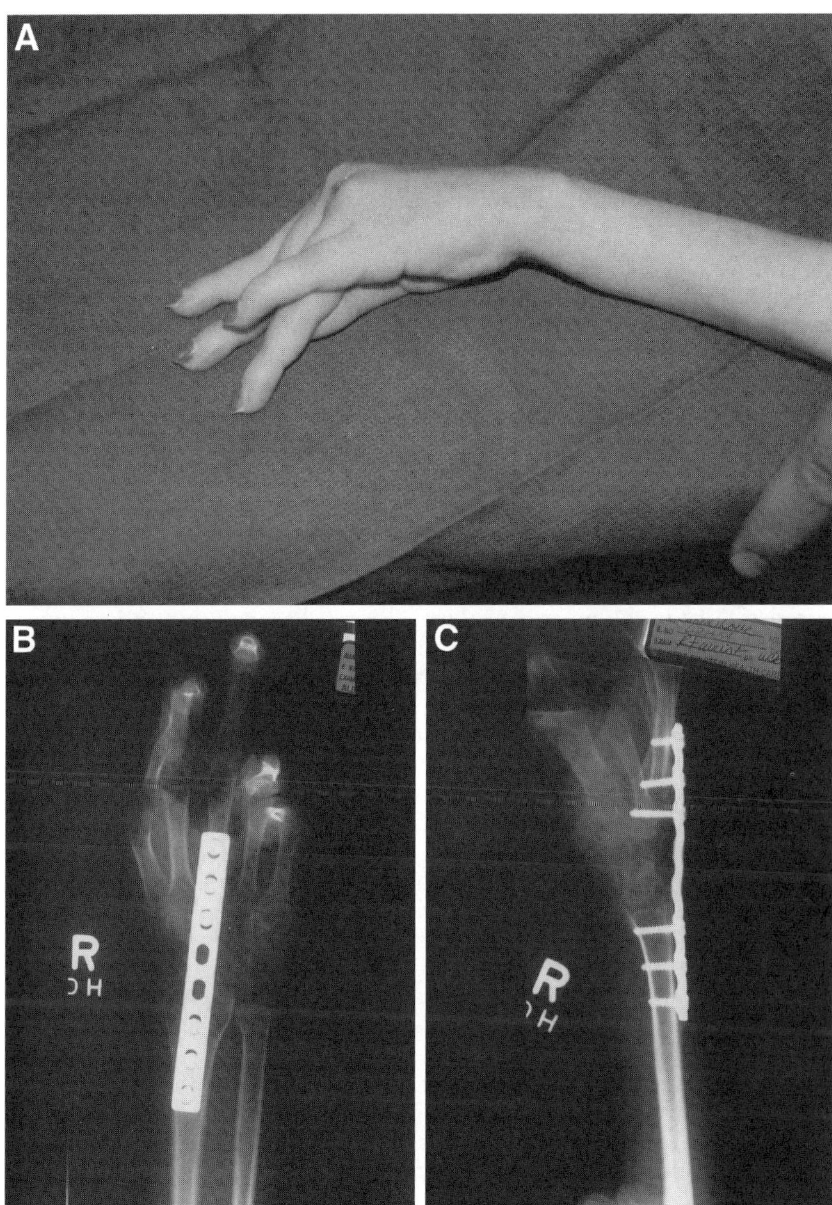

FIGURE 2.—Postoperative correction of patient depicted in Figure 1 in (**A**) anteroposterior and (**B**) lateral and (**C**) posteroanterior radiographic views. (Courtesy of Pomerance JF, Keenan MAE: Correction of severe spastic flexion contractures in the nonfunctional hand. *J Hand Surg [Am]* 21A:828–833, 1996.)

Tendon Transfers and Functional Electrical Stimulation for Restoration of Hand Function in Spinal Cord Injury

Keith MW, Kilgore KL, Peckham PH, et al (Case Western Reserve Univ, Cleveland, Ohio)

J Hand Surg [Am] 21A:89–99, 1996

9–24

Objective.—Electrical stimulation has been shown to restore function in hands of patients with spinal cord injury at C5 and C6 levels. The approach has limited success in patients with lower motor neuron damage to muscles. Results of a study that examined the surgical modification of the biomechanics of the hand, such that functional electrical stimulation of paralyzed but lower motor neuron intact muscles, were reported.

Methods.—Transfers of the palmaris longus, flexor carpi ulnaris, extensor carpi ulnaris, and brachioradialis were performed in 11 patients with cervical spine injuries for optimum range of motion against antagonist and passive forces. Several surgeries were performed on each patient to provide finger flexion, finger extension, wrist extension, and thumb extension. Functional electrical stimulation-powered tendon transfers with side-to-side synchronization of finger flexor and extensor tendons were also performed. Three patients had the Zancolli-Lasso procedure and 5 had arthrodesis of the thumb interphalangeal joint. Preoperative and postoperative grades of muscles, ranges of motion, force vectors produced by the muscles, the joint angle changes, and the function level obtained with electrical stimulation of the motoring muscle were measured.

Results.—When functional electrical stimulation procedures were performed, 38 of 41 demonstrated a functional benefit. There was a loss of muscle force or range of motion in the thumb in 2 patients and in a loss of 20 degrees of thumb extension in 1 patient.

Conclusion.—Most patients with C5 and C6 level spinal cord injury demonstrated increased hand function after restorative surgery, when that surgery is expanded to use appropriate transfers of paralyzed but lower motor neuron intact (LMNI) muscle.

▶ Even among specialists there are specialists, and the niche occupied by these investigators is home to very few. They occupy that interface between the investigational and the clinical where practical usage for today arises from available technology. Functional electrical stimulation associated with tendon transfers for optimal usage of the available muscles (paralyzed but not lower motor neuron damaged) is an exportable technique that should improve the life styles of many patients.

J.H. Dobyns, M.D.

The Angiosomes of the Forearm: Anatomic Study and Clinical Implications

Inoue Y, Taylor GI (Royal Melbourne Hosp, Australia; Univ of Melbourne, Australia)

Plast Reconstr Surg 98:195–210, 1996

9–25

Objective.—Nerve supply, radial or ulnar arteries, and muscle tissue can be transferred from the forearm to provide sensation, shape, and blood supply to donor sites, but the amount of tissue that can safely be harvested is not known. The anatomic contribution of angiosomes derived from arteries to the blood supply of each tissue layer from the skin to the bone was studied.

Anatomic Studies.—Ten cadaver limbs were radiographed to obtain an image of the vascular network of the forearm. Radiographs were taken of all forearm muscles; the arterial branches to the muscles and the source of the arterial branches were noted. Muscles were dissected one at a time and x-ray films were taken. The contribution of each angiosome and its associated artery to the skin, each muscle, radius, and ulna were cataloged.

Results.—Most connections between angiosomes occurred within tissues and originated from the arteries or their branches. Each angiosome is responsible for a specific skin-to-bone territory defined by linked arteries. Most muscles received their blood supply from at least 2 territories, which explains how circulation can be reconstructed after a source artery is damaged (Fig 10). Some muscles were supplied by 1 angiosome, however, which accounts for occurrences of ischemic contractures in some procedures that injure the single blood supply.

Conclusion.—This anatomic information will make it possible to refine the design of forearm flaps. In a muscle group supplied by multiple angiosomes, only a portion of the muscle needs to be harvested. Ischemic damage to the other muscle groups can be avoided if the pathways for reconstructing circulation when 1 source artery is harvested are understood.

▶ To paraphrase Trueta: "Blood is Life." As a consequence, vessels are vital, but their locations, interconnections, and supply territories are less well known to extremity surgeons than are those of the bones, muscles, and nerves of the region. Not only have the authors supplied us with the vascular details of the upper extremity by dint of much old-fashioned anatomy dissection and tedious hard work, but they direct us to some of the important clinical applications of this knowledge.

J.H. Dobyns, M.D.

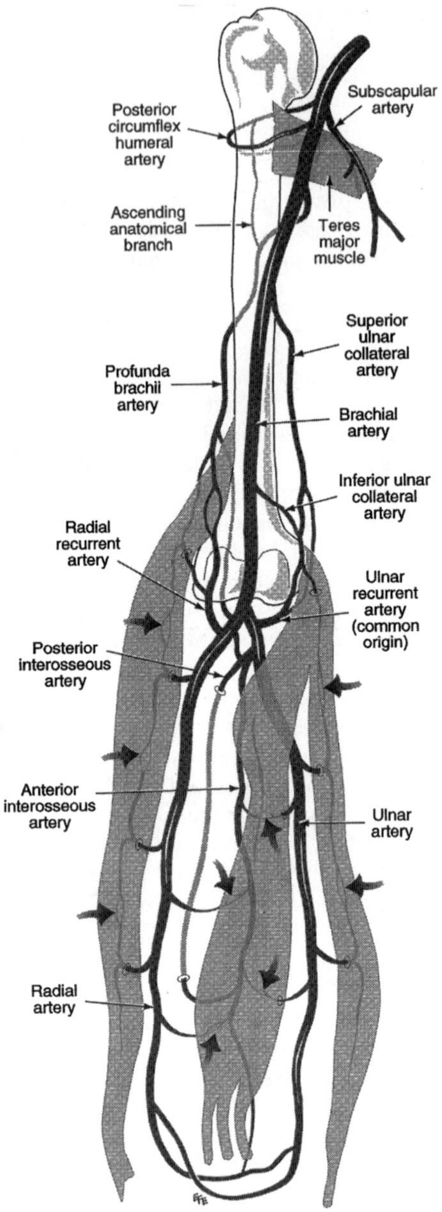

FIGURE 10.—The anastomosis around the right elbow and within the forearm. Note the anastomoses within muscle groups shown schematically and highlighted with *arrows*. (Courtesy of Inoue Y, Taylor GI: The angiosomes of the forearm: Anatomic study and clinical implications. *Plast Reconstr Surg* 98:195–210, 1996.)

The Use of Intra-arterial Urokinase in the Management of Hand Ischemia Secondary to Palmar and Digital Arterial Occlusion
Wheatley MJ, Marx MV (Oregon Health Sciences Univ, Portland; Univ of Michigan, Ann Arbor)
Ann Plast Surg 37:356–363, 1996   9–26

Introduction.—Acute ischemia of the hand and digits secondary to palmar or digital artery occlusion can progress rapidly to gangrene. Aggressive intervention is required to salvage a profoundly ischemic hand. The efficacy of selective intra-arterial urokinase (UK) infusion was evaluated retrospectively in the management of acute vascular occlusion in the hand and digits of 9 patients with severe hand ischemia and impending tissue loss secondary to distal forearm, palmar arch, and digital artery occlusion.

Methods.—Duration of symptoms ranged from less than 24 hours in 4 patients to more than 72 hours in 5 patients. Significant medical history included atrial fibrillation in 2 patients, wrist trauma in 4 patients, and subclavian artery occlusive disease in 2 patients. One patient had no known source of embolism. Patients underwent diagnostic arteriography, which included evaluation of the aortic arch, brachiocephalic vessels, and selective arteriography of the entire affected extremity. Clinical histories and angiography suggested probable causes to be thromboembolism in 3 patients, atheroembolism in 2 patients, and traumatic ulnar artery occlusion in 4 patients. The occlusions were not responsive to the administration of intra-arterial vasodilators and were not considered operable in any patients. Thrombolytic therapy was chosen for treatment after diagnostic arteriogram. The first 6 patients received low-dose UK infused at 60,000–120,000 IU/hr. The last 3 patients were treated using a high-dose/low-dose protocol of 240,000 IU/hr for 2–4 hours, then 80,000–120,000 IU/hr if there was evidence of improvement with the high dose of UK. All patients were therapeutically heparinized. Arteriography was performed at 2- to 12-hour intervals to evaluate progress.

Results.—Hand ischemia was reversed in 3 patients with thromboembolism using intra-arterial UK. All 3 patients had angiographic evidence of clot lysis and clinical improvement or resolution of ischemia. Two patients had normal motor and sensory hand function, and the third subsequently required amputation of the tips of her second through fifth digits. The latter had profound ischemia of her entire hand for nearly 24 hours with no arterial flow beyond the wrist. Digital perfusion was restored, but the fingertips could not be saved because of duration and severity of digital ischemia. The 2 patients with embolism from atherosclerotic lesions of the subclavian artery did not benefit from lytic therapy. One patient was managed with embolectomy, and the other patient had fingertip amputations and carotid-subclavian bypass with exclusion of the ulcerated subclavian stenosis. One of 4 patients with traumatic ulnar occlusion showed angiographic improvement after UK therapy. The patient with improvement and 2 patients in whom no clot lysis was observed had partial or

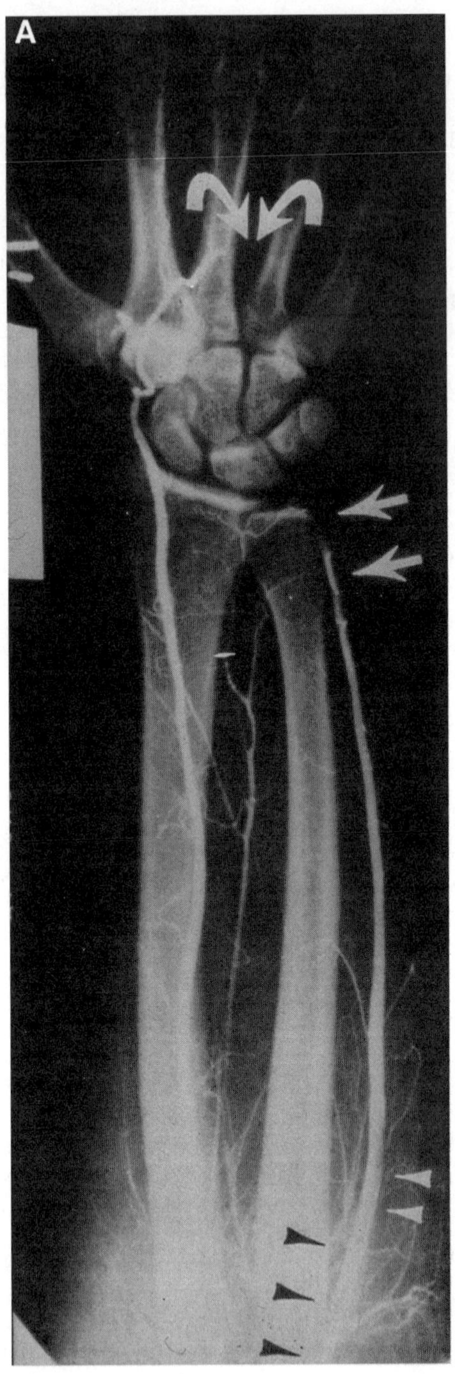

(*Continued*)

FIGURE (cont.)

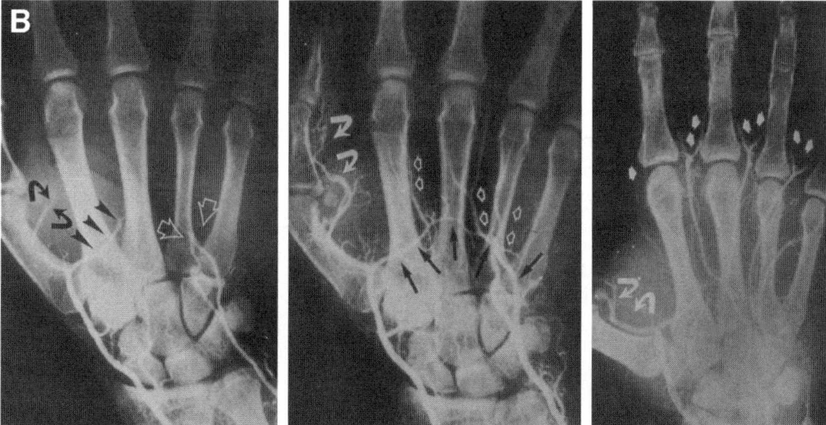

FIGURE.—**A,** complete occlusion of the ulnar and near-complete occlusion of the radial artery after embolization secondary to atrial fibrillation. **B,** after urokinase administration, flow is re-established to the palmar arch, the princeps pollicus, and the digital vessels. (Courtesy of Wheatley MJ, Marx MV: The use of intra-arterial urokinase in the management of hand ischemia secondary to palmar and digital arterial occlusion. *Ann Plast Surg* 37:356–363, 1996. Reprinted from *Annals of Plastic Surgery* by permission of Little, Brown and Company, Inc.)

complete clinical resolution of ischemia. Two patients had no further problems, and 1 patient required amputation of the fifth fingertip. The fourth patient showed no improvement with lytic therapy and underwent ulnar artery resection and bypass. There were 2 complications of UK infusion: pericatheter thrombosis and subcutaneous abscess at the femoral puncture site in a patient who was steroid dependent.

Case Report.—Woman, 72, with a history of atrial fibrillation was seen because of a 24-hour history of a cool, painful hand. Angiography showed a clot in the proximal subclavian artery with complete occlusion of the radial artery and near-complete occlusion of the ulnar artery (Fig A). Blood flow was restored to all hand vessels after 80,000 IU of UK was infused over 30 hours (Fig B). The patient was maintained on Coumadin and had no further problems at 18-month follow-up.

Conclusions.—Infusion of UK in not effective treatment for hand ischemia caused by atheroembolism, but may obviate the need for complex microsurgical reconstruction in patients with thromboemboli or traumatic ulnar artery occlusion. Lytic therapy is safe when properly monitored. Surgical intervention is not precluded by failure of lytic therapy.

▶ Although intra-arterial UK is not quite the miracle drug that we anticipated back in the 70s, it still works so dramatically for impending gangrene of the hand or digits after thromboembolism, and so surprisingly effective after traumatic ulnar (or radial) artery occlusion, that this update of the protocol for the evaluation of acute hand ischemia, beginning with angiography, should be in the reference file of every surgeon dealing with the upper limb.

J.H. Dobyns, M.D.

Compartment Syndromes of the Hand

Ouellette EA, Kelly R (Univ of Miami, Fla)
J Bone Joint Surg (Am) 78A:1515–1522, 1996   9–27

Background.—Compartment syndromes of the hand and forearm can lead to tissue necrosis, resulting in a devastating loss of function. Compartment syndrome of the hand has not been described as well as those of the leg and forearm. The pathophysiology of compartment syndrome of the hand was investigated and its effects on treatment outcomes were determined.

Patients and Findings.—Nineteen patients undergoing fasciotomy because of compartment syndrome of the hand were included in the review. They were 9 children and 10 adults aged 5 months to 67 years. Mean follow-up for 17 patients was 21 months. In all patients, pressure was increased in at least 1 interosseous compartment, and the hand was tense and swollen. Compartment syndrome of the forearm also occurred in 8 patients. Compartment syndromes developed after IV injections (n = 11), gunshot wound (n = 2), crush injury (n = 2), or from complications associated with the use of an arterial line (n = 2), an arthrodesis of the wrist (n = 1), and a crush injury from prolonged pressure on the upper extremity caused by a drug overdose. Fifteen patients had an obtunded sensorium at the time of compartment syndrome recognition. In 8 children and 5 adults, the syndrome was related to a complication from IV or intra-arterial drug administration. Thirteen of the 17 patients followed up had satisfactory outcomes after carpal tunnel release and decompression of the compartments involved. Outcomes in the remaining 4 patients were poor. Two children needed amputation, 1 child had impaired hand function secondary to brain damage, and 1 adult (with extensive forearm involvement) had complete loss of hand function. All 4 had been obtunded when the compartment syndrome developed.

Conclusions.—Clinicians need to maintain a high index of suspicion for compartment syndrome of the hand in critically ill, obtunded patients, especially children, receiving multiple IV or intra-arterial injections. The degree of elevation of the preoperative pressure apparently does not affect outcome.

▶ A more common nightmare for the orthopedist is death of tissue, rather than death of patient. Often tissue death is preventable if we and the medical communication system that alerts us are sufficiently sensitive. In their review of 19 patients, ranging in age from 5 to 67 years, the authors have once more instructed us about this serious problem, so often seen in uncooperative, obtunded, or noncommunicative patients. We must sensitize our colleagues to the insidious nature and serious sequelae of compartment syndromes and to the fact that we are prepared to deal with them, IMMEDIATELY, once informed!

J.H. Dobyns, M.D.

Suggested Reading

ARM, ELBOW, FOREARM, AND WRIST

Gerwin M, Hotchkiss RN, Weiland AJ: Alternative operative exposure of the posterior aspect of the humeral diaphysis (with reference to the radial nerve). *J Bone Joint Surg Am* 78:1690–1695, 1996.
▶ This is another article for the upper limb surgeon's surgical anatomy workbook (must I plead with you again to keep one), but it is a particularly good article because it clearly tells how to accomplish the infrequent but important exposure of the proximal posterior portion of the humerus while keeping the radial nerve in view and protected meanwhile. There is no way an abstract can do justice to this article; you will need to read and file the whole thing, but it is worth your while.

Lintner S, Fischer T: Repair of the distal biceps tendon using suture anchors and an anterior approach. *Clin Orthop* 322:116–119, 1996.
▶ Although cases are few and results testing nonchalant, the implications of this simple, limited dissection approach to a common problem with an unacceptable number of significant treatment complications are important. If the technique continues to be as foolproof for the authors *and others* as it seems to have been to date, it may well become the preferred method of management, at least for the vigorous patient.

Schroeder LE, Horlocker TT, Schroeder DR: The efficacy of axillary block for surgical procedures about the elbow. *Anesth Analg* 83:747–751, 1996.
▶ Useful statistics regarding common regional block procedures for surgery about the distal end of the humerus and elbow are given for a significant group of cases (N = 330 blocks in 260 patients). Bone procedures (N = 156) and soft tissue procedures (N = 174) were covered by adequate surgical anesthesia in 86% of the cases, including 89% of the axillary blocks, 78% of the supraclavicular blocks, and 75% of the interscalene blocks ($P < 0.025$). In axillary blocks a 95% success rate was achieved with the paresthesia technique, 88% of the blocks were successful with a nerve stimulator/motor response technique, success was achieved in 94% of the combination blocks (using paresthesia or a nerve stimulator combined with transarterial injection), and 81% of blocks performed exclusively with a transarterial technique were successful ($P < 0.05$). Axillary blocks performed with mepivacaine had a success rate of 93% as compared with 81% for bupivacaine ($P < 0.01$). There were no patients with perioperative respiratory compromise.

Simpson NS, Goodman LA, Jupiter JB: Contoured LCDC plating of the proximal ulna. *Injury* 27:411–417, 1996.
▶ Even titanium limited-contact dynamic compression plates may not be the ideal support for comminuted, displaced fractures of the proximal end of the ulna (they apparently need some precontouring as well), but they seem to be

what the authors claim, i.e., a better solution than we have had heretofore for these difficult problems. The early range of motion possible afterward is a definite plus. Make no mistake, however; the technique for reducing fragments, aligning joint surfaces, and reducing and holding the dislocation is still more important than the plate. Furthermore, contouring and applying the plate and its variable types of screw fixation are an art form that must be mastered.

Richardson D, Fisher SE, Vaughan ED, et al: Radial forearm flap donor-site complications and morbidity: a prospective study. *Plast Reconstr Surg* 99:109–115, 1997.
▶ Many studies, both retrospective and now prospective, have revealed that radial forearm flap use is not innocuous; this is particularly true of composite flaps that include bone. In this latter group, residual function of the donor arm was affected in 16% of the fasciocutaneous group, 36% of the composite group without fracture, and 100% of the group (17% of the 35 patients who had this procedure) who sustained a fracture of the radius. The combination flap is obviously high risk, and other alternatives, if available, are preferable.

Samuelson M, Reider B, Weiss D: Grip lock injuries to the forearm in male gymnasts. *Am J Sports Med* 24:15–18, 1996.
▶ This fascinating account of another unique injury etiology from the combination of highly skilled performance and a special assistive device adds to the lore that the lifestyle's difficult and repetitive stress testing is provided for the observant. From "bowler's thumb" to "rodeo digit/hand avulsions" there are an array of special-circumstance injuries that are oh-so-slowly being accumulated. Gymnasts have been at the fringe of the just barely possible for the human body for some time, and it is not surprising that another injury pattern has been added to their burden.

McKee MD, Richards RR: Dynamic radio-ulnar convergence after the darrach procedure. *J Bone Joint Surg Br* 78:413–418, 1995.
▶ Although many have condemned the Darrach procedure, there are just as many who have defended it, as these authors do after studying 23 (25 wrists) of their post-Darrach patients at a mean follow-up of more than 75 months. Although their patients were elderly (mean age, > 61 years at surgery) and they did not test them stringently for endurance or heavy provocative usage, the outcomes were good enough that both the physicians and patients were satisfied. An interesting categorization is used for the radiologic postoperative result, that of no convergence, convergence, and impingement. The latter group, of course, was the most symptomatic, and the symptoms related more to excess ulna excision than any other factor.

Pennig D, Gausepohl T: External fixation of the wrist. *Injury* 27:1–15, 1996.
▶ This article is an excellent review of the development, current usage, and suggested techniques for improved results when using external fixators in managing fractures of the distal end of the forearm. The authors rightly indicate that not all such fractures require external fixation and that even when it is indicated, supplemental techniques may also be needed.

Jones WA, Lovell ME: The role of arthroscopy in the investigation of wrist disorders. *J Hand Surg [Br]* 21:442–445, 1996.

▶ This assessment of 48 cases, 28 with concurrent diagnosis both clinically and by arthroscopy, 6 not diagnosed by either method, and 14 diagnosed by one or the other method, suggests that clinical examination and arthroscopy are adequate for diagnosis in most instances. Another study[1] suggests the same, i.e., that arthrography does not supplement clinical findings as well as arthroscopy does.

Reference

1. Chung KC, Zimmerman NB, Travis MT: Wrist arthrography versus arthroscopy: A comparative study of 150 cases. *J Hand Surg [Am]* 21:591–594, 1996.

Schuind F, Alemzadeh S, Stallenberg B, et al: Does the normal contralateral wrist provide the best reference for x-ray film measurements of the pathologic wrist? *J Hand Surg [Am]* 21:24–30, 1996.
▶ Luckily, for those of us who cannot treat without the opposite-side radiograph for guidance, the authors have found that only the normal values for ulnar variance, palmar tilt, and radial inclination can be adequately assessed from databases. Carpal height and carpal angles are best assessed by comparing with the normal wrist. So get a radiograph of the other wrist for the latter, but use it for all comparisons.

DeFiori JP, Puffer JC, Mandelbaum BR, et al: Factors associated with wrist pain in the young gymnast. *Am J Sports Med* 24:9–14, 1996.
▶ Those who still doubt that repetitive stress can cause physiologic harm as well as physiologic adaptation should consider the gymnast's wrist, where physis damage and other wrist problems are common, sometimes from precipitate causes but most often from repetitive stress over prolonged periods of time. This finding is well documented in this study of nonspecific wrist pain in nonelite gymnasts. Wrist pain was present in 73% of the gymnasts (in 47% for more than 6 months) and was related to the intensity of training ($P = 0.036$), age (older than 10 years but less than 14), and age at the onset of training. The authors speculate that there is an "intensity threshold" above which risk is greater but do not have the number or alternate training patterns to prove this.

Lynch NM, Linscheid RL: Corrective osteotomy for scaphoid malunion: Technique and long term follow-up evaluation. *J Hand Surg [Am]* 22:35–43, 1997.
▶ Having seen a number of malunited scaphoids *without* big problems, I was more than content to let Ron Linscheid be the sole investigator of this management method for those who did have problems. He proved to me that there were occasions when it was warranted and that it could succeed. If you run across such a patient (the evidence is usually present early after healing), this is the way to handle it.

Miura H, Uchida Y, Sugioka Y: Radial closing wedge osteotomy for Kienbock's disease. *J Hand Surg [Am]* 21:1029–1034, 1996.
▶ Despite the conflicting laboratory data regarding the effect on the lunate of the various wedge osteotomies of the distal end of the radius, personal experience with closing wedge osteotomy, done with some of my many shortening osteotomies of the radius, convinced me that the multicenter Japanese experience of the beneficial effects of the closing wedge osteotomy was correct. As with the other stress-alteration techniques, lower-stage (Stahl-Lichtman I–IIIA) cases do better, cases without carpal collapse do better, and radioulnar variance should

be neutralized. Perhaps this additional 26 cases with follow-up of over 4 years will force us to give this method of altering lunate stress the attention that it deserves.

Trumble TE, Gilbert M, Vedder N: Isolated tears of the triangular fibrocartilage: management by early arthroscopic repair. *J Hand Surg [Am]* 22:57–65, 1997.
▶ This is a very carefully selected group of patients, beginning with exclusion criteria of (1) Palmer type 1A or 2 tears, (2) radiocarpal arthritis, (3) inflammatory arthritis, (4) prior articular fractures of the wrist joint, (5) prior reconstructive wrist surgery, (6) distal ulna instability, and (7) obvious ulnocarpal impaction (range not given, but the average ulnar variance was 0.2 ± 0.6 mm). In addition, half of the patients had negative arthrograms but had arthroscopic diagnoses of Palmer 1B or 1C lesions, often a difficult diagnosis to make with certainty. Associations of ulnar instability, carpal instability, or ulnocarpal impaction are so common that relatively pure cases of TFCC tear may be few in any one practice. Nevertheless, the basic premise here, i.e., that one can not only diagnose peripheral tears, radial and ulnar, of the TFCC, but also treat them successfully, whether by arthroscopic or open repair, is pure gold.

Siegal JM, Ruby LK: A critical look at intercarpal arthrodeses: review of the literature. *J Hand Surg [Am]* 21:717–723, 1996.
▶ Less than total carpal arthrodeses of various types have enjoyed great popularity in the past 3 decades, and a review of the reported results has been needed. It is not surprising to note that only 47% of these patients had complete relief of pain and that postoperative function seemed to depend more on pain relief than on more objective measurements.

Schiltenwolf M, Martini AK, Mau HC, et al: Further investigations of the intraosseous pressure characteristics in necrotic lunates (Kienböck's disease). *J Hand Surg [Am]* 21:754–758, 1996.
▶ Proof continues to build that abnormalities of intraosseous pressure should receive serious consideration as an etiology, perhaps the principal etiology, of Kienböck's disease, thus placing this condition in the same category with Legg-Perthes disease and other similar skeletal afflictions. So far, there is no correlation between this concept and the various management methods in current usage, nor any suggestion of new treatments based on the concept. These developments, anticipated for the next decade, will be of considerable interest.

Watson HK, Yasuda M, Guidera PM: Lateral lunate morphology: An x-ray study. *J Hand Surg [Am]* 21:759–763, 1996.
▶ More precise studies of differences in lunate morphology have been done (Antonio-Zapico; Stanley), and more precise imaging studies would help this study. Nevertheless, the concept is intriguing, may be valid, and may be one (not the only) reason for the volar-flexed intercalated segment instability of the lunate in some injury settings. As the authors say, the concept warrants further investigation.

Finsen V, Russwurm H: Metacarpal lengthening after traumatic amputation of the thumb. *J Bone Joint Surg Br* 78:133–136, 1996.
▶ Distraction lengthening with bone consolidation by either callotasis or a bone graft is still doing yeoman service for short digits, and as the authors suggest, it

may be possible to improve its chief drawback, the time required for function to be resumed. The opposite problem of a retained thumb skeleton with no soft tissue cover is addressed elsewhere.[1]

Reference

1. Yao J-M, Song J-L, Xu J-H: The second web bilobed island flap for thumb reconstruction. *Br J Plast Surg* 49:103–106, 1996.

HAND

Leijnse JNAL: A graphic analysis of the biomechanics of the Massless articular chain. Application to the proximal bi-articular chain of the human finger. *J Biomech* 29:355–366, 1996.

▶ The original Landsmeer (1955) concept, a biarticular three-tendon chain model without mass or friction, has been used ever since to explain control of the similar, unloaded proximal system of the human finger. The current paper extends this concept to the condition of load and demonstrates that (1) the anatomical position of the extrinsic extensor and flexor determines efficient function, (2) flexion loads are more easily sustained than extension loads, and (3) control is not optimal.

Turowski GA, Zdankiewicz PD, Thompson JG: The results of surgical treatment of trigger finger. *J Hand Surg [Am]* 22:145–149, 1997.

▶ The times are now in balance. As the authors remark, the only other long-term study of this management method was pessimistic, contrary to this report and to the concensus of practicing hand surgeons. However, as was said about the "steroid injection treatment of trigger fingers," the surgical treatment is also very operator dependent.

Benson LS, Ptaszek AJ: Injection versus surgery in the treatment of trigger finger. *J Hand Surg [Am]* 22:138–144, 1997.

▶ In 102 patients (109 fingers) the authors found that about 75% responded well to the first steroid injection and that most of those who did not eventually needed surgery and might as well have had it at the second treatment episode. In general I agree with this postulate, but with 2 provisos. Only *your* injection effort should count, not prior ones performed elsewhere for reasons that I can give by the dozen. Second, if a recurrence of bothersome triggering does not occur for 6 months or more (often several years), I would suggest injection again.

Patel MR, Moradia VJ: Percutaneous release of trigger digits with and without cortisone injection. *J Hand Surg [Am]* 22:150–155, 1997.

▶ In medicine as elsewhere, the simpler, less costly method will always prevail if risk is not increased. A coterie of our colleagues continue to reassure us that needle, percutaneous release of the A1 pulley area of trigger digits fulfills these criteria. The current authors still like cortisone injection before considering surgery and here have even made a case for the use of cortisone with percutaneous release. Were I still in active practice, they just might convince me.

Shaw DL, Wise DI, Holms W: Dupuytren's disease treated by Palmar fasciectomy and an open palm technique. *J Hand Surg [Br]* 21:484–485, 1996.

▶ The "open palm" method for Dupuytren's disease management has stood the time test; many who trash it have probably never tried it. If you are having trouble with your current method, try it; you'll like it and so will your patients.

Tang JB, Shi D, Zhang OG: Biomechanical and histologic evaluation of tendon sheath management. *J Hand Surg [Am]* 21:900–908, 1996.
▶ A strong experimental case is made for a closed but larger sheath of normal or decreased volume with regard to both the strength of healing and the degree of adhesion formation. Whether this chicken result will translate to humans is not yet known, although there are clinicians who think this is true (see the next article by Messina et al.)

Messina A, Messina JC: The direct midlateral approach with lateral enlargement of the pulley system for repair of flexor tendons in the fingers. *J Hand Surg [Br]* 21:463–468, 1996.
▶ This technique-only paper does not prove the advantages claimed, but the approach and the ingenious method of opening the pulley system at its lateral bony margins and repairing it in an expanded version by sliding the retained transverse digital lamina into the pulley defect are attractive enough to warrant a trial.

Whitney TM, Jones NF: Magnetic resonance imaging findings in secretan's disease. *J Hand Surg [Am]* 21:464–466, 1995.
▶ This clinically dramatic and historically well-known condition is so poorly understood that an aura of the factitious hangs over it in many minds. Such has not been my experience, and these authors note that both MRI and histopathology suggest an unusual type of tissue reactivity to injury, particularly in those tissues that contain synovial cells as well as collagen precursor cells.

NEUROVASCULAR

Songcharoen P, Mahaisavariya B, Chotigavanich C: Spinal accessory neurotization for restoration of elbow flexion in avulsion injuries of the brachial plexus. *J Hand Surg [Am]* 21:387–390, 1996.
▶ This brief review, essentially a summary of a massive experience with spinal accessory to musculocutaneous neurotization, will be of little interest to most orthopedists, but such work, the more extensive prior reports upon which it is based, and the developments in progress (rerouting regenerating axons directly to motor fibers) are of extreme interest to those involved in the management of such injuries. Even with the current technique, the results (biceps recovery to MRC III or better in 72.5% of the patients operated on less than 9 months postinjury) are better than those with any other neurotization procedure.

Ihara KI, Doi K, Sakai K, et al: Restoration of sensibility in the hand after complete brachial plexus injury. *J Hand Surg [Am]* 21:381–386, 1996.
▶ Many methods have been attempted over several decades to bring sensibility to the insensate hand of a brachial plexus victim. The length of nerve regeneration required is so long that new methods are badly needed. However, the authors have provided some evidence that use of the lateral cutaneous branches of the third through the sixth intercostal nerves to suture directly to the median nerve gives the best results now obtainable (S2 to a 2+ level of median area sensibility in the hand).

Spinner RJ, Davids JR, Goldner RD: Dislocating medial triceps and ulnar neuropathy in three generations of one family. *J Hand Surg [Am]* 22:132–137, 1997.
▶ This paper may get short shrift since it seems to deal with a syndromic problem, *but* it discusses well the variant medial band of the triceps, which intrudes into the ulnar nerve space *much more often* than our clinical accounts suggest and can be a factor in cubital tunnel syndrome *even when the triceps band is not snapping over the medial epicondyle.* It is easy to manage if it is considered. Consider it always as one of the potential factors in cubital tunnel syndrome!

Weinzweig N, Sharzer LA, Starker I: Replantation and revascularization at the transmetacarpal level: Long term functional results. *J Hand Surg [Am]* 21:877–883, 1996.
▶ Transmetacarpal replantation/revascularization cases are notorious for "poor function" despite viability and adequate sensibility. Destruction and subsequent fibrosis of the intrinsic muscles are largely responsible, and techniques for diminishing this problem are reviewed. Even with the poor function, patients are happy with the stiff and sometimes deformed hand and would opt for the treatment again.

Radecki P: Variability in the median and ulnar nerve latencies: implications for diagnosing entrapment. *J Occup Environ Med* 37:1293–1299, 1995.
▶ Certainly, there is more to the diagnosis of carpal tunnel syndrome than is dreamt of in our usual philosophies. This mix of demographics, anthropometrics, and statistics is almost indigestible, yet it may provide a baseline for meaningful evaluation of the multiple factors that are at play in one of our most common problem diagnosis.

Okutsu I, Hamanaka I, Tanabe T, et al: Complete endoscopic carpal canal decompression. *Am J Orthop* 1:365–368, 1996.
▶ Perhaps no one has had more experience with endoscopic release of the carpal canal than these authors, who have been doing it since 1986. They make a good case for the need to divide transverse fibers (called by others the "deep layer of the midpalmar fascia" or by Cobb et al. the "distal portion of the flexor retinaculum") in order to permit spread of the already divided transverse carpal ligament (TCL) and diminish intracanal pressure (dropped from 50 mm Hg at rest pre-operatively to 6.6 mg Hg after TCL release and to 4.8 mm Hg after release of the transverse fibers). However, these transverse fibers are distal to the TCL and are in the subcutaneous layer; releasing them endoscopically beckons the neophyte toward possible damage. One should conquer the essential TCL release first.

Kluge W, Simpson RG, Nicol AC: Late complications after open carpal tunnel decompression. *J Hand Surg [Br]* 21:205–207, 1996.
▶ This review of the complaints in 89 hands, assessed at 10 months or more postoperatively, is typical (50% with reduced grip, 19% with tender scars, 18% with incomplete relief of symptoms, scar area sensory disturbance in 7%, and "pillar pain" in 4%). As the originator of the term "pillar pain," I find it interesting, although not unexpected, that the term has undergone a change into something new and strange, i.e., "an aching discomfort in the thenar or hypothenar eminences aggravated by gripping." There is indeed such a symptom

complex and I am willing to accept it as "pillar pain 2" or "pillar pain—late." "Pillar pain 1" or "pillar pain—early" is tenderness, to aching, to intolerable discomfort over the healing ligament-fascia masses overlying the bony pillars of the carpal canal, i.e., primarily over the hook of the hamate, the ridge of the trapezium, or the tuberosity of the scaphoid. These areas may be but are not usually directly under the operative scar and can in some instances be confused with scar tenderness and pain. In my experience, "pillar pain 1" may devolve into "pillar pain 2" in about 30% of the cases, but very few instances of persistent "pillar pain 2" are seen after 2 years.

Wang W-Z, Crain GM, Baylis W, et al: Outcome of digital nerve injuries in adults. *J Hand Surg [Am]* 21:138–143, 1996.
▶ With current review and in succinct form the authors reaffirm important precepts from past work with digital nerve repairs in adults, i.e., that (1) patients less than 40 years old do better than those older than 40 years, (2) nerves with simple laceration do better than nerves with crush injuries, (3) nerve grafting to avoid tension (in mild crush or saw injuries) does better than primary repair, and (4) some digits, perhaps as many as 25%, receive overlap from the contralateral, uninjured nerve.

Povlsen B, Tegnell I: Incidence and natural history of touch allodynia after open carpal tunnel release. *Scand J Plast Reconstr Hand Surg* 30:221–225, 1996.
▶ This study of 51 consecutive patients treated by standard open carpal tunnel release confirmed the standard expectations of relief of nocturnal pain and fairly swift resolution of most clinical findings, but the authors were able to detect persistent allodynia to pressure over the thenar and hypothenar eminences (their illustration shows the test site to be almost identical to the trigger sites for the condition known as "pillar pain" in American hand literature). The incidence was rather higher than that usually reported (41% at 1 month) and persisted longer than is usually reported (6% at 12 months). As the originator of the term "pillar pain," it is easy for me to agree with their findings; indeed, there is some pain of this type that persists much longer than 1 year and/or may be severe enough that additional treatment is given.

Brandt K, Khouri R, Upton J: Free flaps as flow-through vascular conduits for simultaneous coverage and revascularization of the hand or digit. *J Plast Reconstr Surg* 98:321–327, 1996.
▶ This potpourri of cases with somewhat anecdotal follow-up is nevertheless worth remembering because all 12 of the cases represent catastrophic problems poorly salvageable or nonsalvageable by the usual methods of hand surgery. There are amputations and other posttraumatic defects, but also included are inadequate vascularization after tumor removal, contracture releases, and deteriorating replants. When one faces such a challenge, this article will become of great interest.

GENERAL

Hadler NM: Repetitive upper-extremity motions in the workplace are not hazardous: A clinical perspective. *J Hand Surg [Am]* 22:19–29, 1997.
▶ If you have given up being puzzled and therefore open-minded and can ignore the increasing basic evidence of the damage that repetitive insults to body tissues can do, then this polemic is for you. The author is a master at setting up the

"paper tigers" of bad research and poor clinical conclusions (with which our literature abounds), destroying them, and then concluding that there is no substance to claims of somatic damage. Once such denial of any possibility of physiologic damage is accepted, it is much easier to also deny the major problems of the "repetitive strain syndrome," i.e., the psychological and socioeconomic parts of the triad. Such an approach can lead to legislative denial, which presumes to be an end point, but neither this nor any similar strategy will keep the pot from boiling!

Bonzani PJ, Millender L, Keelan B, et al: Factors prolonging disability in work-related cumulative trauma disorders. *J Hand Surg [Am]* 22:30–34, 1997.

▶ It seems to be taking forever to realize that cumulative stress pathology *is* a physiologic entity but that the great majority of instances in the workforce suffer from a preponderance of psychological and socioeconomic maladies, or as I have put it on other occasions, "Cumulative stress in the workplace is an amalgam of Soma, (P)syche and Socio-economic factors, which vary in percentage from case to case!" The authors' groupings under diagnosis are merely a way of assessing the relative percentage of the "somatic" in each instance. Their ergonomic grading is principally useful in assessing the potential for changing workplace conditions and therefore has more to do with management than with diagnosis. Their grading of the psychsocial factors lumps psyche and socioeconomic together, which is probably all right for diagnosis but not for treatment. In any event, it is this latter melange of factors that determines the success of management. The sooner that surgeons, hand and other, realize this and put aside the knife until later or not at all, the sooner will society and the medical profession come to grips with this epidemic.

Mackinnon SE, Novak DB: Repetitive strain in the workplace: A clinical perspective. *J Hand Surg [Am]* 22:2–19, 1997.

▶ The historical aspects, clinical findings, and physiologic investigations relating to use-related problems of the body, particularly the upper extremities, are summarized and referenced with due awareness that some studies are of limited value. Probably the best service that the authors give is their perception that surgery is not the answer but that surgeons and their surrogates, the upper limb therapists, should not therefore abandon the patients but should continue to work within the parameters of ergonomics, legalities, and psychosocioeconomic issues to rehabilitate the patients to some, not necessarily the same work situation.

Gonzalez MH, Kay T, Weinzweig N, et al: Necrotizing fasciitis of the upper extremity. *J Hand Surg [Am]* 21:689–692, 1996.

▶ Despite recent media hysterics over "flesh-eating bacteria," necrotizing fasciitis is not new and is probably not increasing in incidence except as the population at risk (immunodeficient, drug using, alcohol using, and diabetic individuals) increases. Nevertheless, the bonfire rapidity of infection spread and the limb- and life-threatening features of the condition make it something to keep in the forefront of the mind.

Amadio PC, Higgs P, Keith M: Prospective comparative clinical trials in the *Journal of Hand Surgery (American)*. *J Hand Surg [Am]* 21:925–929, 1996.
► It is not surprising but it is alarming that only 25 controlled clinical trials and 8 randomized controlled trials were found in 3,107 submissions to the journal. Although we do learn and will always delight in the art and the anecdote of medicine, we must improve the validity of our reporting.

Subject Index*

A

Abducted
  shoulder, capsular restraints to
    anterior-posterior motion of,
    96: 47
Abduction
  glenohumeral, in scapular plane,
    shoulder muscle forces and tendon
    excursions in, *96:* 87
  traction, guided, for congenital hip
    dislocation, *95:* 7
Abductor
  digiti, neurolysis of nerve to, with
    partial plantar fasciectomy for
    plantar fasciitis, *97:* 234
Ablation
  percutaneous radiofrequency, of osteoid
    osteoma, *96:* 235
Abrasion
  glenoid, after débridement in superior
    glenoid labrum injuries, *96:* 53
Abscess
  deep tissue, after varicella, in children,
    97: 332
  epidural, tophaceous gout of lumbar
    spine mimicking, MRI of, *97:* 134
  subperiosteal, ultrasound detection of,
    in children, *96:* 44; *95:* 35
Absorptiometry
  dual-energy x-ray, for stress fracture
    prediction in Marine Corps
    recruits, *97:* 267
Abused infants
  rib fractures in, *97:* 331
Accidents
  road traffic, arthroscopy for acute knee
    hemarthrosis after, *97:* 257
Acetabular
  allograft reconstruction with acetabular
    reinforcement ring during total hip
    revision, *95:* 105
  component in total hip arthroplasty (*see
    under* Arthroplasty, hip, total)
  cups, metal-backed, measurement of
    polyethylene wear in, *96:* 104
  development after early treatment of hip
    dysplasia by Pavlik harness, *95:* 3
  dysplasia and Charcot-Marie-Tooth
    disease in family, *96:* 20
  fracture (*see* Fracture, acetabular)
  procedures, complex, superior gluteal
    artery in, *95:* 110

protrusion in Marfan's syndrome,
  97: 352
reinforcement ring in total hip revision,
  95: 105
Acetabuloplasty
  Dega, combined with intertrochanteric
    osteotomies, in children, *97:* 346
Achilles tendon
  stretching for plantar heel pain,
    long-term follow-up, *95:* 165
Acquired immunodeficiency syndrome
  transmission through musculoskeletal
    allograft transplantation, *96:* 124
Acromioclavicular
  arthritis, arthroscopic resection of distal
    clavicle with superior approach for,
    96: 73
  dislocation
    complete, surgical treatment of,
      96: 70
    ligamentoplasty for, coracoacromial,
      96: 68
  hypermobility, arthroscopic resection of
    distal clavicle with superior
    approach for, *96:* 73
  ligaments, role of, and effect of distal
    clavicle resection on, *97:* 12
  separations
    during alpine skiing, *97:* 3
    arthroscopic resection of distal
      clavicle with superior approach for,
      96: 73
Acromion
  morphologic condition and age-related
    changes, *97:* 27
  morphology, radiographic assessment,
    reliability of, *97:* 29
  -splitting approach for large and
    massive rotator cuff tears, *95:* 58
  structure and rotator cuff tears, *96:* 79
Acromioplasty
  (*See also* Subacromial, decompression)
  anterior
    effect on litigation and workers'
      compensation, *96:* 78
    Neer, for degenerative irreparable
      rotator cuff lesions, *96:* 82
Actinomycin D
  in rhabdomyosarcoma, *96:* 228
Activity
  ordinary, for acute low back pain,
    96: 161

G

M

Mallory-Head hip prosthesis
  health-related quality of life after,
    95: 119
Malunion
  ankle, intraarticular contact stresses in,
    95: 176
  forearm fracture, operative treatment
    of, *96:* 262
  of phalanges in hand, posttraumatic,
    corrective osteotomy for, *97:* 397
  radius fracture, distal
    reconstruction of, early *vs.* late,
      97: 368
    volar-displaced, after internal fixation,
      95: 223
  scaphoid, corrective osteotomy for,
    97: 426
  tibia
    after indirect reduction and composite
      fixation of extraarticular proximal
      fractures, *96:* 347
    after nailing in closed tibial fractures,
      97: 270
    after open shaft fracture treated with
      external fixation followed by
      sequential intramedullary nailing,
      97: 275
Mangled Extremity Severity Score
  in evaluation in severe open fractures of
    lower extremity, *95:* 264
  as guide to treatment of severely injured
    upper extremity, *95:* 266
Manipulation
  gentle passive, for proximal
    interphalangeal joint contracture in
    Dupuytren's disease, *97:* 396
  spinal, in subacute low back pain,
    95: 139
  vs. arthroscopic release for resistant
    frozen shoulder, *96:* 88
Manipulative
  reduction for slipped upper femoral
    epiphysis, long-term results,
    97: 354
Mantle
  cement, in total hip arthroplasty,
    long-term radiographic results,
    95: 87
Manual
  assessment of fracture stiffness, *97:* 314
Marfan's syndrome
  protrusio acetabuli in, *97:* 352
Marine Corps recruits
  stress fracture prediction in, dual-energy
    x-ray absorptiometry for, *97:* 267
Mason-Allen suture
  new modification in rotator cuff repairs,
    mechanical strength of, *95:* 62

Massage
  for back pain, subacute low, *95:* 139
Material
  properties as factor in selection and
    application of splinting materials
    for athletic wrist and hand injuries,
    96: 315
Mayo total ankle arthroplasty
  results, *97:* 246
  survivorship analysis, *95:* 177
McBride procedure
  for hallux valgus, juvenile, *96:* 196
Mechanical
  comparison of dynamic compression
    plate, limited contact-dynamic
    compression plate, and point
    contact fixator (in sheep), *96:* 325
  consequences of bone ingrowth in
    cementless hip prosthesis, *96:* 156
  influences on tissue differentiation at
    bone-cement interfaces, *96:* 451
  properties of articular cartilage in knees
    with unicompartmental
    osteoarthritis, *95:* 358
  strength of rotator cuff repairs, *95:* 60
Median nerve
  displacement through carpal canal,
    95: 255
  fibers, motor, sensory, and sympathetic,
    estimation of axonal loss in carpal
    tunnel syndrome, *96:* 299
  injury after YAG laser carpal tunnel
    release, *96:* 314
  latencies, variability in, *97:* 430
Medical
  back care program, impact on
    utilization of services and primary
    care physician satisfaction in
    HMOs, *96:* 160
  problems, and mobility of transtibial
    amputees, *97:* 291
Medullary
  fixation, press fit, limits in revision knee
    arthroplasty, *96:* 406
  lavage, effect on embolic phenomena
    and cardiopulmonary changes
    during cemented hemiarthroplasty,
    96: 143
Melanoma
  malignant, of foot and ankle, *96:* 204
Melphalan
  interferon-γ and tumor necrosis factor-α
    in isolated limb perfusion with
    nonresectable extremity soft tissue
    sarcomas, *97:* 121
Membrane
  interfacial, of intramedullary nails,
    histologic features of, *97:* 263

Author Index